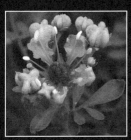
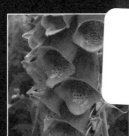

Homeopathy
for Epidemics

Eileen Nauman, DHM (UK)

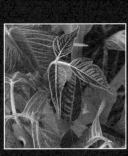
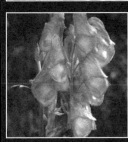
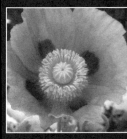
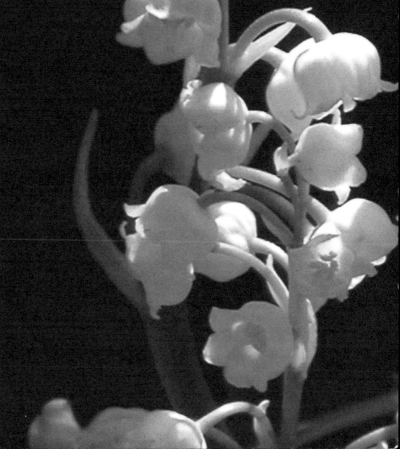

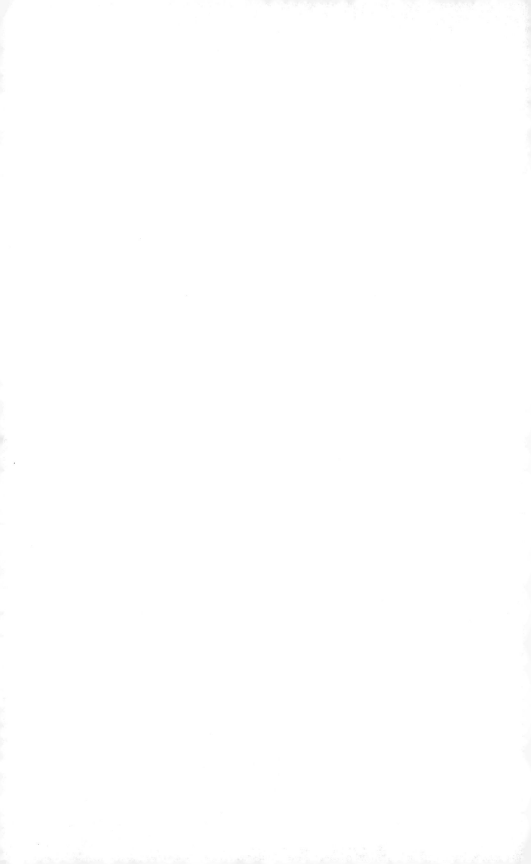

Homeopathy for Epidemics

Homeopathy in Times of Crises

Eileen Nauman

DHM

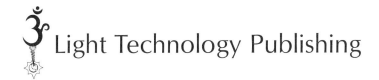

Light Technology Publishing

ISBN 1-891824-42-2
Published by

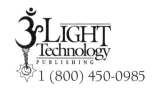

1 (800) 450-0985

Printed by

PO Box 3540
Flagstaff, AZ 86003

All photographs were taken by the author. Photographs on the cover were taken at the following locations: *Ruta graveolens* (yellow flower, garden rue) in De Kruidhof Botanical Gardens; *Foxglove purpurea* (pinkish-purple flower, digitalis) at Barbara Ward's home near Green Island, Dunedin, New Zealand (South Island); *Rhus toxicodendron* (poison oak) at Westfork Creek, Sedona, Arizona; *Aconitum napellus* (blue flower, monkshood) and *Convalaria majalis* (white-flower lily of the valley) in my backyard. The photograph of the gorgeous purple opium poppy was taken "somewhere in Europe."

Dedication

To those who want to be prepared.

Acknowledgments

Many thanks to my publisher, (Melody) O'Ryin Swanson. Without her belief in the information contained here and in the fact that it may well save lives, this book would not have been brought into being.

Thanks also to my homeopathic colleagues Dr. Gail Derin, Doctor of Oriental Medicine and classical homeopath, who worked with me on the hantavirus epidemic to find remedies that would save lives and who helped me with her work on locating the Ebola virus remedies; Dr. Vickie Menear, MD (H), homeopathic teacher at Hahnemann College, Albany, California; and Julian Evinston, homeopathic historian, for their information about remedies used during the 1918 Spanish influenza epidemic.

To Kathy Leonardi and Joanne Matkovich of Cottonwood, Arizona—members of the Kachina Affiliated Study Group of the National Center of Homeopathy—who took the bull by the horns in locating all the known Ebola virus symptoms, collating, researching and digging for them. Without their efforts, we homeopaths would not know which remedies to use to treat this deadly virus.

To my brave, intrepid homeopathic team: Dr. Gail Derin of Sacramento, California; Rosemarie Brown of Cottonwood, Arizona; Ardella Hecht of Phoenix, Arizona; Luanne Somers-Yazzie of Rough Rock, Arizona; and Mary Masuk of Albuquerque, New Mexico. Thank you for your individual and collective contributions, which have, in some way, helped make this book what it is—a life saver. Yahtehay!

To Catherine Creel, medical researcher, who provided a lot of amazing, updated information on SARS and anthrax; and to Debra LeRoy, FBIH, Canadian homeopath, who provided the information on smallpox. Without their contributions, this book would not be as whole as it presently is.

To the botanical gardens around the world where the people so kindly allowed me to photograph their beautiful plants, many of which we use in homeopathy. In particular, I'd like to thank the following: Le Jardine Botanical Garden in St. Triphone, Switzerland; my thanks go to owner William Aviolat. La Thomasia Botanical Garden, Alps of Switzerland; my thanks to Mme. Michèle Burdet, who kindly drove me to this wonderful high-mountain garden and to Le Jardine many times over a four-year period. Dunedin Botanical Garden, Dunedin, New Zealand; thank you, Barbara Ward, for taking me there, driving me around and helping me. De Kruidhof Botanical Garden, Buitenpost, Netherlands; thanks to Dr. Jean Pierre Jansen, homeopath and MD, and his wife, Marina, who so kindly drove there many times from their home in Grøningen. Quail Botanical Gardens, Encinitas, California. Pacific Horticultural Botanical Garden, Victoria, Canada. Naturescape Flower Garden, Langar, Nottinghamshire, England; thanks to David Witko, owner of ISIS homeopathic software, England, for taking me to this lovely spot. Geneva Botanical Garden, Geneva, Switzerland; thanks to Gail Carswell, who patiently helped me that day.

I wish to thank my husband, David Nauman, for spending untold hours helping me as I puttered around in botanical gardens in utter bliss. And thanks go to my intrepid friends who took on the task of helping me find those elusive homeopathic plants: Mme. Michèle Burdet of Chesières, Switzerland, who not only loaned me her chalet to stay at, La Palette, but also her array of flower identification books, a bed, her amazing flower and vegetable garden and a Mac computer—what a friend! On top of that, Michèle took me on numerous hikes in the Alps to find those elusive homeopathic plants—too numerous to count. Some of my most enjoyable times during the research were being out on the trail with her, "on the hunt"!

To Barbara Ward from Dunedin, New Zealand, who took me to the Dunedin Botanical Garden, but the flowers at her home were just as beautiful! To David Witko from Nottingham, England; Jan Dingemans from the Netherlands, who showed me a flower market many years ago where I found real, live *Aconitum napellus* for the first time. To Gail Carswell, friend and photographic carrier and scribe—what would I do without you, sidekick? To Ingrid Kropf of Witte Paarden, Netherlands, who owns her own herbal medicine business and has a beautiful herb garden, for her support and information. And last, but never least, to my New Zealand friend who lives in England, Diana Corrigan, who spent nine days with me at the wonderful Kew Gardens library doing some very serious, heavy, nonstop research—this was her "vacation" and I'm gratefully indebted to her for her love of and passion for flowers, which is equal to my own.

I owe you all much gratitude. Finding homeopathic flowers around the world is not an easy thing to do and it couldn't have been done without a lot of help! I'm sure I have forgotten someone, and to you I owe my apologies. Just know that I truly valued your help.

Disclaimer

The ideas, procedures and suggestions in this book are not intended as a substitute for the medical advice of a trained health professional. All matters regarding our health require medical supervision. Consult your homeopath and your physician before adopting the suggestions in this book or any other suggestions for any condition that may require diagnosis or medical attention. If you are pregnant, do not attempt these techniques without the approval of your physician. The author and publisher disclaim any liability arising directly or indirectly from the use of the techniques suggested in this book.

Contents

Part 3: Epidemic *Materia Medica*

Part 4: Posttraumatic Stress Disorder

Foreword

Homeopathy is a complementary form of medicine practiced around the world. It was discovered as a therapeutic system of medicine by Dr. Samuel Hahnemann, a German doctor, in the early 1700s. It spread rapidly throughout Europe and then went east as far as India and west to the Americas. In 1850 homeopathy was brought to America.

In the 1800s and 1900s, four out of ten doctors in the U.S. were homeopaths, and there were over 100 homeopathic hospitals. Up until 1940, when the discovery of penicillin made such a dramatic entrance, homeopathy was still practiced in the United States. From 1940 through 1970, it was kept alive and well through lay homeopaths and homeopathic study groups. The flame burned dimly, but it was not extinguished thanks to this small, stubborn core of people who recognized homeopathy's almost miraculous ability to cure by inviting the body to heal itself—naturally. In Europe homeopathic remedies now sit side by side with allopathic, over-the-counter drugs at any grocery store or pharmacy. Half the over-the-counter goods bought in France alone are homeopathic. And no wonder!

Homeopathy's philosophy is "like cures like." Let me give you an example of this in everyday terms. Most of us have been stung by a honeybee or bitten by a mosquito. Our skin turns red, there's heat around the bite area and swelling. One of the more than 2,000 homeopathic remedies for bites and stings available in the U.S.—and approved by the FDA—is *Apis mellifica*, honeybee. In homeopathic pharmacies, homeopaths capture a honeybee, place it in alcohol to kill it and then grind it up, which starts the process of making *Apis mellifica*. The honeybee's venom is part and parcel of this remedy. When potentized, or made stronger, it becomes the remedy of choice for honeybee stings, mosquito bites and other skin-related symptoms.

By potentizing a remedy through dilution steps, eventually only the energy signature of the original substance is left in the alcohol carrier. Quantum physics will one day be able to explain why water "has memory"; similarly, homeopaths know that each remedy has its own unique frequency—whether there are molecules of the substance left or not.

A number of remedies from organic sources are well-known poisons. For instance, arsenic is used to create *Arsenicum album*.

If one were to take arsenic in its original, raw state, one would die very quickly. However, when the arsenic is potentized homeopathically, what is left is the energy signature, or frequency, of the compound. Arsenicum is a well-known cure for botulism, food poisoning and asthma plus a number of other ailments. So a *poison can and does heal.*

Here is another example that shows that poisons can heal: Our U.S. homeopathic pharmacopoeia, which is FDA-approved, includes a number of venomous-snake remedies. One of them is rattlesnake or, to give it its Latin name, *Crolatus horridus.* During the 1918 Spanish flu epidemic that swept across the world killing 22 million people worldwide and 500,000 in the U.S., this one remedy alone was responsible for saving the most lives. Going back into the homeopathic archives, we find that *Crolatus horridus* was the remedy of choice given to homeopathic patients during that devastating flu epidemic, along with gelsemium and belladonna.

In fact, out of this epidemic of 1918 emerged some interesting statistics that affect us today. It was shown that 80 percent of patients treated with allopathic drugs during the 1918 epidemic died; 80 percent of those treated with homeopathic remedies—*Crolatus horridus* being the major remedy—lived. It is a stunning testament to the importance of homeopathy during an epidemic, or indeed at any time—whether it be on an acute basis or when dealing with a chronic disease. So a poison, in this case rattlesnake venom, saved hundreds of thousands of lives in the U.S. during the 1918 Spanish influenza epidemic.

There are other snake venoms: coral snake; copperhead; water moccasin; lachesis, from the Surukuku snake of South America; puff adder; bothrops, from the yellow viper, also known as the fer-de-lance, on the Caribbean island of Martinique. There are also naja, which is cobra venom, and Gila monster poison. All of these venoms have been instrumental in hemorrhagic (bleeding) diseases such as typhoid, Lassa fever and, most recently, diseases caused by the filovirus family, which consists of the Ebola Marburg, Ebola Zaire and Ebola Sudan viruses.

Homeopathy also uses poisons from the insect kingdom: honeybee, wasp, black widow, orange spider, tarantula, New Zealand spider, gray spider, Spanish spider, Cuban spider and papal cross spider.

Poisons kill, but they can also heal. If we are sick, aren't we filled with some kind of poison? It's just a question whether we're dealing with a spiritual, mental, emotional or physical poisoning. We can take a case homeopathically and determine the root cause of the "poisoning"—be it in spirit, in mind, in the emotions or from a physical source, such as tainted food, water pollution or something other. Once we collect a patient's unique set of symptoms, we can then match them up with those listed in our repertory, which contains thousands of compiled symptoms. Certain homeopathic remedies have certain sets of symptoms. A homeopath is trained to match your symptoms to the right remedy in our pharmacopoeia, and there's a good chance it will be a poison. But don't be worried. Remember, you're only ingesting the frequency, or energy signature, of this substance, and it's completely safe.

Nowadays, I'm afraid, we live in a very poisoned world. Humans have buried their toxic waste beneath Mother Earth's skin, and they have polluted the air we breathe until people across our globe die from toxic poisons and fumes from our cars and industry. Humans have polluted the water they drink by allowing fertilizer toxins to drain into our groundwater and chemical manufacturers, paper mills and raw sewage sources have turned our pristine waters into poisons. Is it any wonder we become poisoned?

Our world is reaching a crisis in terms of overpopulation, pollution and behavior. Mother Earth is a sentient, living being and she's beginning to speak to us in some deadly terms, telling us to clean up our act or she's going to get rid of the vermin, the humans, who are slowly killing her with toxins of all kinds. Her immune system, if you will, is using viruses and epidemics to destroy the overpopulation of her surface. By reducing the number of humans, she also reduces the amount of toxins that are seriously injuring her biosphere.

We aren't being good, responsible tenants for Mother Earth, and she has no other recourse. Our own immune systems, if invaded by a virus or bacteria, send out soldiers known as white blood cells to kill off what is threatening to kill us; Mother Earth's soldiers on the front lines are her viral epidemics.

One doesn't have to be psychic to know that the epidemics are coming—and soon. Virologists across the world have already sounded the alarm, but the governments of the world aren't listening. The homeopathic community knows that in the past, homeopathic remedies have made the difference between life and death during these global epidemics—a fact that was proven dramatically in 1918. We know homeopathic remedies can make the difference in the forthcoming epidemics. But it's impossible to make the world listen to what we know. All we can do is reach the people who are willing to listen and to apply their commonsense logic to our argument. The information contained in this book can make the difference between living and dying when the epidemics begin.

I'm no stranger to epidemics. My great-grandmother died of the Spanish influenza in 1918. The homeopathic team I assembled to help the Navajo people in 1993, when the hantavirus hit with a 60-percent death rate, gave us some valuable knowledge on how to use homeopathy "in the trenches" to combat a killer virus. My team of intrepid women homeopaths—Dr. Gail Derin; Rosemarie Brown, MSW; and Ardella Hecht—was there and made a difference.

The information contained in this book is divided into several segments. There is a chapter explaining what homeopathy is and how it works—not *why* it works; we'll leave that to the quantum physicists to explain. We only know it *does* work. We are entering a dark phase in our lives with these epidemics hanging in the closet, waiting to come out and begin killing. As this book goes to press, we now have SARS being a global killer and Dengue fever in the United States. The forecast is working, unfortunately. I'm confident, having lived through the hantavirus epidemic as a homeopath, that if each person is armed with the necessary homeopathic remedies, we can survive the coming "cleansing" that Mother Earth's immune system is going to unleash upon us.

Is it any wonder that, given homeopathy's central concept, "like cures like," poisons will have to be used to heal poisoned human beings?

It is my hope that you will pass along the information in this book to your relatives and friends. It may be the greatest gift you ever give them—information that can save their lives.

Eileen Nauman
La Casa de Madre Tierra
Sedona, Arizona
September 2004

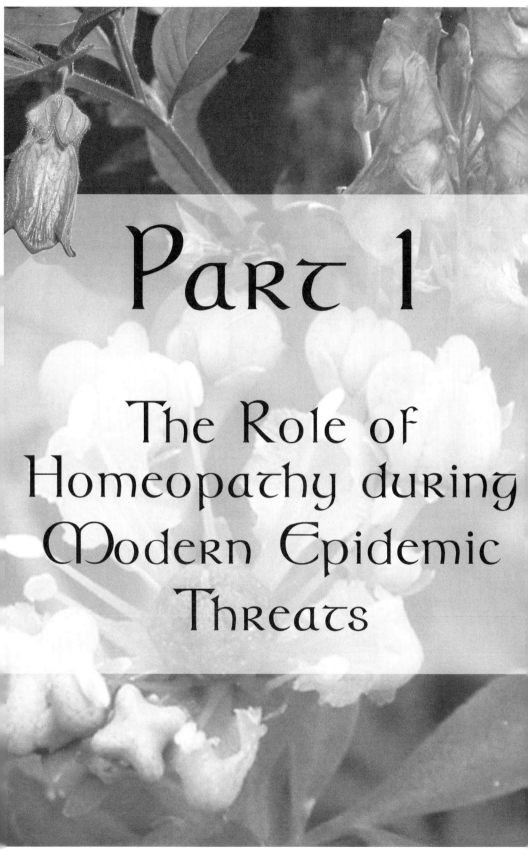

Part 1

The Role of Homeopathy during Modern Epidemic Threats

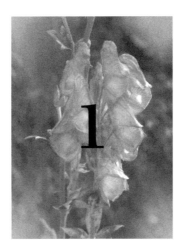

What Is Homeopathy and How Does It Work?

Homeopathy, a complementary form of medicine practiced around the world, is based on the law of similars. The Greek word *homeo* means "similar" and *pathos* means "disease"—similar disease, or "like cures like." Homeopathy utilizes medically active substances at infinitesimal potencies, which makes them safe, non-habit forming, non-addictive, non-allergenic and without side effects.

Let me give you an example of "like cures like" so that you can understand homeopathy in action. Everyone, with few exceptions, has been stung by a bee at some time in his or her life. Everyone has felt that sharp, burning pain from the sting itself. Then the skin rises and turns bright red; there's lots of heat surrounding the area of the sting and the skin usually feels itchy too. Using a more scientific explanation, one can say that your body is "dis-eased" by the sting. We choose a homeopathic remedy that parallels the symptoms of the sting and introduce it, like an artificial disease, into your body. Because the potentized remedy is stronger than the sting, the body or rather, the vital force, gets the signal that something is wrong, reorganizes itself and its systems and focuses its energies on healing the symptoms introduced by the remedy. In doing so, the actual bee sting is cured too.

The vital force is our intrinsic energy that is within and outside of us. It includes our physical, emotional, mental and spiritual states. This force helps us in our daily lives and becomes invaluable when we fall sick. Homeopaths are trained to perceive the vital force and are able to measure this life energy in each of us, to help us get well.

Let's get back to the insect bite. Our homeopath will consult a special reference manual called a *materia medica*, which contains 1,400 hundred FDA-approved remedies. The one potentized remedy whose symptoms most closely match those of swollen insect bite is *Apis mellifica*, crushed honeybee, and is therefore the remedy used for such a sting. The homeopath gives you one medicated sucrose pellet, and within minutes the symptoms of the sting disappear. We've introduced an organic, potentized remedy at an infinitesimal potency into your body. Your body has responded to this remedy, and voilà—you have cured yourself of a sting with all its accompanying symptoms.

The most exciting thing about this process is that your body's own natural healing force creates the cure. There are no side effects, and the body does not become dependent on drugs.

Homeopathic Remedy Preparation and Potency

We have FDA-approved homeopathic pharmacies all over the U.S. and we have the HPUS, the homeopathic pharmacopoeia for the U.S. and our guidebook that tells us exactly how to produce a remedy. Our homeopathic remedies come from three sources: the animal, vegetable and mineral kingdoms. They are made of flowers, plants, roots, trees, insects and minerals, to mention a few sources.

How Is a Homeopathic Remedy Made?

Let me lead you through an example that shows how a homeopathic remedy is made. Almost everyone, especially mothers, is familiar with ipecac, which we keep in our household in case one of our children accidentally becomes poisoned. We know that if they do, we will give them ipecac, an herb that will immediately cause vomiting.

The ipecac root is gathered according to HPUS guidelines, which may state that it must be dug up at a certain time of the year. We then take it to our pharmacy, wash it, sterilize it properly and macerate it, or put it into a machine to tear it up and break it down. We then add a certain amount of ethyl alcohol (also known as "grain" alcohol) and water and place the macerated root into a gallon jar. There it sits for a certain period of time to let the alcohol pull all of the nutrients and chemicals out of the root. At the specified time, we strain the entire contents and throw away the ipecac root. What is left is known as a mother tincture. This comprises the constituents—the vitamins, minerals and chemicals of the ipecac—now suspended in a fluid of alcohol and water.

To keep this simple, let's say we will make an "X" potency, which means that there is one part of the mother tincture to nine parts of alcohol and water. When the parts are measured out, the fluid is placed into the vial a lab assistant has prepared. The vial is corked and then "succussed," which means that its bottom is struck against something solid—but not so hard as to shatter it! This succussion, or jarring, is done 100 times, and we then have Ipecac 1X.

When the contents are succussed, the energy contained in the molecules of ipecac are released. The more jarring that occurs, the more energy is released. The lab assistant will then take a small amount from this first vial of 1X ipecac and place it in a second one, which contains the same parts of alcohol and water. You can see that by doing this, we are putting less of the original mother tincture in the second vial. This vial is also succussed 100 times, and we end up with ipecac 2X. Depending on the potency needed, we can do this upward to 3X, 4X, 5X and so on. When we have the potency desired, we spray the contents of the vial over sucrose (sugar) pellets; they are thus impregnated with the ipecac that has been homeopathically prepared.

Is There a General Homeopathic Potency for Remedies Sold in Health Food Stores That I Can Buy?

Yes. Let's take a closer look at a common, over-the-counter potency that is sold in better health food stores, called a "30C." The C (which stands for 100) means that the mother tincture for the remedy was made of one part of substance and 99 parts of alcohol and water. The 30 means that the remedy was then diluted

30 times and succussed 100 times with each dilution. The higher numbers represent more potent remedies, because the energy released by succussion increases with each dilution.

You may find lower-potency remedies on store shelves, such as 3X or 6X, but generally speaking, FDA laws allow health food stores to sell up to a 30C potency. Anything higher should come directly from a homeopathic practitioner.

Can a 30C Potency Harm Me?

A 30C potency is considered a moderate potency, and it is used in the U.S. because of its gentle and persistent action. However, in some cases, it can cause an "aggravation." In homeopathy, an aggravation is an intensification of the symptoms you already had before taking the remedy; your symptoms may intensify after taking the remedy. An aggravation can last a few moments or hours. If it goes on for more than 24 hours, consult a homeopath immediately.

When you take a low potency, such as 30C, your body's response would be a gentle stimulation of its natural defenses. But if you use a much higher potency, such as a 200C, you could get too much "bang for your buck"—an aggravation. For example, if I took a 30C potency for hot flashes, they would lessen or completely disappear over a period of hours, with no negative physical reaction. But if I took a 200C potency, I might have more intense hot flashes for a period of time before they disappeared—which is highly uncomfortable.

Ideally, you should contact a homeopath in your vicinity and ask her or him about any possible use of any remedy you find in this book. Get a professional opinion. Then, if the homeopath approves, you will be under her or his guidance, which is best. To self-medicate with a homeopathic remedy, even at a 30C potency, is not the best of conditions. If nothing else, if this book inspires you to find out who your local homeopath is, then you are well on your way to better health.

If You Make a High Enough Potency, Is Anything of the Herb Left in the Liquid?

It may seem that we're using less and less of the herbal substance when we're making higher and higher potencies, and you may wonder if there is anything of the herb left in the liquid when we make a high enough potency. In mathematics, which is not my forte, there is a theoretical calculation known as Avogadro's number. Avogadro, an Italian physicist, postulated in 1811 that equal volumes of any chemical substance contain equal numbers of molecules. By this theory, a 24X or 12C homeopathic potency has no molecules left in the liquid. That is true—insofar as his hypothesis goes. However, Dr. Jacques Benveniste, a world-renowned homeopathic researcher from France, proved that water continues to contain a *memory* of that remedy

This is the reason why we call homeopathy "energy medicine." With potencies above 24X or 12C, we are dealing with submolecular materials that continue to retain the memory of the remedy. As we continue to dilute our remedies, there is less and less of the actual substance in the liquid, and at some point, there are no molecules of the original substance left. This is what makes it infinitesimal. No one can explain *why* it works after the molecules are gone. I'm sure that in the years to come, there will be a sufficient scientific explanation and we'll have instruments that can prove this phenomenon adequately. Until then, we must rely on faith, anecdotal case histories and scientific research. No one can see gravity; all we can do is measure its effects upon us. Homeopathy falls into that category.

Is There Proof That Homeopathy Works?

Yes. One kind of proof is anecdotal evidence, which means that doctors or health practitioners have consistently observed a healing effect of a certain drug or treatment in their practices, but no clinical studies have yet been performed to prove exactly how it works. Nonetheless, if such a treatment is known to be safe and effective, doctors will not hesitate to prescribe it. An example is the popular drug Retin-A, which has been scientifically studied and proven only for use as a treatment for acne. However, because anecdotal evidence shows that it works for wrinkles, it is used by thousands of people who haven't seen a pimple for years. Another kind of proof comes from scientific studies.

Anecdotal Evidence That Homeopathy Works

As I said, for homeopathy, there is evidence of both kinds. You'll get plenty of anecdotes by simply asking anyone who uses homeopathy. After people have used a homeopathic remedy, they have seen its often near-miraculous results. In my 30 years of practice, I've seen homeopathy work just like this in thousands of cases.

Here is one highly dramatic case I helped with while attending the Lakota Indians' Sundance ceremony in South Dakota in 1991. Bob, a paramedic who was also attending the event, called me by walkie-talkie to tell me that a family of four was in acute distress. The members of this family were having an allergic reaction to the lime dust spread over the porta-johns. Their throats were swelling, closing, and Bob was afraid that if help didn't come soon, they would suffocate. I raced to their tent, where Bob pointed out a 50-year-old woman seated on a chair, leaning over with her hands on her throat. She was wheezing, her face was gray, and I knew that she was not getting enough oxygen. Reaching for my high-potency homeopathic kit, I took out an appropriate remedy and pushed a couple of pellets into her mouth, telling her she would be all right.

I then looked over at the husband and the oldest daughter. They were both breathing harshly but were in better shape than the mother. The baby, a beautiful little girl, played quietly on a quilt on the floor between us. She didn't display any symptoms at all. Bob, in the meantime, was hovering over the mother. I'm sure he was thinking that he'd have to cut a hole in her throat to allow breathing if this remedy didn't work. I gave Bob the proper dosages for the husband and daughter, and a smaller, preventive dose for the baby.

Within five minutes, the older woman's harsh breathing had evened out. Her hand left her throat, and the gray color began to leave her face. Within fifteen minutes, her allergic reaction was gone. Twenty minutes later, everyone was fine. I walked back to my truck with Bob at my side. He shook his head, saying that he couldn't believe his eyes. He'd been a paramedic in Seattle for 10 years and thought he'd seen it all.

Scientific Evidence That Homeopathy Works

The second kind of evidence, which is most respected by the medical establishment, comes from scientific studies. The best ones are "controlled, double-blind" studies. In this kind of research, a large group of people who are treated with the drug being studied are compared against a similar, untreated group. Those in the untreated group receive a placebo, or pill with no active ingredients. A third control group receives nothing. Nobody knows which group she or he belongs to, though, which prevents subjects from guessing the effects of the treatment or drug and results in a more objective proof.

Studies published in the *Journal of Holistic Medicine* (1993) and the *Journal of the American Institute of Homeopathy* (1968) show that different homeopathic remedies tested at different potencies had distinctive readings of subatomic activity, whereas the placebos did not (see studies by Sacks and Boericke/Smith on page 355).

On October 18, 1986, *Lancet* published results of a double-blind study from the University of Glasgow (Scotland) showing that a homeopathic remedy significantly reduced symptoms of hay fever in patients (see study by Reilly, Taylor and McSherry on page 355).

The results of a double-blind study conducted on patients with dental neurologic pain following tooth extraction were published in the *Journal of the American Institute of Homeopathy* in 1985 (see study by Albertini et al on page 355). It was shown that an impressive 76 percent of those given the homeopathic medicines arnica and hypericum experienced relief of pain.

Why Aren't There More Scientific Studies?

These studies are solid, but you may wonder why there aren't more. It is because homeopathy honors the individual in all respects. It is very tough to devise a statistical return that will show the effectiveness of homeopathic remedies because, for example, everyone's "headache" is different. Headaches can start at the root of the nose, at the temples, at the rear of the skull or on top of the head. The pain associated with a headache is not general either. If you ask your friends to describe the pain associated with their headaches and compare them to your own, you'll see how varying the symptoms really are! Further, headaches occur for differing reasons: some result from stress, whereas others stem from high blood pressure, dehydration, too much sun and so forth. Hence, every headache may need a different remedy.

To try to devise a test of homeopathy that is acceptable to the prevailing scientific establishment is tough because our conventional, or "allopathic," system of medicine generally takes the stance that one kind of drug can treat almost everyone's headache, stomachache or flu. By contrast, homeopathy believes that everyone's headache is different; therefore, a different remedy is needed for each of these individual headaches.

Now you can appreciate our problems in trying to convince the medical establishment! We rely heavily on the millions of people who use homeopathy to prove that it works. But the best proof of all will be your own experience, when you try it yourself.

Was Homeopathy Ever Popular in the United States?

Absolutely! Homeopathy was brought here to us in 1825 by several doctors who had studied in Europe. They taught their colleagues and slowly, schools were established. By the mid-1800s, we had homeopathic medical colleges, including the New England Female Medical College, which was the first medical school in America to admit women.

By 1900 we had 22 homeopathic colleges and one out of every five doctors in the U.S. was a homeopath. Unfortunately, there was a move toward a mechanical model of the body and disease, and homeopathy lost ground—not because it didn't work, but because homeopaths, by nature, weren't politicians, whereas the American Medical Association (AMA), the allopaths, were. By 1910 only 15 homeopathic colleges remained, and by the end of the 1940s, no courses were taught anymore in the United States. Homeopathy was also pushed into the background of America's medical history with the discovery of penicillin and the use of drugs or shots that would give instant relief. That, and the discovery and use of vaccinations, all forced homeopathy further from the minds of the millions who had used it and been cured by it.

Interestingly enough, when we had the Spanish flu epidemic of 1918, when 22 million people died worldwide of this virus, some fascinating facts emerged to show that homeopathy was still a better medicine. Homeopathic doctors used several homeopathic remedies to save lives during this devastating flu epidemic, whereas the allopathic doctors relied on their crude drugs. In the U.S. alone, 500,000 deaths were caused by this epidemic. Afterward, Dean W. A. Pearson of Philadelphia and Hahnemann College collected data on 26,795 cases of influenza treated by homeopathic physicians, which showed a mortality rate of 1.05 percent. The mortality rate among those treated by allopathic medicine was 30 percent.

Because of vigorous and aggressive politicking by the AMA, homeopathy was pushed out of the picture via congressional acts and laws and would have died a certain death in the U.S. if not for the "lay" homeopaths—the ordinary people who had been patients of homeopaths and who picked up the torch and carried it forward. If not for the lay public, who continued not only to use homeopathy but also to teach it to those who were interested, homeopathy would not be enjoying the resurgence it is enjoying today. From 1940 to 1980, the lay public kept homeopathy alive and gave it a second chance.

Over the years since 1980, homeopathy has become the "darling" of the complementary, or alternative, medicines in our country. We have medical doctors as well as doctors of osteopathy and naturopathy taking courses and going to newly established homeopathic colleges. Homeopathy is strutting its stuff once again and proving it where it counts—with the people.

Homeopathy is grassroots medicine. It is about people caring for people. It is about knowing that all things are connected and that natural medicines are not only kinder and gentler but can give profound, equally miraculous help to someone who is ill.

Who Uses Homeopathy?

In the U.S., people from the poorest to the richest utilize homeopathy. Because it is inexpensive, it is within reach for anyone who desires to use it. There is no slide rule to say that only a certain part of our population is drawn to it. Rather, people discover homeopathy because the allopathic, traditional medicine system has failed them or because they have run out of money and therefore can't continue drug treatment.

People who are interested in their health and those who would rather use something other than invasive drugs that cause side effects, cause allergy reactions or in some way inhibit a true quality of life, are the ones who check out homeopathy. Once they've tried it, few ever return to drug treatment or they use drugs more sparingly.

I know mothers who absolutely refuse to have their babies immunized, because they see the deadly spiral of children getting sicker and sicker at a younger and younger age, which wasn't so before the advent of vaccinations. These mothers don't want their children's immune systems compromised with a series of shots from the moment they're born and throughout adolescence, so they turn to homeopathy to strengthen their children's immune systems—naturally and without the side effects of vaccinations. There is mounting evidence that too many vaccinations sensitize a person's—or child's—immune system at a too-high degree. And this is why children are ending up with allergies and asthma, which were practically unheard of before the vaccination generation!

For instance, the DPT shot, which comprises three vaccinations in one, was routinely given to every baby. Unfortunately, over the past decade, there is more than anecdotal evidence that this DPT shot causes epilepsy. A lot of mothers don't want to trade off the DPT shot for epilepsy in their child, so they research alternatives, and homeopathy is certainly a viable answer.

Another example are the Navajo people I care for on their reservation. They dislike and distrust "white man's" medicine. In their realm of thinking and seeing the world, they would rather use homeopathy, because many of the products are herbal in origin and their medicine people use herbs all the time to cure people in ceremonies. Further, they intrinsically understand "energy" medicine like homeopathy, because they believe that all things have energy in and around them. So it's quite easy for them to make the choice between homeopathy and allopathic drug treatment at a hospital.

Can Homeopathy Totally Replace Allopathic Medicine as It Is Practiced in This Country?

No, not entirely. Homeopathy has its limits, just as *every* form of medicine does. Fortunately, homeopaths recognize these limits and refer patients if homeopathy is unable to help a condition. For example, homeopathy cannot replace surgery when it is needed. It can, however, delay or even prevent surgery in some cases. There are also homeopathic remedies that can be given before or after an operation that enable people to heal faster and leave the hospital more quickly.

There are other factors that may not make homeopathy the treatment of choice. One of them is age. Older people (70 years of age and up) are more difficult to treat, often because their vital force may be low or weak. Because homeopathy has limited effects on a weak, faltering vital force, drug intervention may have to be used instead. A homeopath can assess your vital force and your potential for the use of homeopathy.

Homeopathy is also ineffective when an organ is beyond mending. For instance, homeopathy is not able to "fix" cirrhosis of the liver, although the liver is a regenerative organ (the only one in the body). If you have suffered a heart attack, homeopathy cannot replace or fix the dead muscle tissue. What it can do is support the circulatory system and the heart, which, along with diet, can prevent another attack.

Generally speaking, homeopathy can help everyone, to varying degrees. Even if a person has a life-altering disease, homeopathy can make a positive difference. Let a homeopath determine if you're a candidate for homeopathic treatment.

What Happens When I Go to a Homeopath?

First, speak to the homeopath by phone and see if there is good rapport. If you don't feel good about the phone consultation, then seek out another homeopath until you find one who is right for you.

At the homeopath's office, you'll find that "taking your case" may run anywhere from one to many hours. This will be in sharp contrast to the usual 15-minute history taken by an allopathic physician. Your homeopath will take the time to question you about many different levels of yourself, and you may find some of the questions funny or seemingly irrelevant to your problem. However, your homeopath will be looking at you as a *whole* person who has spiritual, mental, emotional and physical needs.

At the end of the case taking, the homeopath will probably give you a remedy to place under your tongue. This may be in form of a few white sugar pellets or a dilution of water, alcohol and the remedy. The homeopath may also tell you to take your remedy home and take it later that day or night. Then you'll be given a follow-up appointment for four or six weeks after you've taken the remedy to see how well it's working. I like to vary this slightly in my practice. I tell my new client to take the remedy home with her and take it just before she goes to bed. Then I ask her to call and check in with me 48 hours after taking the remedy. If I have chosen the right remedy, there are going to be minor signs that it is working to help her.

Some conditions or people may be slow to respond and a homeopath is lucky to see any movement or change for six weeks or more. So be patient after taking the remedy; your symptoms will slowly, subtly change—without you really being aware of it. In chronic diseases, it may take one to three years.

When you check in with your homeopath four or six weeks after your initial visit, you may or may not receive another remedy; it's not unusual if you don't. Regardless, another appointment will be set up for you another four to six weeks later.

Generally speaking, I have found that it takes three months to "clear a case" of, say, menopause complaints. There may be some exceptions to this rule, but under normal circumstances, you should be free and clear of any menopausal symptoms within six months of homeopathic treatment.

If I Have Questions about Homeopathy, Will My Homeopath Answer Them?

In most cases, yes. Many have brochures and pamphlets to give you a more in-depth explanation. Homeopathy is a highly complex form of medicine, and homeopaths don't always have the time they wish they had to answer all of your valid questions. Some homeopaths have a receptionist or lay homeopath who can answer your questions; others do not.

Another way to seek more information is to write or call the National Center for Homeopathy (see page 360 in Appendix B). Also, if you're fortunate, there may be a homeopathic study group in your area. The National Center for Homeopathy is an educational nonprofit corporation with hundreds of affiliated study groups around the United States. You can call and find out if there is a study group in your area. The president or leader of such a group will be exceptionally helpful and enthusiastic in answering any and all of your questions!

What Happens After I Take a Homeopathic Remedy?

Those who take a correctly prescribed remedy will begin to experience a lessening of their symptoms. This can happen gradually, over several weeks, or as quickly as within a few hours; it depends on an individual's vital force and the remedy chosen—some remedies are fast acting, whereas others are exceedingly slow. This is why the homeopath usually sets up the next appointment six weeks from the time the remedy was taken.

Twenty percent of those taking a remedy may experience a very fleeting aggravation—the intensification of symptoms discussed earlier. The aggravation may last seconds, minutes or up to a few hours or even days. For example, let's say you are dealing with menopause and always get hot flashes in the afternoon. After taking the remedy, your hot flashes may become more intense, last longer and be more uncomfortable for a few hours or a day afterward. The aggravation *is* uncomfortable, I won't deny that; I've experienced it myself. However, an aggravation is actually a sign that the correct remedy was chosen, so this is good news. And then, the symptoms all go away shortly after that aggravation.

For some people—a very small percentage—an aggravation may go on for more than the expected time. If this happens, you should get in touch with your homeopath right away. There is no sense in suffering! The homeopath may antidote the remedy and choose another one that usually will not create an aggravation in you. Sometimes the remedy chosen matches your set of symptoms so closely that it creates long-term aggravation. The homeopath will then antidote it and choose another remedy, one that isn't so close to your set of symptoms, and then you won't experience aggravation.

Understanding the Difference between Allopathic Medicine and Homeopathy

Allopathic, or conventional, medicine as practiced in the U.S. treats a condition based on the structure of chemical changes presented. Allopathic doctors may look at the patient's background or try to determine why the structure—cause—appeared in the first place. In other words, they are trained to look only at the pathology or problem presented. This does not include your state of mind, your emotions or an event (root cause) that might be connected with your disease and may have a direct bearing on it. By contrast, a homeopath does consider these aspects of you and your

case. When an allopathic doctor "diagnoses" the problem, it is usually treated with a synthetic drug given in large, continual doses for
a certain period of time; pills will be prescribed for a number of
days. At the end of that time, the pathology or problem should be
gone. The cause, however, may not be gone.

The problem with drugs is not that they are synthetic; rather,
it is that the drug is not a "close fit" to the symptoms. Further, the
drugs may be toxic and won't heal the dynamic problem that is
creating all of the symptoms. But the drug does take away the
symptoms, so people think they are healed—and they are not. A
good example is a woman with a yeast infection who is given
drugs. As long as she takes the drugs, the symptoms are gone.
When she stops taking the drugs, the symptoms come back.
Why? Because the drugs are not addressing the dynamic in her
vital force that is sending out this array of symptoms.

For a homeopathic treatment, you go to a homeopath and get
your case taken. There is no "diagnosis" in homeopathy; rather,
you present a compilation of many, many symptoms. A homeopath then looks up your group of symptoms in a special book
called a *repertory* and finds the single remedy that most closely
matches your particular, individual set of symptoms. You will be
given an initial dose of that potentized remedy just one time,
along with instructions on when to take it again. That might be
several hours later, or days or even months later; only your homeopath can determine the frequency of dosage for you. She or
he does this by retaking your case every four to six weeks and, if
there is a shift in your symptoms, you may be given another dose.
The remedy, which in reality is an artificial disease, is more powerful than the set of symptoms you are currently experiencing, and
your body generates enough resistance to eliminate the new symptoms and your old condition.

Homeopathy uses infinitesimal doses of a potentized remedy,
given only once, to set the body's natural response into action.
Allopathy, on the other hand, hammers away at the symptoms day
after day, with a synthetic drug that the body regards as a poison
and that does not enlist the help of the body's own responses in
any way. When a person takes a drug, it may often suppress the
symptoms. Later the cause of the problem, which was not dealt
with, may create another set of more serious symptoms.

Is There a Time When Drugs Should Be Used Instead Of Homeopathy?

Yes. An example of where drugs should be used is diabetes. Diabetics should always take their shot or pill(s). If a homeopathic remedy is administered, it is an adjunct to this other, primary, process. Also, the medical doctor should be told about the possible use of a homeopathic remedy *before* it is dispensed and used because, in all likelihood, it will lower the sugar level (providing it is the correct remedy) and the doctor needs to know because the medication has to be adjusted accordingly.

Here is an example of a situation where drugs would have been the preferred choice if the first remedy had not taken. I had a call from a client recently and it was obvious over the phone that she had pneumonia. She hates medical doctors and hospitals and turned to homeopathy because it's user-friendly and natural. I told Judy that I would take her collection of symptoms over the phone, repertorize and find a remedy to hopefully halt that pneumonia in its tracks. Her husband came over and picked up the remedy. I told Judy to call me in an hour; if she wasn't obviously improved in that time, she was to get to the emergency room for immediate treatment. With more than 1,400 remedies in our pharmacopoeia, a homeopath can be wrong about which remedy to use. Homeopaths are only human and as such can error on the choice of remedy. However, in most circumstances, the right remedy is found by the second or third try. In Judy's case, her pneumonia had struck her so hard and fast that I knew I didn't have time to try a second or third remedy if I didn't choose correctly the first time. I wasn't about to let my client suffer at my hands. Fortunately, the remedy I chose for her was correct and within 24 hours, she was up and around, without pneumonia symptoms. It took us three days of intense, close work together to clean it up completely, but it was done without drug intervention.

There is a right time and a wrong time to use homeopathy. A homeopathic prescriber knows which occasions are going to need allopathic intervention. The bottom line is this: your life, your health, comes first; the medical philosophy shouldn't count—your survival does. An example is a client who steps on a rusty nail. In that case, I automatically tell that person to go to an allopathic doctor and get a tetanus shot. I then give a homeopathic remedy after the shot, but basically, tetanus is something that doesn't always respond well to homeopathic treatment.

With lethal epidemics, my opinion is that we cannot risk *not* going to our medical doctors and get whatever help they can give us—and that includes a prescription drug if necessary. Homeopathy can work right alongside a prescription drug, with excellent results. So in epidemics or terrorist threats, always go to your medical doctor first and then call your homeopath for a remedy. Luckily for us, most symptoms *do* respond beautifully to homeopathic treatment.

What Is Hering's Law of Cure and How Does It Affect Me?

Homeopaths discovered more than 250 years ago that when they gave a remedy to a client, there was always a very definite, clear curative path that rarely wavered or fluctuated from person to person; it followed almost always the same pattern. Dr. Constantine Hering, one of our great homeopaths, brought the collection of curative path insights and observations together, and the healing path has since been known as Hering's Law of Cure.

Hering's Law of Cure states that once you take a homeopathic remedy, your vital force engages with this substance. (Your vital force consists of you, your physical energy; your aura, or electromagnetic energy; and your spirit. It's also known as the inner, organizing force or energy that generates your strength, endurance and so on.) There will be a noticeable change in your symptoms shortly afterward. A remedy works with the vital force, and in its own innate wisdom, cure begins following this pattern:

1. From the Top Down

The remedy works from the top of your head moving down your body to the tip of your toes; cure usually has a very specific direction, from the top down, so to speak, and this includes your mind, emotions, mental state and spiritual state as well. It also means that if there are any problems, injuries or traumas to your head or brain, they will be addressed first by the remedy and vital force. (I have seen some cases where it started elsewhere, like the chest or the extremities; it then moved up to the head and began its unaltering downward path to the toes.)

If, after taking a remedy, you get a headache and the next day experience a pain in your left arm, then a minor ache in your right knee, this is the remedy working in tandem with your body to create balance and health within you. You may see a slight change or alleviation of your symptoms in general regarding your head. Once things are "fixed" there before the cure moves down to your neck, shoulders, chest, abdomen and so forth, until it finally reaches your toes. Interestingly enough, any little fleeting aches and pains you may get will be transitory, so don't worry.

2. From the Most Important to the Least Important

At the same time, the remedy and vital force address the most important organs in your body first and the least important last. They deal with any injury or trauma connected with your brain and heart first, for without those two being in good health, one can die. The last organ of the body to be addressed is our skin. Frequently, a person will develop a rash somewhere on her or his body during the treatment for an amount of time. The homeopath is thrilled to hear this, because it means that the remedy is pushing the last of the poisons and toxins out via the skin, which is our major eliminative organ! The skin rash will disappear within a few days or weeks on its own and is nothing to worry about.

If the person is deeply disturbed on the mental or emotional level, the remedy and vital force will work there first, leaving the physical body and its problems until last. For example, if a person is suffering anxiety attacks due to trauma experienced, the remedy and vital force would deal with that before dealing with their sinus headaches or injured knee. The vital force knows that if we are in a state of imbalance mentally or emotionally, we need fixing there first in most cases.

3. Addressing Old Symptoms: Retracing

Any old symptoms you've had in the past or if you've taken an allopathic (traditional) drug—whether it be aspirin or prescription drugs—are addressed by the remedy and by the vital force in the reverse order of their occurrence.

Here is an example: Let's say you are 52 right now. At age 50, you got allergies; at age 45, you got sinus headaches; at age 20, you had a miscarriage; and at age 5, you broke your arm. When you take the remedy, the vital force goes backward in time and age until it encounters some symptom or a set of symptoms. Your old symptoms arise, and they may be just like you experienced them in the past—only this time, they won't be as intense, painful or last as long. The vital force goes back to age 50 and work on your allergies. Once they are cured, it continues to go into your past, looking for the next symptom(s). In this case, at age 45, you get your old sinus headaches back for a while until the remedy can cure them—permanently. Then the vital force continues to forage and hunt around for the next symptom, which in this example comes at age 20 when you experienced that miscarriage. As a result, a lot of suppressed emotions, such as grief or anger, might rise up or your menses may change for a couple months. Whatever is left or not worked through completely will be gone over one more time, the last time, during retracing. Once that is cleared up, the remedy and vital force address the broken arm you had at age 5. You get similar pain in that region where the break occurred for a few days, and then there is no more discomfort.

Can Anything I Eat or Drink Antidote My Homeopathic Remedy?

Yes, there is quite a list. Go to Appendix A for specific items that will antidote your remedy. One of the biggest is coffee, and it doesn't matter whether it's "real" coffee or decaffeinated. There is an oil in the coffee that will antidote your remedy. Another one is camphor, usually in the form of eucalyptus. Mint, which contains camphor, also is an antidote. Most people brush their teeth with a mint toothpaste and this will antidote the remedy. It is better to brush with baking soda. Besides, baking soda gets rid of gingivitis, so this is an extra bonus.

Another area of possible antidoting is dental drilling. The spinning of the drill creates a frequency that may instantly antidote a homeopathic remedy. So if you are slated for dental work, get it done first and take the remedy afterward. Of course, if you crack a tooth or develop tooth pain, go see your dentist right away. It's better to get this taken care of rather than worry about antidoting your homeopathic remedy. (Novocain is also known to antidote a homeopathic remedy.)

Right now, aromatherapy is big, and any strong oil or essence (or even perfume from the cosmetics counter in a department store!) placed on your skin, or simply you being in the room where it's kept and inhaled, will antidote your remedy. If you get a massage, use an oil without fragrance or strong odor.

Ask your homeopath if your remedy can be antidoted by anything other than what's on the list in Appendix A. Some remedies, such as *Hepar sulphuris*, are easily antidoted by taking vinegar in any form—even in salad dressings! *Crolatus horridus* is antidoted by drinking any beverage containing alcohol.

Homeopaths don't like to keep giving you a remedy every time you antidote it. A great deal of caution on your part must be maintained, along with the responsibility to make sure you stay away from items that will antidote your remedy. Some homeopaths will even refuse to re-dose you if you've antidoted. Homeopathic remedies strike your vital force, and to keep striking it isn't good for your health either. This means you have to pay some "watch-dog" attention to this list so that you don't antidote your remedy.

Something else that may disrupt your remedy is any other form of energy work, such as hands-on healing, Rolfing, Reiki, acupuncture, chakra balancing and so forth. Even electric blankets or electric heaters to warm a water bed are out! They too will antidote a remedy in some people.

Sometimes, no matter what you do, something new will come up and antidote a remedy. One of my clients, a singer, was working in his room setting up for yet another gig, when an extremely high, intense shriek from one of the microphones filled the air. He called to tell me that within five minutes, his asthma symptoms had started to return! So he took another dose of his remedy, and the asthma symptoms went away. This was the first time I'd heard of a piercing sound rupturing a remedy, but it makes sense because the remedies are high frequencies of energy—and any other source of high frequency sound could, in essence, antidote it. And there is the possibility that the fright from this sound antidoted his remedy. Any powerful, sudden emotion can do it too.

If you think you've antidoted your remedy, get in touch with your homeopath. A gradual return of some of your old symptoms will be the signal that it was, unfortunately, antidoted.

Are Homeopathic Remedies Dangerous?

They can be if you are self-prescribing. For instance, many homeopathic remedies sold over the counter do not put on their label a warning: "Stop taking the remedy as soon as your symp-toms go away." But you should!

The desire to take a homeopathic remedy without professional help during an epidemic or terrorist threat is going to be very invit-ing, but don't do it. This book is designed to help you get to a ho-meopath nearest you, to establish a long-term relationship with her or him and have that person be of critical help during such upset-ting times in your life. The best course of treatment is to find a ho-meopathic practitioner where you live, and information to help you do that is provided starting on page 360 in Appendix B. Do not try to dose yourself.

Go to a professional and avoid a potential situation where you might take a homeopathic remedy for weeks on end and cause a "proving" in you. This means that all of the old symptoms you got rid of initially with the remedy have come back—and there may be more symptoms than you originally had! You will feel far more mis-erable than you did before you took the remedy in the first place.

What Is a Proving?

A proving is a collection of symptoms. When we as homeopaths want to find out what kind of symptoms a remedy will cause in a person who is healthy, we give it to 10, 20 or 30 people who are volunteers, both men and women, willing to take the remedy to find out. There is a proving case manager who oversees the dispensing of the homeopathic remedy to the volunteers, who do *not* know what the remedy is. The volunteers are given a "proving log" to jot down all their symptoms: spiritual, mental, emotional and physical. Over a period of weeks or months (however long the case manager has decided this proving will go on), s/he keeps detailed lists of all the symptoms via the proving logs that are mailed to him or her on a regular basis. All of the symptoms caused by taking this remedy over a period of time will show the proving case manager what it can address. By hav-ing proving symptoms for a remedy, we can then match our cli-ents' symptoms when they come into our office, complaining of pain, for example.

The collections of symptoms are compiled into *materia medicas*, which have been created on and around provings by thousands of people for the past 200 years. "Like cures like" applies: A remedy that creates certain symptoms in a healthy person can cure a sick person whose symptoms parallel those symptoms that are listed in the *materia medica*. That is why provings are so important.

Provings are written in a funny way. They are not straightforward; rather, they are very detailed and usually stated in short, abrupt sentences. Proving sentences will never pass muster under an editor's eye, that's for sure! They are descriptive. A proving symptom has to show where it occurs in the body, and it has to describe the sensation, location or movement of it as well. Further, if something makes the symptom better (ameliorates) or worse (aggravates), that is also included in the proving description. Here's an example of a proving symptom for *Magnolia grandiflorus* (that beautiful Southern tree):

"**Head**: Headache, with gripping in abdomen with flushes of heat, congestive throbbing."

Wow! A mouthful, isn't it? Yet it is a symptom that one of the provers had while taking this remedy. As you can see, everything is very explicit and detailed. The prover had a headache with a gripping (think of a fist grabbing your abdomen) in the abdomen. "With flushes of heat" means the person experienced sudden heat. Just ask a woman about a hot flash, and you get the picture! The "congestive throbbing" means the prover had a sensation of congestion in his head and it was throbbing.

So you see, proving symptoms can be very tough to understand. In this book, I've attempted to make them 21st century and easier to read, but I cannot actually change the language. Why? Because a proving symptom is exactly that—a detailed symptom actually experienced by a person. And homeopaths do not like to change meanings because we didn't have the symptom, and to arrogantly change it could change the entire context of the proving symptom, which is a big no-no in our industry.

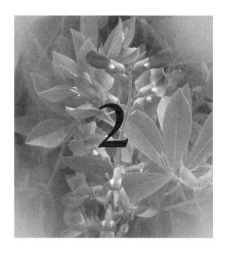

Homeopathic
Standard Operating Procedures

What Do We Do during an
Epidemic or a Terrorist Attack?

Unfortunately, here in the U.S., we have no official homeo-pathic "disaster plan" created and implemented by our national organization or any statewide homeopathic association so that we could hand out a set of protocols to you and say, "Follow this." However, homeopathic organizations have gotten together to hammer out a blueprint for disasters of this type in the future that could then filter down to each state and each professional homeopath so that people who are interested in homeopathic treatment can get it.

Your *best defense* is to contact a homeopath in your immediate area. If you don't know a homeopath, go to Appendix B; starting on page 360, there is information that helps you find the nearest homeopath to where you live. Your *second-best defense* is to be in touch with your medical doctor and pharmacist. I can't stress this enough. You will need antibiotics or other prescription drugs first, so see your medical doctor about this. Your *third-best defense* is to have certain homeopathic remedies on hand. See Appendix B and page 387 in Appendix C for information on obtaining a homeopathic home kit.

This chapter talks about the homeopathic remedies you should have on hand in case of an epidemic or a terrorist attack of chemical or biological nature in your area. It also outlines when to take the remedies and how often. Again, if you have a homeopath, talk this situation over with her or him or take this text to her or him and discuss it. Follow whatever your homeopath advises in lieu of this text.

Taking Your Constitutional Remedy

If you are fortunate enough to know what your constitutional remedy is, get your homeopath's approval and take it *one time.* This will help strengthen your immune system immeasurably, and it will help you in general through this very highly stressful time.

To find your constitutional remedy, you need to go to a professional homeopath, who then looks at all your symptoms and finds one remedy that best parallels them—like cures like. Constitutional case taking is complex and only a professional can do it. Usually, it takes one to three years to get you back to a reasonable state of health.

Nosode Homeopathic Remedies
Your Homeopath Needs to Keep on Hand

- For anthrax: *Anthracinum*
- For plague: *Pestinum*
- For *E-coli,* food poisoning, *Clostridium botulinum* toxin: *Botulinum*
- For smallpox: *Variolinum*
- For hemorrhagic fevers (including Ebola): *Crolatus horridus*

One other category A biological disease is *Francisella tularensis* (tularemia). At this time, I don't know of anyone who has this, but you might check with Ainsworth Homeopathic Pharmacy in England. Ideally, your homeopath has all the nosodes for epidemics as well as chemical and biological attacks on hand. Be sure to ask him or her!

Some Frequently Asked Questions

Where Can I Get Information on Attacks?

Your best resources are your health department, which is on the front line of defense and is at all times in direct contact with the Centers for Disease Control (CDC); your local hospital(s); your local radio station; your county's disaster planning department; and your fire station and police department. Your medical doctor is also an asset. Call locally first. If you don't get the answers you need, then go directly to the CDC at http://www.cdc.gov.

When Should I Take a Remedy?

If you live within 20 miles of a *known* terrorist attack via chemical or biological release, you should call your homeopath and with her approval, take the remedy she has chosen for you as well as the antibiotic or prescription drug your medical doctor has prescribed *simultaneously*. In the world of homeopathy, traditional medical drugs are usually looked down upon, but in such a scenario, we are going to need everything we can bring to the fight to survive this. Antibiotics are essential in such an event. Under no circumstances should you replace medical, prescribed drugs with a homeopathic remedy. Use both of them.

What Remedy Do I Take?

Take whatever remedy addresses the particular attack you have just undergone. This means that you must first find out what chemical or biological bacteria, virus or spore was released upon you.

For example, let's say anthrax has been determined to have been flown and released over your area. You would *first* go to your doctor for antibiotics and *then* call your homeopath and take whatever remedy s/he feels best suits your symptoms. It is *imperative* that you know what was released so you know what to tell your homeopath. Only your local authorities and hospitals or the CDC will have that answer. So call them!

Under no circumstances guess and, out of panic, decide to pop a homeopathic pellet. *Do not do this!* Wait with this and find out first. Let the proper officials alert you and others. Call your doctor too and see what you can find out. And then call your homeopath.

What Else Can I Do?

If you find yourself under attack, we suggest Rescue Remedy every 10 to 15 minutes (four drops beneath the tongue) to help with your anxiety and panic reactions. Once you settle down, you can stop taking it. After that, take Rescue Remedy on an "as needed" basis.

We can't stress enough the communication between you and your medical doctor. If things get bad, there is going to be panic, so you need to have your own house in order, have your homeopathic kit, your remedies and your instructions, as well as phone numbers of your homeopath and your medical doctor. Panic serves no one. Be prepared. Talk all possibilities over with your medical doctor and your homeopath well beforehand.

What About My Animals?

You need to try and contact your veterinarian. Talk to her or him about terrorist assaults and what strategy s/he has for such a scenario. Ask for the appropriate drugs of choice for each type of scenario. Keep these drugs on hand and give them to your pet(s) as directed by your veterinarian. Again, be prepared.

Can My Animals Take the Same Homeopathic Remedies I Do?

Yes and no. Pets weigh a lot less than us humans; consequently, the potency and dosage would change considerably. There are so many possibilities with this that it is impossible to cover all possible scenarios. You are best off with your veterinarian's intervention, information and drug of choice.

We would *not* recommend homeopathic treatment out-of-hand for pets at this time. If you can locate a homeopath, call and ask if s/he is willing to treat pets; many are. There are a few homeopathic veterinarians around, but not many and certainly not enough to serve the U.S. at large. Again, good communication with your veterinarian now is essential.

Stay Calm and Focused

Having been in many disasters and events, I can tell you that the best thing you can do is stay calm—calm and thinking through the panic or anxiety around you. Rescue Remedy is a remarkable flower essence, and I highly recommend it. The calmer you are, the better your chances of surviving this.

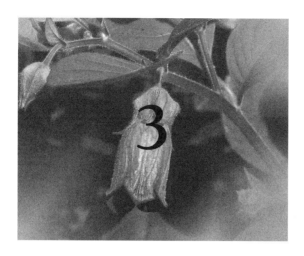

The History of Pandemics and the Ebola Virus

Killer Bugs and Viruses:
The Black Plague of the Twentieth Century

In the Middle Ages, the black plague was the scourge of Europe and millions died; it was Europe's pandemic. Back then, antibiotics weren't known—and neither was homeopathy.

In 1918, after World War I ended, a virulent form of influenza, or flu, virus swept across our globe and 22 million lives—more than all those killed during the war—were lost to this lethal virus, commonly called the grippe or influenza. In the U.S., homeopathy was on the decline at that time because politically, allopathic medicine was taking a larger role in our country's system of medicine; allopathic medicine was put to a test when this deadly flu virus arrived.

An interesting statistic emerged from this trial of allopathic versus homeopathic treatment during a killer epidemic. Eighty percent of those who contracted the flu and used allopathic medicine in any form, died. Eighty percent of those who were treated by a homeopathic physician with a homeopathic remedy, lived. Old journals mention the six homeopathic remedies that were known to save lives; some of the most prominent were *Crolatus horridus*, baptisia, *Gelsemium* and *Eupatorium perfoliatum*. It was one of the few times when two entirely different forms of medicine were put to the test against something so deadly—and homeopathy won hands down.

So what are superbugs? There's been a spate of information on what is happening worldwide with bacteria. Antibiotics have been used since 1940 to get rid of bacterial infections such as streptococcus (as in strep throat, gangrene, impetigo, meningitis, pneumonia, rheumatic fever, scarlet fever, tonsillitis, wound and skin infections, sore throats, blood poisoning [septicemia] and so forth) or staphylococcus (causes innumerable ailments throughout the body, including cholera, syphilis, tuberculosis, toxic shock syndrome, pneumonia, impetigo, food poisoning, endocarditis and cellulitis). Other disease agents include viruses such as smallpox, HIV/AIDS, SARS and hepatitis B, to name a few. Protozoa, the third type, causes such illnesses as malaria.

Our reliance is on only one form of medicine in the U.S., and that is allopathic medicine. In allopathic medicine, large doses of a crude drug are used to overwhelm the liver's defenses, killing a small part of the liver in the process, to get into the bloodstream to kill the bacteria or protozoa. Unfortunately, viruses are not as easily killed by antibiotics. Usually, something that can kill a virus will also kill the host—in this case, the human being carrying the virus.

There are very few antiviral drugs in the world. The biggest weapon against viruses have always been preventive vaccines, and lately we've seen that they don't work either. For instance, look at those who took the polio vaccine, the DPT (diphtheria, pertussis and tetanus) shot or the measles vaccine only to find that they don't really work; if they did, our children wouldn't be coming down with measles and these other illnesses in such huge numbers.

We're coming to a point in our development where we will have to pay for having blinders on and using only one form of medicine to keep us healthy. From a homeopathic standpoint, vaccines and antibiotics are suppressive to the human being, and at some point, perhaps years or decades later, the disease that was supposedly "cured" by the antibiotic or vaccine will remanifest within the person. None are better examples of this than those who contracted polio as children, went through allopathic drug treatment and now, decades later, have the polio remanifesting in them. The medical professionals are throwing up their hands saying that they can't explain it, nor do they have a drug to "fix it" again.

I wish that polio victims could be treated homeopathically. I know that by gently stimulating their own natural systems with a homeopathic remedy, they could get relief from this returning ailment or perhaps, in some cases, a complete cure. Polio is a virus; all the allopathic drug treatment does is suppress it. As per homeopathic philosophy, the virus is then free to come back—and it has. The polio virus incubates quite comfortably in these people. Allopathic drugs might put it to "sleep" for decades, but like every virus, it can wake up and begin to wreak its symptomatic havoc again.

The beauty of homeopathy is that once the patient is seen and all the symptoms are gathered, a remedy can be given to force the virus to run its natural and *entire* course. Once this is done, the virus will die and the person will never be bothered by those viral symptoms again. No allopathic antiviral or antibiotic can force a virus to run its complete course and leave the body. All it can do, at best, is anesthetize it so it will "hibernate" somewhere in the person's body. The problems begin all over again when the virus wakes up.

In my personal opinion, the world is tottering on a precipice where billions of people could be killed by superbugs, and it is only a matter of time before these deadly bacteria and viruses sweep across countries, killing millions upon millions of people. The great flu epidemic of 1918 will be considered minor in comparison to what is going to happen within the next decade. The black plague will also seem to have been minor, because there weren't nearly the population numbers in the Middle Ages that we have now.

The worst part of this nightmare unfolding before our eyes is that allopathic medicine no longer has antibiotics that can halt these scourges once they start. As a medical astrologer, I predicted the AIDS virus three years before it actually manifested. I spoke at many national astrological conferences, warning astrologers that a reproductive disease of a proportion that we'd never seen before—except for the black plague—would manifest on our planet. And it did.

The people of our country have been running to a doctor for every cold and flu, asking for and receiving antibiotics. Those in the medical community are not innocent either, for they have abused antibiotics for decades. Between these two camps, bacteria have gotten smarter faster than their human counterparts. For instance, earaches in children are routinely treated with antibiotics. Children might receive a dozen rounds of antibiotics before the physician suggests surgery to correct the condition. If these children would have gone to a homeopath, they would have received a remedy—usually belladonna—and the entire earache cycle would have been broken forever, with no returning symptoms. Any parent whose child has this problem should see a homeopath first before considering surgery for a child's continual ear infections.

When an antibiotic is used against a colony of bacteria, most of the microbes are killed. However, there may be one microbe in that colony that mutates because of the antibiotic given and it goes on to replicate itself, until a new colony exists that is resistant to that antibiotic. A bacterium can, in some cases, reproduce a new generation in just 20 minutes! There is no way drug makers will be able to keep up with such swiftly reproducing, smart bacteria; sooner or later, the bacteria will be resistant to all forms of drugs. At that point, a bacterium can become a merciless killer of millions of people, for there will be nothing left in the drug maker's arsenal to stop it.

Another way bacteria become drug resistant is when a harmless, drug-resistant microbe in us attaches itself to a harmful microbe. This creates a "tube," or connection, between the two microbes, a phenomenon referred to as conjugation. At this point, a copy of the genetic structure of the drug-resistant microbe is passed both ways from each individual microbe. As Dr. George Curlin of the National Institute of Allergy and Infectious Diseases says, "The more you use antibiotics, the more rapidly Mother Nature adapts to them." (Healthtrak Infosource, "Colostrum: Nature's Infectious Disease Fighter," *Healthtrak Infosource,* http://www.colostruminfo.com/articles/ disease_fighters.html.)

And speaking of Mother Earth, a living, viable entity in herself, she has gone into a defensive mode against human beings. Why? If you accept the premise that Gaia, Mother Earth, is a living entity who has a brain and emotions, then she also has an immune system, just like us. Humans have done great damage to her in the past five decades by polluting her water (her blood) and her air (the air she breathes like we do) and by putting toxic waste in her soil (her skin). Because we are killing her, her immune system is going to rise up and kill the invader who is sickening her daily—us, the humans who live upon her. She will create deadly viruses and bacteria to infect the humans who are doing her damage.

Long ago I attended a homeopathic conference with Dr. Edward Whitmont, an MD and Jungian therapist. Now deceased, he had worked with Carl Jung for a number of years and, as a homeopath, he had made a fascinating discovery. He did worldwide research on where Lyme disease, a then recent phenomenon carried by ticks, was manifesting, and in every instance, Lyme disease cropped up around cities and suburbs. But if he went out in the forest, away from the cities and suburbs, there was no Lyme disease! He felt this was Mother Earth's way of trying to get rid of the encroachers who were replacing her forests with cities, and she had manifested the Lyme disease through one of her allies, the ticks. In other words, she was trying to get rid of the "bug" that was trying to hurt her—the human being.

Mother Earth's Defense Mechanism

Another area on which humans are encroaching mindlessly is the Amazon rain forest, a literal womb of humidity where we find a triple canopy of trees, life-saving herbs, molds, bacteria, wildlife and viruses. The world's overpopulation and overcutting have begun to destroy the natural old forests, but Mother Earth is fighting back—with deadly viruses that have lain dormant for thousands or millions of years but are awakening as humanity comes in and disturbs them. These viruses or bacteria have been carried by animals that are not harmed by them, but as humans assault Mother Earth, she activates the transfer of these deadly bacteria and viruses that attack the encroachers and kill them quite quickly.

There is proof of this already happening. One instance is the rain forest region of Zaire, where the overpopulation had been cutting into the forests for years until a very swift and deadly virus known as the Ebola virus attacked the people. Several days after contracting this virus, the typical victim's eyes turn red, his head aches, red spots pop out on his flesh and become a rash of small blisters; and then his skin begins to rip open. Blood flows from every orifice in his body. The victim coughs up black, bloody vomit and in the process, parts of his tongue, throat and windpipe slough off. Every organ fills with blood and at some point ceases to function. The victim has seizures and that way spreads the virus to others. Within days, the victim is dead; the tissue is actually liquefied.

From the rain forest of the Amazon come at least 50 viruses that scientists know can make people sick or even kill them. The most lethal thus far discovered in South America are the Junin, Machupo and Sabia viruses. Sabia was unknown in Brazil until it killed a woman there in 1990; it had lived benignly in rodents in Brazil until then. Now the virus, much like the hantavirus of the Four Corners region, is transferring from animal to human. In Africa is a virus known as X, which came out of the rain forest in southern Sudan in 1989 and killed thousands before it disappeared. No one knows when or if it will come out and attack again.

All of these attacks occurred when populations overflowed from the cities into the country and began hacking back old forest growth. Richard Preston, in his new book *Hot Zone*, writes about what would happen if one of these killer viruses went on a rampage and attacked more than just those city dwellers who come to destroy Mother Earth's forests. In *Time* magazine, he warns that "the rain forest has its own defenses. . . . The Earth's immune system . . . is starting to kick in. . . . The Earth is attempting to rid itself of an infection by the human parasite." (Richard Preston, "A Deadly Virus Escapes," *Time Magazine*, September 5, 1994: 66.)

To make matters worse, certain viruses are more deadly than others. For instance, the Arena virus family, which includes the Sabia, Junin, Machupo and Guanarito in South America and the Ebola, Marburg and Lassa in Africa, kills in a horrible way: high fever; hemorrhaging all over the body, including the organs; shock; and finally, death. The liver turns yellow and decomposes rapidly, and blood leaks from every orifice of the body, including the eyes as well as the skin.

New viruses are moving from animal hosts to human hosts. Nowhere has this been more clearly illustrated than with the hantavirus, which erupted in 1992 in the Four Corners region of the Southwest. As a homeopath who lives in Arizona, I was very interested in this viral upper respiratory illness that can kill within 48 to 72 hours; the victim's lungs literally fill with fluid and s/he suffocates due to the kidneys shutting down. The hantavirus has been found in 25 percent of all chipmunks and in smaller percentages of deer mice and other rodents. The interesting thing is that these animals had carried this virus benignly for years, perhaps decades, and never spread it to humans. Now they are spreading it, and scientists haven't figured out why.

In 2003 a virus jumped from chickens to humans. Called the bird flu virus, this is a potential killer worldwide. It started in China and spread to Southeast Asia. By January 2004, millions of chickens infected with this virus were killed so that it could not leap to humans. It is rare that a virus will jump from animal to human, but it has occurred in the past. This one is quite lethal and the CDC and major health organizations around the globe are continuing to watch for it spreading.

AIDS is said to have been carried benignly by monkeys in Africa before it began to infect villagers and then spread worldwide. Many people who contracted AIDS (not HIV) die within two years of onset. But the AIDS virus is a long-term killer in comparison to the new viruses that are now being transmitted from animals to humans. Lyme disease, which is transmitted from deer to ticks to humans, is one example.

Science isn't necessarily helping things. In 1989 at a U.S. Army laboratory on the East Coast where researchers were studying a group of contaminated African monkeys, the Ebola Reston virus spread throughout the lab. The army had a potentially major disaster on their hands and ended up killing all the monkeys to prevent the spread of this virus to the American people. They had to shut down and abandon the entire facility as a result.

At Yale University this summer, a scientist had a test tube containing the deadly Sabia virus break during a spin in a high-speed centrifuge. He followed all procedures for cleaning up after this break but neglected to report the accident to the Centers for Disease Control. A few days later, this scientist came down with the virus and nearly died. In the meantime, he'd infected 75 other people, including his family. Yale Arbovirus Research Unit, where the break and escape of the virus occurred, is looking at how to halt such accidents.

Recurring Viruses

Things are heating up worldwide with bacteria and viruses that are fighting back. In Gloucester, England, the flesh-eating variety of streptobacillus known as strep A has flared up. Strep A claims thousands of lives each year in the U.S. and Europe, and if it is not detected within hours and treated, the victim can lose a limb—or die. This necrotic, or flesh-eating, strain of bacteria is a swift-moving killer and is now appearing more often than in the past. Puppeteer Jim Henson died unexpectedly of strep A.

Tuberculosis is also on the rise worldwide. After a 16-year-old Vietnamese immigrant brought the airborne disease into a high school in Westminster, California, 400 students (30 percent of the school's students) were infected. At least 12 of these students have a variety of TB that is antibiotic resistant. Tuberculosis, generally speaking, is now antibiotic resistant.

Between 1979 and 1992, only 352 cases of pertussis (whooping cough) were reported in Cincinnati. In 1994 there was an epidemic, and 542 cases were reported. The twist to this was that all the children had been vaccinated against pertussis! Furthermore, there were 6,500 cases of Pertussis reported nationwide in 1994—more than in any other year over the previous 26 years. Again we're seeing that vaccinations aren't working. Even though the whooping cough vaccine is given routinely, infants are still getting this disease. According to Brian Pascual, CDC public health specialist, 9,771 cases were reported in 2002. That is the most since 1964. Further, 15 deaths were caused by whooping cough. What is even more disturbing is that officials believe that only about 10 percent of the actual whooping cough cases get reported.

Lyme disease, which is prominent in the northeast portion of our country, has just evolved a new and more lethal strain. Twenty-five people in Wisconsin and Minnesota were bitten by ticks carrying the new strain, *Ehrlichia*, which is life threatening and drug resistant. Two of those people died. Doctors are worried that this new strain might be misdiagnosed as the regular type of Lyme disease—or as just a cold.

In my own town of Cottonwood, a year after the hantavirus outbreak, Dr. Gail Derin, the other local professional homeopath, and I observed a spin-off flu virus that we're certain was a result of the hantavirus. In January and February of 1993, the entire Southwest was swept by a frightening flu virus that within 48 hours would send a victim to the hospital with a full-blown case of pneumonia! Forty-eight hours! The hantavirus, in that same time, would not only create pneumonia-like symptoms, but would kill the victim.

The flu that swept our region in 1993, the year after the hantavirus outbreak, wasn't to be taken lightly. Gail and I spent untold hours on the phone with our patients who had contracted this upper respiratory flu virus. We got little sleep in those two months, but the outcome was good: Our patients responded well to three homeopathic remedies. The remedy used depended upon how soon they called us after they started experiencing symptoms.

The flu virus hit suddenly, with a high fever; a ralelike, nonstop cough; and fluid settling quickly into the lungs—within 48 hours. If the patient called us at the outset, when experiencing high fever and cough, belladonna took care of it quickly and knocked out the flu virus. If patients waited those 48 hours, they would get serious pneumonia symptoms, but *Hepar sulphuris* handled those symptoms and kept them out of the hospital and away from the antibiotic route. In some cases, the flu would hang on and people would have a cough that did not go away for weeks or months afterward although the fluid in the lungs was gone. We prescribed *Gelsemium sempervirens* (the great flu epidemic remedy that saved so many lives in 1918) to mop up and get rid of the last vestiges of the virus.

Interestingly, Gail Derin and I found four homeopathic remedies to address the known symptoms of the hantavirus picture: *Pyrogenium*, *Baptisia tinctoria*, *Eupatorium perfoliatum* and *Rhus toxicodendron*. All these are well-known influenza remedies for serious flulike symptoms.

The Coming Pandemics

On May 19, 1995, we saw the reemergence of the deadly Ebola virus in Zaire, Africa. This Ebola virus is a member of the filovirus family, a new strain that had lain dormant for some time. Perhaps it's not as new as the scientific world thinks it might be. After all, the electron microscope has only recently been invented. Fifty years ago, the epidemics sweeping the world were routinely called "flu" or "influenza," because no one had the capability to see the viruses; one could just see the damage they inflicted. I know this strain of viruses will sweep the world, much like the black death, the bubonic plague, swept through the Old World.

The plague, as it is commonly known, seems to have had its roots somewhere in China between 1330 and the 1340s. It then got Europe's attention by showing up in 1346 in the Crimean area of Turkey. This killer virus was not a filovirus, but bacteria carried through rats (similar to the hantavirus here in the western U.S., which is carried by mice, squirrels and chipmunks).

The plague did an interesting thing. If you imagine a straight line that suddenly forks, with the right fork going clockwise in a curling motion and the left fork going counterclockwise also in a curling motion, you get an idea what the plague did as it came out of the Crimea. The counterclockwise rotation hit lower Egypt in 1347, Cyprus/Rhodes in 1348 and Baghdad and Armenia in 1349. The clockwise rotation struck Alexandria in 1347 and then, in 1348, it roared mercilessly into Spain and up to Paris. In 1349 it struck England, and in 1350 it turned eastward once again and ravaged Germany. The Balkans and Poland were hit in 1351 before the plague's deadly attack finally ended in Moscow in 1353.

Countless millions died from the plague. It would ravage a city, then quiet down and suddenly pop up in another city or region. It seemed to respond in a wavelike motion, curling to gather force and then rushing forward at stunning speed, engulfing a region and killing hundreds of thousands in startlingly short time. And then, like a wave receding from the shore, it would suddenly stop its forward motion, gather more force and energy and, seemingly out of nowhere, strike again.

From a medical astrology standpoint, I'm always interested in pandemics such as the plague. Influenza or flu epidemics swept through Europe in 1729-30 and 1732-33, then again in 1761-62 and 1781-82. The 1781-82 pandemic in Europe was considered one of the greatest manifestations of disease in all history. This influenza made two-thirds of the people of Rome ill, and three-quarters of Britain's population fell to their knees. That year the killer influenza quickly swept to North America, the West Indies and Spanish America.

There were three more influenza pandemics, in 1830-1831, 1833 and 1889-1890. The 1889 pandemic in Europe, known as the Russian flu, killed (by a conservative estimate) 250,000 people; virologists who study pandemics suggest that this particular pandemic flu killed a two to three times greater number. All told, influenza killed more people in Europe during the 19th century than did cholera.

The lulls between these pandemics are of particular interest to virologists. From 1847 to 1889, Europe saw only a few minor upsurges (and certainly nothing on the epidemic level) of influenza. Again, it's as if the viruses pull back to gather energy and force, like an ocean wave withdrawing from the shore, and then they come crashing down and rush forward again at dizzying speed. This is when they take on pandemic proportions.

The Spanish Influenza

On U.S. shores, we've had a number of killer epidemics during our short 200-year history. For instance, there have been several influenza epidemics. In 1918, at a military camp in Kansas, a soldier returning from Europe shortly before the end of World War I came down with what was known as the Spanish influenza. This strain of flu had its origins in Spain, and so the name stuck.

The Spanish influenza first went eastward and, just like the plague, it would reach out with dizzying speed and strike a city, and thousands of inhabitants would suddenly die of the flu. Then it would seem to stop, but a week or two later it would strike out again, this time in another city. Overall, this pandemic killed 500,000 of our people in 1918 and 1919. A great-grandmother on my mother's side who lived in Ohio at that time died of it. In the winter of 1920, a second wave of the Spanish influenza virus struck. In terms of deaths, this was the second-worst influenza strike of all time, after the 1918-19 epidemic.

The killer aspects of the Spanish influenza are astounding if you look at the world population at that time. When the pandemic finally wore itself out after a two-year attack around the world, 22 million people—one percent of the Earth's entire population—were dead from this one killer influenza attack. The segment of the population that suffered the greatest losses was the younger adults (half of those who died were between 20 and 40 years old). The virus had a nasty upper-respiratory kick to it that sent people down with violent, pneumonia-like symptoms, choking the victims with inflammation and edema.

The Spanish flu did most of its killing around the world over a six-month period. This is particularly shocking when you consider that in 1918 airplane travel wasn't available, only ship or train travel, which certainly wasn't that fast. Yet the Spanish flu killed 7,542 Samoan people, out of a population of 38,302, in just two months!

We've had other, less deadly influenza-like epidemics in 1900, 1957, 1968, 1977 and in 2003. We've had SARS appear along with one of our most deadly flu seasons since the killer flu of 1968. Since then, influenza pandemics in the U.S. have been missing. But "missing" doesn't mean gone or guaranteed not to happen again.

Other U.S. epidemics include:
- Cholera in New York, Boston and Philadelphia in July/August of 1832, which killed 2,251, though 5,835 contracted the disease.
- Yellow fever, which struck Philadelphia between August and November 1793; 4,000 people died.
- Polio in Vermont between June and September 1894; 123 cases were reported.
- Smallpox in Boston, Massachusetts, starting on May 26, 1721. It killed between 12 and 24 percent of the city's population.

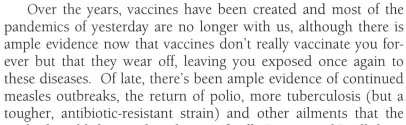

Over the years, vaccines have been created and most of the pandemics of yesterday are no longer with us, although there is ample evidence now that vaccines don't really vaccinate you forever but that they wear off, leaving you exposed once again to these diseases. Of late, there's been ample evidence of continued measles outbreaks, the return of polio, more tuberculosis (but a tougher, antibiotic-resistant strain) and other ailments that the medical establishment thought were finally "conquered." All these "conquered" diseases are mutating into stronger, vaccine- and antibiotic-resistant strains that will kill us instead of just causing a week's worth of discomfort, as a case of measles will do.

The Filovirus Family

This leads to what is staring us in the face right now: a virus that's ready to inflict global damage of untold proportions, the filovirus family. There are a number of filoviruses and, interestingly, they all look like long snakes or worms under a microscope. Among the members of this family are Ebola Sudan, Marburg and Zaire filoviruses—much like brothers and sisters in the same family.

The first notice we were given about filoviruses occurred in 1967 when a simultaneous outbreak of hemorrhagic fever occurred in Marburg and Frankfurt, Germany and in Belgrade, Yugoslavia. Lab workers in these two countries had been processing kidneys from Ugandan green monkeys for cell-culture production. Thirty-eight people became infected with this unknown filovirus and seven died. It then became known as the Marburg virus.

After this first attack, the filovirus disappeared—until 1975, when three cases of the Marburg hemorrhagic fever were reported in Johannesburg, South Africa. The man who first contracted it had traveled to Zimbabwe and died after a 12-day illness. His traveling companion and a nurse contracted it as well, but they survived.

In 1976 the second attack erupted. This time it was severe: 550 cases, with 430 deaths, occurred simultaneously in Zaire and the Sudan. It was at this time that it was realized that the Marburg and the newly coined Ebola virus were the *same filovirus*—with outbreaks in different locations. Later, virologists would consider the Marburg virus one type of filovirus, with the Ebola having two subtypes, the Sudan and Zaire varieties.

In 1979 in the Sudan, another outbreak of 34 cases and 22 fatalities was reported. Then, in 1980, a Kenya man died of the Ebola virus; a doctor was infected by it, and further spreading was prevented only by careful nursing procedures. The Kenya man who died of it had been in Uganda, in the same area the green monkeys had come from. Still, virologists didn't think that these monkeys were the carriers for the filoviruses.

In fact, investigations have still failed to identify the source of the Ebola virus. No antibody or virus has ever been found in thousands of specimens of animals, and this includes 200 monkeys collected in Zaire and Sudan. So scientists and virologists are puzzled; they have no idea where this virus originated. One thing is for sure: Ebola is the most lethal killer the world has ever seen, and it makes the plague look like an infant in comparison. There is no *known* medical treatment available for filoviruses, none. There is no vaccine, and antibiotics have proven useless.

The Spread of the Ebola Virus

This leads us to the possibility of the next devastating around-the-world pandemic: a filovirus that will "jump" from Africa and begin a world tour, killing off millions. And it's not going to be a long time in coming if my astrological calculations are correct.

Pandemics, by their very nature, seem to be fostered by hot, moist conditions; for example, in 1918 the Spanish flu made its presence known in the U.S. in August. Prime targets of the Ebola virus are the environments of the larger cities. The reasons are obvious: the more human beings per square inch and the more garbage, the easier it is for a virus to be transmitted from one person to another. If you live out in the country, your chances of avoiding it are better, but you're not completely safe. I believe the next outbreak will occur during a hot and moist season.

The April 1995 Ebola virus epidemic broke out in Zaire and an infected man took an airplane trip from Africa to Canada; he was stopped and quarantined in Canada—we almost had Ebola at our front door. In 1990 Ebola cases were discovered on the docks of Philadelphia and quarantined. Next time I don't believe we're going to be so lucky, and to stick our heads in the sand and think that some alert official at an airport is going to catch every Ebola-infected person is idealism that will get us killed.

With airlines making it possible for people to hop from city to city around the world and considering that Ebola has a 7- to 21-day incubation period, one person can infect many others and not even know it. An example of this is the Sabia virus I spoke of earlier. The scientist who accidentally exposed himself to the Sabia virus infected 75 people, including his family members. All of them were eventually quarantined, which effectively stopped the spread of this South American cousin to the Ebola virus in Boston. We aren't always going to be so lucky. Someone who has been in the Amazon jungle could be a carrier of one of these viruses, take a plane, land in the U.S. and potentially do a lot more damage than the scientist who unknowingly infected so many people.

Homeopathic Remedies

The good news is that there are several homeopathic remedies; one in particular mirrors the filovirus symptoms almost perfectly, at nearly 95 percent. What is very interesting is that *Crolatus horridus* (rattlesnake venom), which was one of the five major remedies used in saving 80 percent of the people treated by homeopaths in the U.S. during the Spanish flu pandemic, is the same remedy that will stop the filoviruses of today!

Crolatus horridus saved so many lives in the U.S. alone via homeopaths who treated patients with Spanish flu symptoms, that I believe keeping this remedy in your medicine cabinet may mean the difference between life and death. It's reassuring to know we've got a homeopathic remedy that can help save lives in such a pandemic.

Here's more information on the Ebola virus, thanks to members of the Kachina Study Group in Cottonwood, Arizona, Cathy Leonardi, Joanne Matkovich and Dr. Gail Derin, who made an exhaustive and detailed search for specific symptoms of the Ebola virus. Without good, useful and specific symptoms, we could not have arrived at the correct remedy to deal with this disease.

- Ebola Zaire: 90 percent fatal.
- Ebola Sudan: 50 percent fatal.
- Ebola Marburg: 25 percent fatal.
- Ebola Reston: monkeys only; cannot affect human beings.

Ebola is distantly related to measles, mumps and rabies; it's related to the parainfluenza virus (causes colds in children) and the respiratory syncytial virus (which causes fatal pneumonia in AIDS patients). Ebola symptoms include an overall body rash (like measles), psychosis, a madness similar to rabies and bad cold symptoms. Ebola consists of seven proteins that are large molecules. Four of the seven are unknown in both structure and function. They seem to explosively target the immune system. The other three proteins are only vaguely understood. Incubation for Ebola is 3 to 14 days; it can work through the body in 10 days, whereas it can take AIDS patients 10 years to destruct. It is transmitted from the dead to the living through touch, direct contact with blood or other body fluids, and through the air via coughing and sneezing.

Ebola Zaire

A man, 56 years old, a loner, contracted Ebola Zaire. On the seventh day of his exposure to this filovirus, he got a headache (throbbing behind the eyeballs, aching temples and pain circling around inside his head) and then a severe backache.

On the third day of the headache, he also got nausea and a spiked fever and began vomiting, which became intense and turned into dry heaves. After that, he became very passive; his face lost all appearance of life (was masklike); and his eyeballs were fixed, paralytic and staring, although his eyelids were droopy. His eyes seemed to be popping out, yet they were half closed at the same time. His eyes seemed frozen in their sockets and the white areas turned bright red. The skin of his face turned yellow, with red, starlike speckles. His personality changed; he became sullen, resentful and angry. Although he had no memory, he was not delirious.

At this point, he was taken to a doctor, who told him to fly to Nairobi to a bigger hospital. The following occurred on the flight:

1. He vomited blood with black specks in it and his lips became slippery and red with blood.
2. His eyes turned the color of rubies, a bright red.
3. His face was masklike, expressionless, and contained many bruises.
4. The skin on his head began turning black and blue.
5. The muscles of his face drooped (a slack expression).
6. He had continuous vomiting and filled many airsickness bags; the vomit turned either black or red with black flecks in it.
7. He had massive interior degeneration in the intestinal areas and the brain.

He died at the Nairobi hospital after being treated by a doctor. In the end there was blood coming out of every orifice of his body—nose, ears, eyes, mouth, anus and urethra.

Some of the patient's blood spattered into the doctor's eyes while he treated him. The doctor became ill nine days after exposure. His symptoms were backache, with the ache spreading throughout his body, eyes turning red and fever. He took malaria pills but to no effect. The nurse gave him a shot, but the pain of the injection was very severe for him. He experienced abdominal pain and developed jaundice (a liver condition that makes the skin turn yellow). This doctor was then examined by a second doctor, who diagnosed fever, red eyes, jaundice and abdominal pain. She ordered an ultrasound, which showed an enlarged liver. The patient's face became an expressionless mask. Exploratory surgery showed his liver to be swollen, red and unhealthy-looking. There was no sign of gallstones. Bleeding would not stop during the surgery. A third doctor watched as the man continued to deteriorate. He took blood samples from the patient and sent them off to the lab. It was then that Ebola Zaire was discovered.

General Symptoms

- The intestines fill with blood.
- The abdominal wall lining sloughs off into the bowel and is expelled with large amounts of blood.
- In women, the labia around the vagina turn a livid blue color due to massive internal vaginal bleeding.
- The brain may experience grand-mal epileptic seizures. (Some philosophize that in this way the virus, which wants to live, propagates itself by being splattered on someone nearby who is trying to help the person with the seizure.)
- Infected cells become crystalline blocks of packed virus particles known as "bricks."
- There may be a hemispherical stroke; one whole side of the body may become paralyzed, leading to death.
- The blood thickens and slows. Clots begin to stick to the walls of the blood vessels. The clots thicken and then drift into capillaries, shutting off the blood supply to different parts of the body. This leads to "dead spots" in the brain, liver, kidneys, lungs, intestines, testicles, breast tissue (both male and female) and skin.
- The blood streaming out of the body will not clot. Under a microscope, the blood cells show broken and dead, as if they have been buzzed with a blender.
- The skin shows a creeping, spotty necrosis (dying).
- The liver bulges and swells, turns yellow, begins to liquefy, cracks apart, dies and goes putrid.
- The kidneys jam with blood clots and dead cells and finally fail. When the kidneys stop working, the bloodstream becomes toxic with urine/toxins/poisons that can no longer be excreted from the body.
- The spleen turns large and hard with blood. In one patient, the clot in the spleen was the size of a baseball.
- The Ebola proteins chew up the body's collagen material (collagen is the cartilage that holds our joints together) and turn it to mush.
- Layers of the skin die and liquefy.
- The skin bubbles into a sea of tiny white blisters mixed with red spots (maculopapular rash). This leads to rips in the skin, with hemorrhaging following and blood pouring forth. The red spots on the skin grow, spread and merge into huge, spontaneous

bruises. The skin becomes soft and pulpy and tears off easily.
- The mouth and the gums bleed. The salivary glands within the mouth hemorrhage and bleed.
- The tongue turns red and sloughs off.
- The throat and lining of the windpipe may slough off.
- The heart bleeds into itself and the heart muscle softens.
- The brain becomes clogged with dead cells.
- Ebola attacks the eyeball lining and the eyes fill with blood—the "ruby-colored" eyes.
- The skin develops red spots called petechiae (small, purplish, hemorrhagic spots on the skin or spots that look like flea bites).

Ebola Zaire, which attacks every organ and tissue except skeletal muscle and bone, was first discovered in early September 1976; the first case was never identified. It's twice as lethal as Ebola Sudan.

Transmission

Transmission of the Ebola Zaire virus occurs through any of the following ways:
- Grieving relatives kissing and embracing the dead become contaminated and infected; direct contact with blood or body fluids.
- Ebola Zaire feeds on primates (monkeys) and it can jump back and forth from monkeys to humans. (This is not true for Ebola Reston.)
- It is suspected that it is airborne, probably due to secretions coming from coughing or sneezing.

Ebola Sudan

The first case involved a man from Nzara, Sudan. The cause of the infection is unknown, although it jumped quickly and viciously. It "amplified" (multiplied) in a hospital in Maridi. The fatality rate is 50 percent (twice that of Ebola Marburg, the mildest filovirus form of Ebola). The outbreak spread through the Sudan and as far as Cairo, then subsided and literally vanished. The people involved had no knowledge of the virus being airborne, but heat accelerated the infection, perhaps causing people to die so quickly that they couldn't infect anyone else.

General Symptoms

- Mental derangement.
- Psychosis.
- Depersonalization.
- Zombielike behavior.

Transmission

Same as for Ebola Zaire.

Ebola Marburg

This strain of the Ebola filovirus was named after the German city Marburg. A person flew from Africa to Marburg, where the disease "amplified" and was diagnosed. It is the "gentlest" of the three deadly filoviruses and affects humans in a way similar to exposure to nuclear radiation. The Marburg filovirus strands sometimes roll into loops and look like Cheerios. It is the only ring-shaped virus known. (From an archetypal standpoint, it fits the Uroboros symbol of a snake eating its tail.)

General Symptoms

- On the seventh day after exposure there are headaches, raging fever, clotting, spurts of blood and terminal shock that damages all body tissues and internal organs.
- Attacks connective tissue.
- Attacks the intestines and skin.
- Hair loss; hair dies at the roots and falls off in clumps.
- Hemorrhaging from all orifices.

Transmission

Same as for Ebola Zaire.

Survivor Recovery Period Symptoms

- Skin peels off face, hands, feet and genitals.
- In males, the testicles swell and rot.
- The virus lingers in the fluid of the eyeballs.
- Behavior of some patients is sullen, slightly aggressive and negative in outlook.

Ebola Reston

This strain of Ebola virus is new and different. It affects and kills monkeys but does not leap to humans. Theoretically, there is a difference in one of the seven mysterious proteins, a small, molecular, structural change that makes it harmless to humans while killing the monkeys. Ebola Reston virus is described as wormlike and longer than the Ebola Marburg variety, a spaghettilike filovirus. (From a symbolic standpoint, it is a snake.)

On October 4, 1989, 100 monkeys from the Philippines were brought to Virginia by Hazelton Research Products, a division of Corning Incorporated. They were held at the Reston Primate Quarantine Unit for one month to prevent the spread of infectious diseases. These were crab-eating monkeys. Two arrived dead, and over the following three weeks an unusual number of monkeys started to die; 29 of the 100 monkeys died between October 4 and November 1, 1989. (It should also be noted that Reston, Virginia, has cold temperatures from November to December.)

Workers at the Reston Army Works reported coming down with the coldlike symptoms of the Ebola virus but nothing more. One worker, a man, convulsed, vomited again and again and doubled over, gasping and choking. He was pale, shaky and faint and had dry heaves with a fever of 101° F. He was hospitalized in isolation. When he had been working with the "hot" monkeys, he had worn only rubber gloves, a gown and a surgical mask, which does not offer much protection. He recovered.

The monkeys' symptoms were fever, runny nose, droopy eyelids, a squint in the eyes; there was a dead, glassy stare to the eyes, which were half open. In autopsy, the spleen was swollen hard as a rock and was tangerine-sized and leathery. (Under normal conditions, a monkey's spleen would have been like a soft sack, with a red center, and the size of a walnut.) The spleen had become a solid blood clot.

What Can We Do?

Locate your nearest homeopathic practitioner. Have her or him read this chapter and order the remedies s/he feels you need, in the potencies you need. Your homeopath can instruct you on how and when to take them. If you have no homeopath in your area, then your only defense is to homeopathically take the symptoms we've been able to garner and find out what remedy or remedies can be used to mimic the Ebola virus.

Dr. Gail Derin collated the symptoms of Ebola Zaire, the most deadly of the three that can infect human beings. Vickie Menear, MD and homeopath, found that the remedy that most closely fit the symptoms of the 1918 flu virus, *Crolatus horridus*, is the remedy that matches the Ebola virus nearly 95 percent in terms of symptoms! Thanks go to these doctors for coming up with the following remedies:

- *Crolatus horridus* (rattlesnake venom)
- *Lachesis muta* (bushmaster snake venom)
- Phosphorus
- *Mercurius corrosivus*

Where Can I Order These Remedies?

If you are not in the U.S., you must locate your closest homeopathic practitioner and ask him or her to order these remedies for you from Hahnemann Pharmacy (see Appendix B). If your country's laws allow you to call a homeopathic pharmacy directly, do so. In any case be *sure* to find a homeopathic practitioner you can work with. Do not try to take care of yourself without the further education and experience a homeopath can give you. Take this information with you to your homeopath and let her or him read it and assess the information. Your homeopath will then instruct you on the use of these remedies.

We are once again faced with a virus crisis that is poised to sweep our country. Homeopathy can help us survive. Find your nearest homeopathic practitioner, get the remedies ordered and wait.

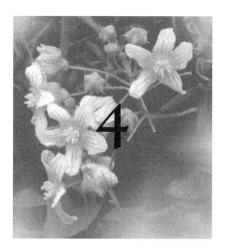

Homeopathic Remedies for the Flu and Colds

Instead of a flu shot next winter, why not think about a homeopathic remedy? It's certainly cheaper, it's natural and it has no side effects. Flu vaccinations have been known to paralyze people or even kill them. Why risk this? To me, the risk isn't worth it. In addition, I don't want to pulverize my immune system any more than I have to.

Aconitum napellus

One great pre-flu remedy is *Aconitum napellus*, or aconite. You can get a 30C potency, and it will serve you well. If you can catch the flu or cold while it's in what I call its "quasi" stage—no true symptoms have yet appeared—then take aconite, one dose every hour for three hours in a row. That should stop the cold or flu in its tracks and you won't get it. Sounds simple, doesn't it? Almost unbelievable, right? Yes, but it works.

The trick, again, is to realize you're feeling a little down, maybe having less energy, feeling less perky or a little mentally dull, followed by the arrival of specific symptoms such as a headache, fever or sniffles. If you take the aconite *after* any of these symptoms have manifested, then it won't stop the flu or cold at all.

Gelsemium sempervirens

Gelsemium sempervirens is a premier flu remedy and, as a matter of fact, it's one of the remedies that saved thousands of lives during the great flu epidemic of 1918 when over 500,000 people died. Want another statistic? During that time, homeopathy was on a decline, thanks to the politicking of the American Medical Association (AMA), and allopathic medicine (what is practiced in this country now) was on the rise. When the flu epidemic ravaged this country, both allopathic and homeopathic physicians attended their ill patients. Here are the facts: 80 percent of the patients treated with allopathic drugs died; 80 percent of the patients treated homeopathically lived. That's a pretty obvious difference between the effects of two forms of medicine.

Gelsemium is yellow jasmine. It is of great use for flu symptoms that have taken one or two days to come on. The person will usually feel lethargic and fatigued, be sleeping more than usual, be less chipper or alert than usual or just feel "draggy"—without any flu symptoms yet. Once the flu does arrive, the person feels like a serious couch potato, not wanting to move but just sitting like a lump, eyes partly closed and feeling absolutely fatigued. The person may say her or his arms and legs feel as if they were weighted down.

Here are other keynote symptoms to tell you *Gelsemium sempervirens* is the flu/cold remedy you need:
• Chills running up and down the back.
• Aching and stiffness in the neck which extend to the forehead.
• Chills beginning in the hands or feet.
• Heaviness or trembling of the limbs, especially the legs.
• Improvement of symptoms after urination.
• Headache that begins at the rear of the skull and moves to the forehead.
• Sensation of a tight band around the head.
• Soreness of the scalp.
• Summer colds with sneezing, fever and watery mucus/discharge.
• Chills alternating with heat up and down the back.

Eupatorium perfoliatum

Eupatorium perfoliatum is another one of the premier flu remedies, and it saved thousands of lives in 1918. Aching bone pain with fever is the hallmark symptom of this remedy. All of us have gotten the type of flu that makes us feel as if our bones are so tender and brittle that they will break with pain.

Here are the other keynote symptoms that would guide you to take this remedy if you get the flu:

- High fever preceded by chills, around 7 AM to 9 AM.
- A craving for cold foods such as ice cream.
- Excruciating back pain.
- Great thirst for cold drinks during chills.
- Head feeling heavy during headache.
- Nausea and vomiting that are worse during chills and during motion.
- High fever with chills.
- Restlessness with intense aching of bones and muscles; stiffness and achiness.

Baptisia tinctoria

Baptisia is another great flu remedy; it is especially good when the person appears to be drunk without having been drinking; it's just the severity of the flu symptoms that makes the person seem "besotted."

Here are some of the keynotes symptoms. If they fit what you're experiencing, try this remedy:

- Great mental confusion, dullness of mental faculties; stupor; comalike.
- Swift onset of flu.
- Offensive odors of the mouth, stool and perspiration.
- Bruised pains that are uncomfortable, no matter what position you try; the bed feels too hard.
- Red, dusky congestion of face.
- Ulcerated and red throat that is pain-free, even upon swallowing.
- Soreness all over body, especially the part on which you lie.
- Thickness of tongue with slurred speech; inability to put intelligible sentences together.

Dosage for any of the above remedies is 30C, usually once an hour for three hours; that should arrest the worst of your flu symptoms. If it does not, it is the wrong remedy and you should *stop taking it*. Ideally, if you have a homeopath, call her or him first and s/he will suggest a remedy that is correct for you. It's better than having the flu and certainly better than getting a vaccination that can bludgeon the immune system. However, as always, consult your local homeopath for your best personal choice of the remedy that is best suited to your unique symptoms.

Headaches with Flu or a Cold

Many types of flu viruses have a headache as a symptom, and most colds do too. Below are some reasons for these symptoms and some homeopathic remedies that may help.

Headaches can be caused by a multitude of things, and in homeopathy, the prescriber will always check out your surroundings, your environment, to see if this is contributing to your headache (or other ache) problem. Part of getting well is not only taking the correct homeopathic remedy but also setting right what is wrong with your lifestyle, your environment or the foods you consume, since all these things either contribute to or take away from your health.

A headache can be caused by something as simple as a vertebra that is out of alignment in your spine, so a chiropractor might need to be consulted. Or the muscles in your neck might tighten up so much that seeing a masseuse might be part of the answer. Migraines, which are a breed apart, are about the blood vessels in your neck suddenly shutting down, or closing up, so that the blood congests in the area; as the muscles tighten, they press upon and squeeze the blood vessels, creating a damming effect, which then causes the migraine's warning symptoms to come on. After the migraine starts, the muscles will suddenly relax and pressure is off the blood vessels so blood rushes into the brain again, causing even more pain.

Allergies can cause headaches, and they can come from the foods you eat or air pollution or water pollution. Sometimes it's as simple as ingesting too much caffeine by drinking too much coffee or soda pop. Headaches can be caused by eyestrain resulting from sitting in front of a computer monitor or reading for too long. Fevers will cause a headache, as will hypoglycemia. Premenstrual tension will create headaches, and so will high blood pressure. Sometimes a spate of headaches follows an attack of shingles. Dehydration can also cause a headache, and this is a little investigated area. Many people do not drink enough fluids. Homeopathically, they are referred to as "thirstless" individuals. These people are prone to dehydration types of headaches. Further, people who consume a lot of alcohol can also dehydrate.

In a worst-case scenario, headaches can be a symptom of damage to the blood vessels in and around the brain, or perhaps an infection in the brain tissue that surrounds the brain matter itself or the spinal cord. In cases like these, quick doctor intervention is a must; it then can be followed up with homeopathic treatment.

A person who has suffered a concussion or brain injury might later go on to have horrendous, nonstop headaches. If you know of a person who has struck his/her head, be on the lookout for drowsiness, nausea and/or vomiting. These are all signs of bleeding taking place in the brain, and that individual should be rushed to the emergency room immediately—and given a dose of arnica on the way!

Another reason for headaches is the light; many people hate fluorescent lights, which are a major creator of headaches. Anxiety can cause a headache, and we have a lot of high-anxiety demands on us at the workplace as well as at home now—for both genders—and headaches are certainly in vogue more than usual because of this!

If a headache continues for more than 48 hours, consult your physician immediately.

Aconitum napellus

The kind of headache you want to treat with *Aconitum napellus* (aconite) is caused by getting damp, getting a chill, even just from a gust of cold wind; the headache will come on afterward. It might feel like a tight binding around your head or as if your brain was going to be forced out of your skull. You might feel anxious or apprehensive. Another cause of this kind of headache is anxiety. If you're nervous or upset about a coming confrontation or a stressful day or event, then consider aconite for relief.

Apis mellifica

Headaches you want to treat with *Apis mellifica* can be caused by allergies, notably in people who have been stung by an insect and get a resultant headache. However, many other types of allergy headaches are helped by this remedy. Symptoms for this type of headache have a stinging, stabbing or burning pain associated with it. The entire head—and perhaps even the rest of the body—feels bruised and/or tender. The headache pain is always worse when the person is indoors in a stuffy, unventilated room; it always gets better out of doors, in the fresh air.

Arnica montana

Arnica montana (arnica) treats the kind of headache that makes the person suffering from it not want to get touched—and this is a keynote reason to give this remedy. If you lift your hand to touch the aching head, s/he will wince and move away from you, step back or growl at you to avoid being touched. The symptoms are a bruised, aching pain in the head that sometimes will become a sharp pain. If the sufferer stoops down or leans over, the headache pain increases.

Arnica is also a concussion remedy. Remember to take arnica on the way to the emergency room, because a concussion-caused headache is nothing to play around with—it could be deadly.

Belladonna atropa

Belladonna treats "cluster" headaches and migraines that come on with a swift, sudden vengeance. This is a keynote of this remedy: It is fast. There is such throbbing pain that the person feels as if hammers are striking inside her or his skull. The face becomes flushed and very red looking and the pupils dilate. The headache gets even worse if the affected person moves into direct sunlight. Belladonna is an excellent migraine remedy, especially in cases of swift, sudden onset of the headache.

Bryonia alba

Bryonia alba is another preeminent migraine remedy. With the type of headache for which bryonia is the remedy, the head will feel very bruised. The pain is sharp and stabbing and made worse by any kind of eye or body movement. There is also nausea accompanying this headache. Once a person gets this type of headache, s/he wants to be left completely alone. The person doesn't want to be touched or have people around. S/he wants the room dark and quiet and won't move an inch because every movement increases the pain in the head or the nausea in the stomach.

Chamomilla matricaria

The person with the type of headache that asks for treatment with *Chamomilla matricaria* is extremely crabby and irritable, literally a "bear" to be around; s/he wants to be left alone. This headache is like the bryonia type, but the crabbiness is even worse and more caustic.

Coffea cruda

Use *Coffea cruda* for a headache that makes the scalp and head feel supersensitive and where the mind is like a "squirrel's cage" that can't be turned off. There are so many thoughts, millions of them, crowding into the brain, and this causes the headache. There is no way to turn this off, and tea or coffee makes the headache worse.

Gelsemium sempervirens

Gelsemium sempervirens is one of my personal favorites as a headache remedy. It addresses pre-jitter headaches, that is, anxiety headaches caused by the stress of having to speak out in public, take a school test of any kind or indeed any sort of test. This is a stress headache/migraine remedy par excellence. Anytime you get a headache because your nervous system is stressed, this is the remedy to take.

Symptoms of the headache you want to treat with gelsemium include a full feeling in the head, as if the brain was swollen and too large for the skull. The face may be red or purple, perhaps flushed or congested looking. The person's expression is dopey-looking. The eyes may be half closed, with the eyes themselves dull or lackluster, and the mouth might hang partly open. This person doesn't want to move and sits like a lumpy couch potato wherever s/he is, lacking the strength to move anywhere at all. The eyes may become dilated—but not always—and s/he might feel extremely weak (which is why the person sits like a round mound) and even shaky.

Glonoinum

Very often a person who has been out in the sun too long or gets overheated (watch for heatstroke or sunstroke here) will get a headache. This remedy, glonoinum, works on violent headaches that seem to throb in beat with the heart rate. In fact, the person might feel the beat of the heart in her or his head. The pain is made worse by either stooping forward or shaking the head.

Hypericum perforatum

Hypericum perforatum is for people who get headaches in foggy, damp weather—be it rain, fog or winter weather. This headache is a bursting pain and the scalp is hypersensitive to the touch. In fact, those with this type of headache may tell you it hurts for them to even touch their scalp very lightly with their fingers.

Ignatia amara

Headaches that can be treated with *Ignatia amara* might be caused by grief of some sort, for example, grief over the loss of a loved one or perhaps the loss of a job or relationship. The symptoms of such a headache are the sensation of a tight band around the forehead, and the person might tell you that it feels like a nail is being driven out through the side of the head.

Nux vomica

This is the alcohol or drug hangover remedy. Anyone who has been out on a drinking binge or who has taken too many recreational drugs and gets a headache then or afterward should take this remedy. The *Nux vomica* headache makes the person irritable and dizzy and s/he tells you her or his head feels bruised. It is always worse in the morning but will get markedly better if s/he gets up and moves around.

Pulsatilla nigricans

Pulsatilla nigricans is for people who get a headache when they eat too much rich food, or "pig out" and simply eat too much. (*Nux vomica* will also help this). The headache makes the person feel like s/he is on an emotional roller coaster; s/he will get weepy and cry, want company and want to be pampered and held.

Ruta graveolens

Use *Ruta graveolens* to treat the type of headache that has a pressing, bruising pain to it and is most often associated with fatigue of some kind—be it from sitting at the computer monitor too long, looking over endless columns of numbers or reading too much. The headache is made worse by reading and is alleviated by rest and not reading or using the eyes.

Other considerations may be going to an osteopath to help stop the headaches by receiving cranial manipulation. If you are taking a lot of vitamin A (more than 4,000 IU three times a week), you might have A toxemia, which is known to cause headaches. Simply stop taking the A, and in a few days these headaches and the toxic condition in your system will go away.

Cold Remedies

Colds are the bane of humanity's existence. There has never been a cure for colds. Some of the old-fashioned "grandma's remedies" come close, but they don't quite make it. In the homeopathic arsenal of remedies are a number of what are known as cold remedies, and I have at times seen a cold stopped in its tracks. The provision is this: If you catch the cold as it is forming, then you can stop it from occurring at all. However, once the cold gets fired up, it's tough to chase it down.

An interesting phenomenon occurs if one has the patience to chase down a cold. Often it will change character after the first remedy is taken, and then you have to reexamine your case by noting what symptoms are left and whether any new ones have appeared. After a remedy has been taken, the character of a cold can change within 20 minutes! Then a new remedy has to be taken. Other colds will go away if you take the one remedy that most closely resembles the major symptoms. I find this to be particularly true of the aconite and gelsemium types of colds.

Below are the most popular homeopathic cold remedies. If the bulk of your symptoms fits one of these remedy pictures, try it. Your cold might be cured within a couple of hours of taking the remedy. Often a homeopathic remedy will nip the cold so it will be shorter, or it will take away some of the most obnoxious symptoms and leave you with a very mild version of the cold. Either of these options is preferable to the misery of having a cold for days.

Aconitum napellus

Aconitum napellus (aconite) should be considered in two specific situations. First, if you are in that period of a couple of hours or a day before the cold symptoms initially appear, aconite can stop the cold before it starts and completely short-circuit it. The key here is to notice that you are beginning to feel a little more tired than usual; perhaps you notice a hint of a headache coming on or a low-grade fever, or perhaps you are just feeling "blah." That's when you should take one dose of aconite 30C. The cold will disappear and so will the tiredness and lethargy. By the next morning, you'll feel like your old self and have your energy back.

The second situation in which to use aconite is if you've taken a chill or been caught in a draft, or if it has been hot and a summer storm drops the temperature 30 or 40 degrees. Remember how Mom used to insist we put on a coat, a hat and our galoshes before we went out in the rain or snow? And remember how, if we resisted, we often caught that blasted cold she was nagging us about? Well, that's an aconite situation. So if you have children like this and they come in from play looking a little peaked or they start sleeping more or are off their feed just a tad, give them a dose of aconite to stop the cold before it starts.

Aconite colds come on suddenly. They may occur only an hour after you experience the chill. There is a lot of sneezing, a burning sensation in the throat and restlessness. The symptoms are always worse at night.

Allium cepa

Allium cepa colds are indicated by discharges running from the eyes and nose simultaneously. The keynote here is that the tears or discharge from the eyes is bland in nature, whereas the discharge from the nose is burning, which means your nose will get very raw very quickly. So if your eyes and nose are nonstop leaky faucets during the cold, this is the remedy for you.

Belladonna atropa

Belladonna is another terrific cold remedy, especially for infants and children, although adults can certainly use it too. Use it for the cold that comes on suddenly, along with a high fever. The skin is dry and hot and burning. Light hurts the eyes a lot, so you squint or put a hand up to shade your eyes. There is a marked sore throat and if you look at it, the back of the throat is a bright, strawberry-red color; usually, it is a right-sided sore throat. There is a tickle that makes you cough. A belladonna cold creates great thirst. Some other, more subtle signs of a belladonna cold are that frequently the face will be flushed bright red and the eyes can appear to be extremely bright and shiny, with dilated pupils. These are the key symptoms that are especially useful with young children who can't communicate their symptoms.

Euphrasia officinalis

Euphrasia officinalis is closely related to Allium cepa, but you use it to treat a cold with just the opposite symptoms: The tears/discharge from the eyes are burning, scalding, acidlike, and the discharge from the nose is bland. Also, the euphrasia cold is always worse at night.

Ferrum phosphoricum

Ferrum phosphoricum is the remedy for another cold that comes on slowly, like a gelsemium cold. With this cold, usually everything is mild—a mild cough, a mild fever, mild sneezing. But there may also be a nosebleed just before the cold comes on or during it, and this is a particular keynote for this remedy. Usually, you are very pale but flush easily. You feel better if you place a cold cloth on your aching head. You may have red spots on your cheeks. There is hoarseness or even laryngitis and a cough that is dry and hacking as well as pain in the chest. The symptoms are more marked and dramatic between 4 AM and 6 AM. Gentle exercise or moving about definitely helps.

A person suffering from a Ferrum phosphoricum cold doesn't like being jarred, lying on the right side or becoming too hot during the cold. Your flushed face may become bright red, just as with the belladonna cold, but the difference here is that the person suffering from the Ferrum phosphoricum cold won't have bright, shiny, dilated eyes.

Gelsemium sempervirens

Gelsemium sempervirens colds come on very slowly, and it may take two or three days of feeling that you are dragging, are more tired than normal and a little out of sorts, but not yet suffering any obvious cold symptoms. This is a powerful message to tell you that you may have a gelsemium cold stalking you. If you arrest it at this stage, you can cure yourself completely. Other symptoms of the type of cold you can treat with *Gelsemium sempervirens* are that it becomes flulike; you feel sluggish and shivery; your arms and legs get especially chilled and feel weighted down or heavier than normal. Frequently, you feel like a lump of coal or a sack of potatoes and you just don't have the energy or inclination to move very much at all. I call *Gelsemium sempervirens* the "couch potato" remedy.

With this kind of cold comes a good deal of achiness that you feel in the muscles of the arms and particularly the legs. You can have chills up and down your back and watery sneezing, along with a nasty taste in the mouth. Your limbs may tremble a bit too. Your scalp will feel very sore to the touch, and the headache that comes with this type of cold may feel like a tight band is wrapped around your head. You will always feel better after urinating, which lessens some of the symptoms. A big keynote of this kind of cold is that you are always thirstless.

There is a particular look of dullness to the facial features: half-closed eyes, partly open mouth, rounded shoulders. You look like a big lump sitting there. The four Ds of an indication to use gelsemium are dull, drowsy, dumb and droopy looking.

Hepar sulphuris

Hepar sulphuris is for colds that spread mucus from the throat to the ears or from the ears to the throat. There is tremendous involvement of the sinus cavities, and the mucus is always a thick, yellow green discharge that is constant. Heavy mucus being coughed up or blown from the nose calls for this remedy. Also, you are very irritable, chilly and supersensitive to drafts of any kind. You have a splinterlike sensation in the throat area, which is what makes you continue to cough. You also break out in a heavy sweat that has a distinct, sour-smelling odor.

This is a sinusitis remedy par excellence—so long as there is lots of nasal discharge that is yellow green and thick. You might also get cold sores at the corners of your lips. There can be hoarseness and loss of voice. Usually, the cough is worse between 6 PM and midnight. The cough can be hoarse and dry, but if it moves down to the chest, it becomes loose and rattling.

Another keynote symptom of a *Hepar sulphuris* cold is that whenever you swallow, there can be pain in the ears, with that splinterlike or fishbonelike sticking sensation occurring simultaneously in the throat.

Natrum muriaticum

Natrum muriaticum is good for the early stage of a cold or for a cold where the sneezing is worse in the morning hours and mucus or nasal discharge looks like raw egg whites. The nose is stuffed up and blocked, and cold sores develop in and around the nostrils. If you have a *Natrum muriaticum* cold, you don't want to be fussed over or taken care of. You reject the sympathy of others and just want to be left alone to go about your business, cold or no cold.

The headache, if there is one, starts at the base of your skull and comes up and over the top of the head. All the symptoms are usually worse around 10 AM or 11 AM. You prefer to have fresh air, an open window, but don't want to be talked to, jarred, touched or have bright lights or music/sound. Usually, if you have such a cold, you are pretty stoic and noncomplaining about your illness.

Pulsatilla nigricans

Pulsatilla nigricans is another wonderful children's or infants' cold remedy. When they catch a cold, they always want extra attention; they want to be fussed over, held and kissed and don't want to be left alone. If left in a bedroom alone, they will drag their favorite blanket out with them and lie on the couch to be near someone. Emotionally, they show just the opposite symptoms of a *Natrum muriaticum* cold.

Symptoms of a cold that can be treated with *Pulsatilla nigricans* include lack of thirst, headaches centered above the eyes and yellow, runny nasal discharge. During the day, the nose runs like a faucet, and at night both nostrils block up completely. You always want fresh air and hate being in a warm, stuffy room. No matter how sick you are, you want a door left open or even a window cracked to allow in fresh air, even in the middle of winter!

You get worse if you take a hot bath or shower to sweat it out. You have a decided loss of smell. The cough may produce green mucus, and it will be a loose-sounding type of cough. One of the best things for a pulsatilla cold is an extra hug or two. It's surprising what touch can do to speed up the healing process—even more than a homeopathic remedy! Pulsatilla children may get far more emotional and weepy than usual when they have a cold.

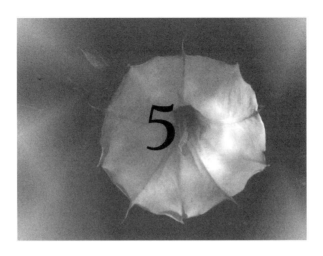

SARS: Pandemic of the 21st Century?

Severe acute respiratory syndrome (SARS) is a viral respiratory illness caused by a coronavirus called SARS-associated coronavirus (SARS-CoV). SARS was first reported in Asia in February 2003. Over the next few months, the illness spread to more than two dozen countries in North America, South America, Europe and Asia. The global SARS outbreak of 2003 was contained; however, it is possible that the disease could reemerge. What is most telling—and new—about this new virus is that most people who contract it get pneumonia, and pneumonia is a killer for many.

The SARS Outbreak

According to the World Health Organization (WHO), a total of 8,098 people worldwide became sick with SARS during the SARS outbreak of 2003; of these, 774 died. In the U.S., there were 192 cases of SARS, and all of the patients got better. Through July 2003, laboratory evidence of SARS-CoV infection had been detected in only eight U.S. cases. Most of the U.S. SARS cases were among travelers returning from parts of the world with SARS. There were very few U.S. cases caused by close contacts with travelers, including health care workers and family members. SARS did not spread more widely in communities in the United States.

In general, SARS begins with a high fever (temperature greater than 100.4°F). Other symptoms, as stated by the Centers for Disease Control, may include headache, an overall feeling of discomfort and bodyaches. Some people also have mild respiratory symptoms at the outset. About 10 to 20 percent of patients have diarrhea. After two to seven days, SARS patients may develop a dry cough. Most patients develop pneumonia.

How SARS Spreads

The main way SARS seems to spread is by close person-to-person contact. The virus that causes SARS is thought to be transmitted most readily by respiratory droplets ("droplet spread") produced when an infected person coughs or sneezes. Droplet spread can happen when droplets from the cough or sneeze of an infected person are propelled a short distance (generally up to three feet) through the air and deposited on the mucous membranes of the mouth, nose or eyes of persons who are nearby. The virus can also spread when a person touches a surface or object contaminated with infectious droplets and then touches his or her mouth, nose or eye(s). In addition, it is possible that the SARS virus might spread more broadly through the air ("airborne spread") or by other ways that are not yet known.

What Does "Close Contact" Mean?

In the context of SARS, close contact means caring for or living with someone with SARS or having direct contact with respiratory secretions or body fluids of a patient with SARS. Examples of close contact include kissing or hugging, sharing eating or drinking utensils, talking to someone at a distance of up to three feet and touching someone directly. Close contact does not include activities like walking by a person or sitting across someone in a waiting room or office for a brief time.

Symptoms of SARS

Here are the latest symptoms that could be gathered. I'm sure more will come to light as SARS travels around the world again in the near future, but for now, this is the array of symptoms. From these symptoms, I have developed a list of homeopathic remedies that may be instrumental in helping to support a person toward living. Also remember: Get to your physician *first* and get on whatever prescribed antibiotics s/he recommends. Utilize homeopathy as a secondary support system that will work hand in hand with your antibiotic treatment. Because SARS is so virulent and potentially deadly, it is *absolutely mandatory* that you have a professional homeopath care for you and choose the correct remedy for you based upon your unique set of symptoms.

SARS Symptoms

- Rapid onset of high fever (greater than 100.4°F), followed by muscleaches. Fever is not present in some patients.
- Respiratory distress to the extent of requiring oxygen.
- Dry cough.
- Pneumonia.
- Diarrhea.
- Confusion.
- Muscular stiffness/pain.
- Headache.
- Leucopenia (low white blood cell count).
- Thrombopenia (low platelet count).
- Rash.
- Chills.
- Rigors.
- Sore throat.
- Relapse after two to three days of getting better (chills and rigors with high fever).
- Acute respiratory distress accompanying the relapse, sometimes to a point where mechanical breathing aid is required.
- Chest x-ray may initially be clear, but changes start on day three or four (bases in particular). Chest x-rays continue to worsen, and most patients demonstrate bilateral changes with interstitial infiltrations (fluid build-up between cells in the lungs). These infiltrations produce x-rays with a characteristic cloudy appearance.
- Malaise.

- Loss of appetite.
- Gastrointestinal upset.
- Pleuritic chest pain.
- Excessive mucus in windpipe.
- Lightheadedness.
- Hemoptysis (coughing up of blood).
- Some elevation in transaminases (AST/ALT/GGT 1, 3 times).
- Possible elevations in creatine kinase.
- Bone pain.
- Elevated CRP (C-reactive protein, used to assess an acute phase reaction in inflammatory and infective processes with an elevated value interpreted as an indication of an acute phase response or active disease).
- Patients invariably have an elevated creatine phosphokinase (CPK).
- Inability to move.
- Extreme weakness.
- Extreme weight loss.
- Myocarditis.
- Severe shooting pain all through body.
- Coma.
- Sepsis.
- Septic shock.
- Inability to oxygenate, resulting in lung failure.

Homeopathic Remedies

The remedies presented in this section may be helpful during a SARS outbreak. Always *check with your medical doctor first* and your homeopath second to receive the correct homeopathic prescription and homeopathic remedy.

How to Use This Information

It is impossible to go into all the rules of homeopathy in this book, which is intended to be utilized with the help and guidance of a professional homeopath. This is not a "how to" book on homeopathy. Rather, it is about looking at potential remedies that *might* be of assistance to you during an epidemic.

Below you will find remedies and symptoms these remedies will help. Provers take a remedy and detail the symptoms they experience.

The collection of symptoms is then correlated to a particular remedy, and that is how we find out which symptoms a remedy can help with.

Ideally, you want to find a perfect match for your symptoms. The more symptoms for a particular remedy parallel yours, the greater the possibility that it can be utilized to help you. Please understand that you should not be dosing yourself. Rather, once you think you've found the correct remedy based upon your unique collection of symptoms, pick up the phone and call your homeopath to discuss it. The homeopath will either allow you to take this remedy or suggest another one that is even more closely aligned with your symptoms.

The remedies listed here are not the only ones that can help you. However, they are the most frequently used based upon the symptoms of the virus.

Bromium

Bromium is made from bromine and is an important remedy for laryngeal affections, as well as for scrofulous and tubercular affections of the glands. Use it to treat croupy, rough, barking or whistling cough that is excited by tickling in the throat and, as if by vapor of sulphur, without expectoration. Further symptoms are:
- Aggravation in daytime, deep respiration, violent motion.
- Great heat in the bed.
- Craves sour food and milk.
- Aggravation from tobacco smoke.

Concomitants

These are symptoms that occur with the other symptoms mentioned above.
- Depression and melancholy; wailing and crying with a hoarse tone.
- Lachrymation (tears in eyes).
- Paleness of the face.
- Salivation.
- Inflammation of the face with reticulated redness and denuded patches.
- Much frothy mucus in the mouth.
- Water tastes salty.
- Nausea and retching.
- Yellow, green or blackish diarrhea.
- Fluent coryza, with scabby nostrils.

- Attacks of suffocation as if from vapor of sulphur.
- Great labored breathing.
- Gasping for air.
- Soreness in the larynx.
- Sensation of coldness in the larynx.
- The air inhaled feels very cold.
- Oppression of the chest with palpitation; convulsions.
- Great weakness; yawning and sleepiness.
- Accelerated pulse.
- Chilliness, with shuddering; sweat after the chill.

Physical Symptoms
Cough
- Croupy, dry, rough, barking or whistling cough.
- Tickling in the throat as if from sulphur vapor; sensation of coldness in the larynx; for blond-haired people.
- Has a remarkable action upon the glandular system and respiratory organs.

Asthma
- Suffocating cough, with hoarse wheezing and gasping, with a false membrane in the trachea, especially where the larynx and trachea are inflamed.
- Great rattling of mucus in the larynx and trachea when coughing.
- Great nervous prostration, remaining after all other symptoms have gone.
- Aggravation in the evening.
- Long, continued, obstinate coryza, with soreness beneath the nose and on the margin of the nose.
- Cold sensation in the larynx, with a cold feeling when inspiring.
- Scraping and rawness in the larynx, provoking cough.
- Hoarseness, loss of voice; cannot speak clearly.
- Cough, with paroxysms of suffocation suddenly on swallowing.
- Icy coldness of the forearms.
- Affections of the glands, without suppuration.
- Pulse very much accelerated.
- Thirst seems to be wanting.
- No delirium.
- Nose discharge generally fluent.
- Respiration with dry sound.

- Expectoration infrequent.
- Saliva increased.
- Complaints of right lung.
- Rock-hard cervical glands; left-sided affections.
- Other glands are affected, for example: thyroid indurated, hard goiter
- Summer colds begin in larynx, extend up or down.
- Asthma on leaving sea, better by the sea.
- Larynx affected (and trachea).
- Croup with rattling, no expectoration.
- Worse in warmth, overheating.
- Inhaled air feels cold; acrid coryza.
- Cobweb sensation on face.
- Croup with great rattling of mucus, but no expectoration; there seems to be a great danger of suffocating from accumulation of mucus in the larynx.
- Dizziness when lying down, with headache, especially in the evening.
- Suffocative fits; he starts up choked with croupy or wheezing cough.
- Spasm of the glottis.
- Labored breathing, cannot inspire deep enough as if breathing through a sponge or as if the air passages were full of smoke or vapor of sulphur; rattling, sawing; voice inaudible.
- Thick, white expectoration.

It should be remembered in fluent nasal discharge that when there is long, continued sneezing, the margin of the nose and parts under the nose are corroded, painful and bleeding when wiped.

Pulse
- Small and weak.
- Skin cool and clammy.

Sensations
- Coppery taste in throat, with dry cough.
- Smoothness and emptiness at a spot in the larynx.
- Coldness in larynx; cold feeling when inspiring.
- Weakens from sleeping gasping for breath.
- Constriction of chest, without cough.

Modalities
- *Worse:* Particularly in the evening, until midnight; when swallowing drink; but less frequently when swallowing food or saliva;

with cold foods or drinks; in wet weather and when bending the diseased limb.
- *Better:* In dry weather, after bodily exertion, riding, drinking coffee and eating.

Naphthalinum

Naphthalinum is made from tar camphor, or naphthalene, a chemical found in coal tar. It has been found to be a valuable remedy for hay fever, and many inveterate cases seem to have been entirely arrested. You can use it to treat symptoms that include sneezing, inflamed and painful eyes, a hot head; it also treats spasmodic bronchitis and ameliorates asthma. Secretions are highly acrid.

More symptoms that can be treated with naphthalinum are soreness in chest and stomach (has to loosen the clothing) in open air and pulmonary emphysema with labored breathing, sighing inspiration. Naphthalinum ameliorates violent motion—it seems as if the person cannot get air out of the chest.

Physical Symptoms
Cough
- Constant sneezing.
- Long, continued paroxysms of convulsive cough, cannot get breath, with bladder irritation. Has been much used in this affliction, in lower potencies, with good results.

Whooping Cough
- Long, continued paroxysms of coughing; unable to get a respiration.
- During the paroxysms, the face becomes purple, the perspiration starts and a quantity of thick, tenacious mucus is expectorated.
- Spasmodic asthma.
- Soreness in the chest and stomach.
- Emphysema.
- Great breathing problems, with a sighing respiration.
- Black urine.
- Terribly offensive odor of the decomposing (ammoniacal) urine.

Respiration
- Labored and irregular, asthmatic.
- Cough in incessant paroxysms, almost arresting breath.
- Night cough preventing sleep.
- Cough with blue or purple face.

Expectoration
- Free, thick, tenacious, almost absent.
- Cough in violent paroxysms compelling the patient to hold his head for the pain.

Modalities
- *Worse*: During night and while urinating.
- *Better:* In the open air and from loosening clothing.

Kreosotum

Kreosotum (cresol) is made from beech creosote. It is a mixture of phenols obtained from distillation of wood tar, and the solution is in rectified spirit. It focuses on the person's circulation, kidneys, mucus membranes, nerves and skin, and symptoms are usually found on the right side of the body.

Mental and Emotional State

When sick, individuals may exhibit euphoria and someone may think they are drunk or on recreational drugs, but they are not. They are nonstop talkers and use their hands and arms a lot as they speak. They become very expansive, wanting to embrace the world. They can also revert to childish behavior. Always restless, they will turn in bed constantly or want to get up and walk around, no matter how bad they are feeling. When very sick, they get confused, although we may be fooled into believing that they are thinking deeply about something. Often they will repeat themselves, a sign that they are in the midst of this confusion due to fever. They will always want a window open or be near outdoor air; they hate stuffy, warm rooms.

Physical Symptoms

There are some outstanding characteristics that may show the use of this remedy. The sick individuals have bleeding gums and will complain of a bitter taste in their mouths. There is a great deal more salivation than normal. Further, they have bad breath upon waking. Their cough is dry and they feel they are suffocating. Further, the expectoration (mucus) they cough up has a very acidic taste to it. When sick, they appear to have skin like leather; some would characterize this as "parchment" skin.

There is a yellow brown discoloration to the skin tone in general when they are ill.

Abdomen
- Painful sensation of coldness in abdomen; icy coldness in epigastrium.
- Diarrhea with vomiting, continued vomiting; straining to vomit predominates and a child resists tightening of anything around abdomen with increased restlessness and pain.

Back
- Small of back feels as if it will break; worse at rest, better in motion.
- Drawing pain along coccyx (tailbone) to rectum and vagina, where a spasmodic, contractive pain is felt.

Breathing
- Shortness of breath as if sternum crushes in.
- Cough, with concussion of abdomen and escape of urine.
- Cough, aggravated from exhaling.
- Asthma, jarring of abdomen; retching; discharge of urine.
- Chills and headache; sleepiness.
- Cough of old people; winter cough of old people; spasmodic turns at night.
- Pain or pressure referable to sternum; better with pressure.
- Dreadful burning in chest, constriction.
- Coughing spells with expectoration of greenish pus, blood, black blood.

Eyes
- Chronic swelling of eyelids and their margins.
- Agglutination of eyelids.

Fever
- Fever and inability to lie on one side.
- Emaciation; intense, hectic fever; night sweats.
- Shortness of breath; dry, teasing cough.
- Great debility (very weak).

General
- Wants to be in motion all the time.
- In turning quickly, danger of falling.
- Tosses all night without apparent cause.
- Great drowsiness, frequent yawning.
- Starts when scarcely asleep, laughs in sleep.

- Burning pains in eyes, ears, bowels, genitalia, back and lower abdomen, chest and small of back.
- Heaviness, stiffness, numbness, tingling, crawling, itching.

Heart
- Anxiety at heart, stitches.
- Pulsation in all arteries when at rest.

Mouth
- Putrid odor from mouth.
- Water, after it is swallowed, tastes bitter.
- Protruding gums infiltrated with dark, watery fluid.
- Absorption of gums and alveolar process.

Stomach
- Painful hard spot, at or to left of stomach.
- Keen appetite, especially for meat; craves smoked meat.
- Stomachaches from acid food.
- Deep and lasting disgust for food in convalescence.
- Cold feeling, epigastrium, as if cold or ice was there.
- Malignant induration, fungus and ulcers of stomach, ulcerative pain with hematemesis (blood mixed with food).

Skin
- Itching, toward evening so violent as to drive one almost wild.

Throat
- Black softening and decomposition of mucus membrane of throat, with atony and extension of softening, especially toward esophagus, in diphtheria.

Urination
- Frequent urge to urinate, with copious pale discharge; cannot get out of bed quick enough at night.
- Urinates six or seven times a day, always with great haste and passing a great deal.

Vomiting
- Of sweetish water, undigested food, with dimness of vision.
- Of large quantities of sour, acrid fluid or white, foamy mucus.

Phosphorus

Phosphorus is an element and is considered a deep-acting homeopathic remedy. One of the major symptoms of this remedy are weakness, fainting, sweating, prostration and burning sensations.

Mental and Emotional State

- Violent delirium (with intense yellow color of the skin); the patient forgot to pass water, respiration was very difficult, the pulse was very small; skin was dry, tongue brown.
- Delirium in which the patient got out of bed and was found lying on the floor, screaming frightfully and tossing about.
- Extreme excitement, with very great heat, great thirst.
- Patient apathetic; at times tossing about the bed and moaning.
- Spasmodic laughing and weeping.
- Sadness and melancholy, as if some misfortune had happened.
- Sadness in the twilight for several evenings in succession, at the same hour.
- Filled with gloomy forebodings.
- Great sadness.
- Weary of life.
- Mental depression and a most uncommon fearfulness or timidity, with a great sense of fatigue. "My mind was greatly oppressed with melancholy; tears would start without cause; a feeling of dread, as if awaiting something terrible, yet unable to resist or move."
- Anxiety restlessness, with much sweat on the forehead and heat of the head.
- Great anxiety and irritability when alone.
- Fear and dread, in the evening.
- Did not like to be alone.
- Person feels nervous, as if s/he was going to die.
- Very irritable and fretful mood.
- Feels exceedingly petulant all day; nothing goes right; feels as dissatisfied with themselves as with others; it seems as if everybody says or does something to provoke them.
- Disinclined to work and unhappy, though without confusion of the head.
- Disinclination for any type of work.
- Forgetful and stupid, so that a person does something quite different from what s/he wishes.
- Loss of senses, as if the person could not grasp any thought, with headache.

Physical Symptoms

Chest

- The respiratory organs become rapidly involved and the lungs rapidly suppurate.
- Frequent sharp pains, as though a knife was pushed into the lungs.
- Frequent stitches of pain through the lungs, especially upon breathing in deeply.
- Cannot fill my lungs as usual (worse on left side).
- Weakness of the chest.
- Heat in the chest.
- Great oppression of the chest, so that the patient, during the attack of cough and in order to expectorate, must sit up in bed; experiences great pain, with a constrictive sensation under the sternum; mucous rattling.
- Tightness of the chest.
- The chest is constantly tense, as if a band was around it.

Chilliness

- Severe chill followed by a fever, flushed cheeks, the left one much more than the right; fever with headache, but no chill (second day); considerable fever in the evening.
- Chilliness in the hands, though they are warm; hands are red and the veins are distended.
- Chilliness, with anxiety, in the evening.
- Person feels so chilly that s/he trembles all over, even by a warm stove.
- Violent, shaking chill at night, with looseness of the bowels four times, followed by great heat and perspiration all over and preceded by perspiration before midnight for several nights.
- Violent, shaking chill, followed by sweat at night; great restlessness on the previous days.
- Coldness of the limbs.

Choking

- Rawness in the voice box and windpipe, with frequent, hacking cough and hawking.
- Very considerable mucous accumulation in the windpipe, with some hoarseness.
- After waking at night, the person has a feeling of contraction in

the voice box and windpipe, as though s/he must suffocate.
- Irritability in the lower portion of the windpipe, with suffocative pressure in the upper part of the chest.

Cough and Expectoration
- Violent cough with expectoration of mucus that can wake the person up in the early AM.
- Frequent cough with much expectoration, even at night.
- Tickling cough.
- Constant cough with much expectoration of mucus, with tensive pain in the chest.
- Spasmodic cough with oppression of chest and some expectoration of mucus.
- Cough hollow, mostly dry, with pressure in the pit of the stomach, so that the person cannot sleep all night.
- Hollow cough, mostly in the morning in bed and also at night; it prevents the person from falling asleep.
- Frequent irritable cough, from scratching in the throat.
- Loose, rattling cough when eating, as in old people.
- Loose cough without expectoration, with pain and a feeling of soreness in the chest, so that the person dreads to cough.
- Dry, intolerable cough with violent bronchial mucus; afterward the cough can be associated with a slimy, purulent expectoration, with rapid respiration, violent oppression of the chest; often the person is obliged to sit up when coughing.
- Cough without expectoration.
- Cough with difficult respiration and violent bronchitis, at first without fever, with remarkably soft pulse; great prostration and emaciation.
- Expectoration of tenacious mucus.
- Expectoration of flakes of mucus, with smarting burning behind the sternum.
- Streaks of blood in the mucous expectoration from the chest.
- Expectoration contained streaks of blood (seventh day).

Heat
- Violent fever, with red, hot face.
- Fever from five to six PM; first violent chill, so that person cannot get warm, followed by heat with thirst and internal chilliness; after

the latter passes off, heat and perspiration all night, till morning (after eight hours).
- Fever in the afternoon, for many days; heat, with or without previous chill.
- Perspiration smelling of sulphur.
- Perspiration all over every morning, exhausting the person (after 24 hours).
- Perspiration during sleep, after midnight, lasting till morning, without thirst.

Respiration
- Breathing rather hurried.
- Respiration always very short after coughing.
- Short respiration.
- Mucous rales are easily distinguishable in different portions of both lungs, but more noticeable in the lower lobes.
- Can breathe only with a loud, rattling noise.
- Anxious, short and hurried respiration, with elevation of the whole thorax, especially of the left side.
- Patient complains of want of air, though s/he frequently takes a deep breath.
- Feeling of suffocation.
- Labored breathing on taking a deep breath.

Skin
- Numerous red spots on the body, associated with great weakness, recognized as purpura; oldest spots can become brownish red the following day, whereas the newest spots are bright red.
- Some red spots on the arms, which disappear on pressure.
- Red points, with corrosive itching, in a spot as large as the hand in the bend of the right elbow.
- Bluish red spots under the skin, especially on the leg; bleeding from the leech bites was very difficult to stop; it was necessary to keep then constantly and tightly bound.

Pulsatilla nigricans

Pulsatilla nigricans is a beautiful flower of the anemone family and is found all over in Europe. It has dark purple petals. This plant remedy is useful in so many ways, but it is especially helpful to people who are "drama kings and queens," emotionally speaking.

Mental and Emotional State

- Nervous excitement.
- When evening comes, he begins to dread ghosts, four evenings in succession; during the day anxiety and flushing heat over the whole body, though the hands and face are cold and pale.
- The child longs now for this, now for that, even with a good humor.
- Extremely capricious and peevish at everything, even at himself.
- Everything disgusts him; he seems averse to everything.
- Anxiety in the evening, after going to sleep, with a rush of ideas and determination of blood to the head, which forces him to get up.
- A tremulous anxiety, aggravated during rest, while sitting and lying; relieved by motion.
- Anxiety in the region of the heart, even to suicide, in the evening, associated with a sensation of nausea in the pit of the stomach.
- Anxiety, as if he would have apoplexy, in the evening, after lying down, with chilliness, sounds in the ears like music, with twitching in the fingers of the right hand (after half an hour).
- Extremely ill-humored and fretful.
- Shuns business, is irresolute, with sighing respiration and a feeling as if he was beside himself.
- A great many wandering thoughts in his head.

Physical Symptoms

Chest

- Lungs ulcerated, eroded, with constant fever and bloody and purulent expectoration.
- Oppression of the chest with cough, without expectoration.
- Pressure upon the chest and soreness.
- Constriction across the chest.
- Scraping in the chest (windpipe), causing cough.

Front and Sides of Chest

- A small spot in the region of the sternum is painful, as if the breath pressed against it.
- Pressure on the middle of the chest.
- Pain in the left wall of the chest, preventing respiration.

Chilliness

- Chilliness on going from a warm room into the cold air.

- Constant chilliness throughout the whole body but especially in the back, with cold hands.
- Chilliness with pains in the evening.
- Chilliness in the house in the evening.
- Chilliness in the evening after lying down; afterward slight heat.
- Febrile chill without thirst; thirst during the heat.
- Shivering running up the back all day, without thirst.
- Creeping shivering over the arms, with heat of the cheeks; the air of the room seems too hot.
- Cold hands and feet; they seem dead.

Cough
- Violent cough, with difficult, scanty expectoration of a little tenacious mucus.
- Dry cough with difficult expectoration.
- Dry cough at night; it disappears upon sitting up in bed but returns when lying down.
- Cough with expectoration of black pieces of clotted blood, lasting till evening.
- Cough with expectoration of yellow mucus.
- Cough with bitter expectoration.
- The mucus expectorated by coughing has a biting, burnt taste, almost like the taste of crab's broth or the juice of an old pipe.

Heat
- With her clothes on she was too warm, and on taking them off she was chilly.
- Heat of the whole body, with the exception of the hands, which are cool; pressive headache above the orbits of the eyes and anxious lamentations.
- Heat of the whole body for an hour in the afternoon.
- Very feverish and thirsty.
- Intolerable dry heat at night in bed.
- Sensation of warmth, as if in too hot a room.
- Heat, followed by shivering.
- Fever; repeated shivering in the afternoon and in the evening; general burning heat and violent thirst; frightful starting-up preventing sleep; pain like wandering labor pains; painfulness of the whole body so that she could not turn over in bed; and watery diarrhea.

- Fever; very violent chill in the evening, with external coldness, without shivering and without thirst; in the morning a sensation of heat, as if sweat would break out (which does not), without thirst and without external heat, though with hot hands and aversion to uncovering.
- Profuse sweat in the morning.

Respiratory
- Violent tickling and scraping in the voice box, bringing tears into the eyes and causing dry cough.
- Tickling in the region of the thyroid and a short cough caused thereby (hacking).
- The person chokes after coughing.
- Oppression in the air passages as if they were pressed from without and constricted so that for a moment the person cannot get her or his breath, in the evening; while standing entirely without cough.
- Shortness of breath immediately after dinner, lasting several hours.
- Want of breath on attempting to breathe through the nose, not through the mouth.
- Sensation of labored breathing in the lower portion of the chest, as if it were too full and tight, in the morning.
- Shortness of breath in the evening, followed by slumbering; then waking with a paroxysm of suffocation, short or hacking cough; tearing frontal headache, extending through the eyes; crawling on the tongue; cold feet, cold sweat on the face and much belching.

Skin
- A (burning) itching over the whole body on becoming warm in bed, before midnight, aggravated by scratching; is unable to sleep on account of it; less during the day, and then only after becoming heated from walking or after rubbing; there is no appearance of an eruption.
- Biting, itching here and there in the skin.

Voice
- Hoarseness, inability to speak a loud word.

Rhus toxicodendron

Known as poison oak, it is made from fresh leaves gathered at sunset just before flowering. It is well known to help with joint symptoms.

Mental and Emotional State

- Full of sad thoughts, anxious and fearful, wherewith she gradually lost strength and was obliged to lie down for hours in order to regain energy.
- Extremely low-spirited, with sense of tiredness; she could not prevent herself from crying.
- Depression and discouragement as well as dissatisfaction with the world in the evening.
- Apprehensive, anxious and tremulous.
- Inexpressible anxiety, with pressure at the heart and tearinglike pain in the small of the back.
- Anxiety; while sitting, she was obliged to take hold of something because she did not think she could keep up on account of the pain (beating and drawing pains in the limbs).
- Anxiety at night; he would flee from bed and seek help on account of an indescribable distressing sensation.
- Anxiety, with loss of strength as if he would die, more after midnight than before.
- Anxiety and apprehension as if he wished to take his own life, for an hour in the twilight, toward evening.
- Forgetfulness; he could not recollect what had just taken place.
- Memory is very dull; he can recall things and names with difficulty, even the most familiar; though sometimes the memory is quite clear and distinct, if he has no chill.

Physical Symptoms

Chest

- Oppression of the chest at night, with sticking pains, especially on breathing.
- Pain in the chest, as if the sternum was pressed inward, in the morning, in bed; disappears after rising.
- Tickling and itching in the chest.

Front and Sides of Chest

- Pressure near the middle of the sternum, on the left side.
- Deep stitches on both sides of the sternum while sitting bent over.
- Frequent stitches of pain in the sides.
- On swallowing moderately cold water transient burning and

pressive pain at the middle of the lower side of the left clavicle (collarbone).

Chilliness

- Chilliness toward evening; he was obliged to lie down and cover up, after which he became warmer.
- Chilliness with dry lips and less thirst than hunger.
- Chilliness in the house toward evening; creeping coldness all over.
- Chilliness and heat in the evening; the face seemed very hot, though the cheeks were cold to the touch and pale; the breath came very hot from the mouth two afternoons in succession.
- Pinching chill in the feet and between the shoulders; a quarter of an hour afterward much external heat with burning pain in the left arm and on the left side of the upper part of the body, with redness of the cheeks.
- Chilliness in the back and head, heat on the anterior part of the body.
- Sensation of internal coldness in the limbs (as from deadness in one finger, as if the limb would full asleep or like a distressing sensation of coldness in the limbs internally, at the onset of a paroxysm of ague), though there was no trace of external coldness.
- Extremely cold hands and feet all day.

Cough and Expectoration

- Cough with a disagreeable tension on the chest.
- Cough immediately after eating.
- A tickling cough that causes dryness in the throat, especially in the evening.
- Some cough with a black, glutinous expectoration, especially in the morning.
- Very fatiguing cough, with expectoration of white mucus day and night.
- He is unable to sleep at night on account of a cough that torments him excessively.
- Spasmodic cough that shatters the head.
- Cough about three in the morning, most violent after waking.
- Short, anxious, painful cough that frequently awakens her from sleep before midnight, with very short breath.
- Coughs night and morning.
- Frequent hacking cough in the evening, after lying down, with bitter taste in the throat till he falls asleep; in the morning a similar

hacking cough and a similar taste in the throat, lasting till he rises from bed.

Heat

- Fever about five in the afternoon, stretching of the limbs, shivering over the whole body with much thirst, cold hands, heat and redness of the face; also again in the evening in bed shivering; in the morning, perspiration over the whole body, with pressure in the temples.
- A high state of fever attended the erysipelas (lesions on skin that are shiny red, swollen and tender—caused by streptococci).
- Heat with great thirst.

Respiratory

- Frequent tickling irritability in the air passages, as if it would provoke cough, that makes the breath short; disappears on moderate exertion.
- Hoarseness, causing a scraping, raw sensation in the voice box.
- Respiration hurried.
- Feels a sensation of choking at times.
- Shortness of breath, especially on going to stool.
- For four days inclination to take a deep breath, with dull pain and oppression at stomach.
- Oppression and anxiety, as if she could not get her breath.
- The breath became difficult after walking a little.
- She is unable to sit up; is obliged to take a deep breath, as if she would suffocate, especially after eating.
- During sleep expiration was light and snoring, inspiration inaudible.
- Very short breath at night.

Sweat

- Sweat all over when coughing.
- Sweat all over the body during sleep, without odor and not exhausting, about three to four o'clock in the morning.
- Sweat from warm drinks.
- Profuse sweat in the morning.
- Sour-smelling sweat in the morning with cold, sweaty cheeks.
- The skin is moist and the hair of the head is wet.
- Sweat before midnight.
- Night sweat, especially about the neck.

Throat

- She was obliged to clear the throat much in the morning; the more she rinsed out the mouth, the worse the mucus in the throat became.
- Profuse hawking of mucus in the morning.
- Sensation of dryness in the throat.
- Sensation of swelling in the throat, associated with a bruised pain when talking and when not; but on swallowing, a pressive, swollen pain with sticking, as if something sharp was penetrating.
- Sore throat, swallowing difficult, with stitching pains; throat much swollen externally as if the maxillary and parotid glands were greatly enlarged.
- She is unable to drink; on every swallow, the drink chokes her as if the back of throat was inactive or paralyzed; associated with a sensation of dryness in the throat posteriorly.
- Parotid glands (neck region) and glands beneath the lower jaw hard and swollen.

Sepia officinalis

Sepia is made from the ink of the cuttlefish, a beautiful and very shy ocean creature. It is actually a member of the cephalaspid family, like the octopus. Sepia is a wonderful remedy for a person who is vastly overworked. Many women who balance work, motherhood and spousal duties and suffer from exhaustion use this remedy.

Mental and Emotional State

- He becomes angry over every trifle.
- Nervous irritability.
- Tried to study but became nervous and confused.
- Nerves very sensitive to the least noise.
- Great internal restlessness for many days, with hastiness; when he has scarcely begun a work, he wishes it were done.
- Great sadness and frequent attacks of weeping, which she can scarcely suppress.
- Very sad, with unusual lassitude.
- Sad and gloomy mood, mostly when walking in the open air.
- Doesn't want company.
- So gloomy she felt as if she could weep over everything, without cause.
- Gloominess; she feels unfortunate, without cause.

- Dark forebodings about his disease in regard to the future.
- He feels oppressed in sultry weather but becomes more cheerful when it storms (lightning and thunder) and feels better.
- Anxiety toward evening.
- He dare not be alone for a moment.
- Very easily frightened and fearful.
- Highly emotional and irritable.
- Very easily offended.
- Impatience when sitting, like an uneasiness in the bones.
- Great indifference toward everything; no proper sense of life.
- Indisposition for mental labor, which aggravates the headache.
- Language comes very slowly; I have to drag out the words to express ideas and forget the chief points.
- I am becoming thickheaded, for it seems as if I could not remember the things that I knew yesterday; it is hard work for me to think or study; it seems as if my mind were hedged in, as if it were circumscribed; for instance, I cannot compare two things; it seems as if my mind was gone.
- Weak memory.

Physical Symptoms
Chest
- Lungs felt slightly sore, but no cough and no expectoration except now and then to clear the throat of a little phlegm.
- A gurgling sound in the chest.
- Feeling of heaviness in the chest, as from outward pressure.
- He cannot take a deep breath on account of contracted feeling around the lower part of the chest.
- Chest is quite raw, owing to much cough and expectoration.
- Throbbing through chest and abdomen as if the heart occupied the whole body.

Front and Sides of Chest
- Severe burning pain in the sternum.
- Pain in the right side of the chest, especially on stooping and lying on the right side.
- Pressure on the right chest in waves, relieved by burping.
- A sharp, piercing pain in the lower lobe of the right lung, coming on in paroxysms and so severe as to almost make me cry out.

- Violent tearing in the lower right ribs.
- Stitches in the right side of chest and shoulder blade during breathing in and coughing.
- Stitching pain in the left chest when coughing.

Chilliness

- Violent, shaking chill for one hour, then great heat with inability to collect one's senses; then profuse sweat in the evening; the urine is brown and of acrid smell.
- The chilliness is felt in evening only, for five days.
- Chilliness for many nights.
- Coldness over the whole body.
- Very cold feet with headache, especially toward evening and in the morning.
- Feet cold and damp all day, feeling as though I stood in cold water up to my ankles (my feet are usually dry).
- Icy-cold feet, particularly in the evening; even for a long time after going to bed I cannot warm them.

Cough

- Cough, awaking at night.
- Cough, mostly in the evening, in bed, with vomiting.
- Cough from tickling in the voice box, without expectoration (after five days).
- The irritation to cough frequently comes on so suddenly and violently that he cannot take breath quick enough and it produces a spasmodic contraction of the chest.
- After rattling of mucus in the chest severe cough with expectoration, producing raw and sore pain in the throat still felt one half hour after the cough.
- Spasmodic cough.
- Severe cough with little expectoration but mostly with bitter vomiting, yet only evenings, when lying in bed.
- Severe cough in the evening.
- Expectoration of blood when coughing every morning, without pain in the chest.
- Gray and yellowish expectoration from cough.
- Yellow expectoration, tasting like rotten eggs.
- Very salty-tasting expectoration from chest.

Heat

- Intermittent fever, returning frequently during the day at indefinite periods; first general heat with sweat in the face, violent thirst and bitterness of the mouth; then chill with general coldness even in the face, with inclination to vomit; pressure in the forehead extending into the temples; during the heat vertigo as if he would fall.
- Fever with pressing fist in the temples at intervals of several minutes; short breath, as from internal heat, the whole night through; following this, in the morning, weakness in the lower limbs, thirst, want of appetite, sleepiness; during the day feverish shivering, pain in the throat and swelling of area beneath the lower jaw.
- Feverish, weak and with hot urine.
- High fever with rash.
- Flushes of heat in the evening, then itching.
- At night heat and, from this, restlessness.
- Painful heat in the head, frequently with flushes of heat over the body.

Sweat

- Much sweat during sleep, particularly on the head.
- Profuse sweat while walking, especially in the bends of the joints.

Voice Box (Larynx)

- Accumulation of much mucus in the voice box that is difficult to cough up but easy to swallow, even with deep breathing.
- Dryness of the voice box in the morning.
- Feeling of dryness in the windpipe.
- Sudden hoarseness.

Respiration

- Loud snoring sounds while inhaling.
- Breathing difficult rather than short.
- Oppression of breathing in the evening, from pain under the right short ribs, which prevents the slightest motion.
- Short breath when walking, as if the chest were full.
- Breathing much shorter.
- Loss of breath caused by every motion, even the slightest one.
- He awakes in the morning with great, labored breathing and covered with sweat lasting four hours.
- Labored breathing, with mucus in the chest difficult to loosen.

Throat

- Hawking up phlegm and a quantity of bloody mucus in the morning.

- Constant accumulation of mucus in the throat, which almost suffocates her.
- Much mucus in the throat; he must hawk much.
- Throat red and dry.
- Throat dry, worse in the evening.
- Dryness of the throat the whole day.
- Dryness and soreness in throat; at night it feels quite parched.
- Pressure in the throat in the region of the tonsils, as if the neck cloth were tied too tight.
- Pressure and cutting in the throat when swallowing, with a coating of mucus in the throat; on attempting to hawk up the mucus the pressure and cutting are aggravated, with a sensation as if the throat were cut with shears, followed by bleeding.
- Throat feels as if it had been skinned.
- Sticking pain in the uvula (a small, soft structure hanging down in the back of the mouth), with redness on both sides of the throat; very sensitive on swallowing, with shaking chill and accumulation of mucus that cannot be loosened.

Sulphur

Sulphur is an element and is also known as sublimed sulphur or "flowers of sulphur." The ancient term for it is "brimstone." It is one of our greatest and deepest-acting remedies in homeopathy, and some of its characteristics are quick temper, nervousness and sensitivity.

Mental and Emotional State
- The child was intolerably violent and difficult and quiet.
- Very much excited and very passionate on violent motion.
- Numerous morbid ideas, extremely disagreeable, causing rancor.
- During the nightly cough, the boy fell into long weeping, with great physical restlessness.
- Greatly inclined to weep without cause.
- Extremely sensitive and weeping easily on the slightest unpleasantness.
- Greatly depressed, hypochondriac and sighing, so that he could not speak a loud word.
- Depressed about her illness and out of humor.
- Sad, without courage.

- She does not know what to do with herself on account of internal discouragement.
- In the afternoon in the open air, great depression of spirits without any cause.
- Great anxiety in the evening in bed, at the time of the full moon.
- So obstinate and morose that he answers no one and will not tolerate anyone about him; he cannot obtain quickly enough whatever he desires.
- Aversion to every business.
- The slightest work is irksome to him.
- Disinclination to talk.
- Very forgetful.
- So forgetful that what has just happened is only vaguely remembered.
- Remarkable forgetfulness, especially for proper names.
- Seems stupid, senseless, confused; avoids conversation.

Physical Symptoms

Chest

- When coughing, a feeling as if the lungs rested against the back.
- Anxious feeling in the chest; he can hardly expand it during inhalation.
- Violent rush of blood to the chest, like a boiling, with nausea amounting to faintness; trembling of the right arm.
- Great weakness of the chest, especially troublesome on getting into bed at night so that he cannot lie long on one side and is longing for morning.
- Such fullness in the chest before the menses that she was frequently obliged to take a deep breath.
- Sensation as if mucus were seated in the chest, after raising of which the respiration was freer; the whole day some mucus was coughed up, less in the afternoon and evening than in the morning.
- Painful constriction of the chest, frequently on motion.
- Rattling sounds in the chest at night.
- Rattling and snoring sounds in the chest, relieved by expectoration.

Chilliness

- Early the next morning, she complained of being cold; the head soon became hot and the extremities cold. A few hours later, she experienced a severe chill, succeeded by fever and perspiration that lasted eight or ten hours; the chill then came on more severely than before.

- Chilliness every evening, not relieved by the warmth of the stove; in the bed great warmth and sour perspiration every morning.
- Shuddering over the whole body in the evening in bed, like a shuddering through the skin.
- Shivering in the evening, with thirst, followed by heat of the face and hands.
- Chilly, creeping sensations up the back, relieved by the warmth of the stove in the evening.
- Febrile heat, first on the face, with a sensation as if she had passed through a severe illness; immediately followed by some chilliness with much thirst (after four days).
- At night feeling of heat in the whole body, especially in the palms of the hands.
- Heat and burning in the face, with a few, chiefly red, spots between the eye and ear.
- Dry heat in the thighs and small of the back with coldness of the back.

Cough and Expectoration
- Some cough, caused by roughness of the throat.
- He wanted to cough and could not; it became black before his eyes.
- Inclination to cough after eating, so violent that he cannot cough soon enough; it draws his chest spasmodically together and he retches as if he would vomit.
- Provocation to cough, in two or three attacks, with every breath; worse in the afternoon.
- Frequent coughing with the sore throat.
- Short cough in the evening while sitting, asleep.
- Much cough when going to sleep, with heat in the head and face and with cold hands.
- Cough only at night.
- Dry cough that did not permit him to sleep, only at night.
- Short, dry, violent cough, with pain in the sternum or with stitches in the chest.
- Cough lasted, with slight remissions, for one month.
- Loose cough, with a sensation of soreness or pressure upon the chest and expectoration of thick mucus, also with rattling in the windpipe and hoarseness.
- Coughs up greenish plugs of a sweetish taste.

- Pieces of hard mucus, like starch, are expectorated by hawking.
- Expectoration of bloody saliva, with a sweet taste in the throat.
- Expectoration of blood at night, with fatty, sweetish taste in the mouth.

Respiration
- Exhaled air feels hot.
- Short breathing, relieved by sitting up.
- Shortness of breath from talking much.
- Shortness of breath when walking in the open air.
- Difficulty breathing; he is obliged to take a deep breath, more while sitting than while walking.
- Spasmodic want of breath at night.
- Labored breathing, with the sore throat.

Skin
- Nettle rash with fever.
- Nettle rash eruption.
- Violent, biting rash on the face, arms and lower extremities.
- Heat rash on the back.
- Nettle rash eruption under the hips.
- Nettle rash eruption on the back of the hand.
- A scaly eruption, which had been driven away by external applications and reappeared after scratching, with violent burning, itching.
- Itching hives over the whole body, hands and feet.

Sweat
- On awaking in the morning, he had to change his linen on account of profuse perspiration smelling of sulphur.
- Profuse perspiration in the morning, only on itching parts.
- Toward morning general, warm perspiration with anxiety, causing him to throw off the bedclothes.
- Morning sweat, always after waking at about six or seven o'clock.
- Perspiration in the morning during sleep, disappearing on waking.
- Night sweat of a sour, burnt odor.
- Profuse, sour night sweats, immediately from the evening on.
- Much perspiration while walking in the open air.
- Inclined to perspire on the slightest motion.

Voice
- Hoarseness in the evening.
- Hoarseness and roughness of the voice, with dryness of the throat and burning on swallowing.

- Talking takes a very great effort and causes pain.

Voice Box
- The voice box feels swollen.
- Swollen gland on the thyroid (center of throat area) that is painful to touch.
- Drawing and dryness in the voice box at times.
- Sensation as if mucus was stuck in throat.

Other Possible SARS Remedies

The homeopathic remedies below should be considered by a professional homeopath during a SARS epidemic if none of the other remedies listed seem to fit a client's symptoms.

Tuberculinum aviaire

You should know that *Tuberculinum aviaire* is a nosode, which means that diseased material was used to make a homeopathic remedy. In this case, the diseased material comes from the lungs of chicken that had mycobacterium tuberculosis.

Tuberculinum aviaire is only available through a professional homeopath. This remedy may have some far-reaching ramifications and should only be used if no other remedy can be found to help a person with SARS. Little is known about it, but it could end up being highly useful if nothing else works as well.

Tuberculinum aviaire has been shown to help the following conditions: bronchitis, colds, influenza, measles, pneumonia, tuberculosis, asthenia, anorexia, emaciation, cervical micro-adenopathy, broken-down condition of Bernand-Jacquelin type (tubercular condition of old homoeopaths).

What Is It?

This remedy is a nosode; it is made from the lungs of a chicken that had tuberculosis and acts on the apices (top) of the lungs. The remedy was introduced by Dr. Cartier and other homeopaths of Paris. Dr. Cartier gave an account of this nosode in his paper read at the International Homeopathic Congress, 1896 (Transactions, Part "Essays and Communications," p. 187). *Tuberculinum aviaire* has proved to be an excellent remedy in influenzal bronchitis with symptoms similar to tuberculosis. It relieves the debility, diminishes the cough, improves the appetite and braces up the whole organism.

Tuberculinum aviaire acts most prominently on the lungs and it corresponds most closely to the bronchitis of influenza, which simulates tuberculosis. It has cured several hopeless-looking cases and has also performed excellently in some cases of bronchitis following measles. The bacillus of avian tuberculosis has been identified with that of human tuberculosis, but the clinical properties of the two nosodes are not identical.

Physical Symptoms

Cough
- Acute broncho-pulmonary diseases of children.
- Itching of palms and ears.
- Acute, inflammatory, irritating, incessant and tickling cough.
- Loss of strength and appetite.

Eyes
- Mucous membranes of the eyelids are congested, with tears.

Ears
- Earache with suppuration and pus.
- Mastoiditis.

Head
- Frontal headache with hot forehead; the root of the nose is painful.
- Troubles of perception with an impaired or confused state of mind.
- Meningeal convulsive attacks.

Heart
- Abnormal rapidity of heart action (tachycardia) with rapid and bounding pulse.
- Cold fingers and hands, may be bluish or grayish in color.
- Cyanosis.
- Circulatory troubles.
- Fever with general uneasiness accompanied by chill, diffused muscular pain.

Lungs
- Pleura (pleurisy).
- Pain in the upper part of the lungs.
- Thoracic wall painful.
- Dry and painful cough.

Nose
- Flaring of nostrils, cyanosis and obstruction in the nose.
- Pain in the root of the nose.
- Loss of sense of smell.
- Continual sneezing with a lot of watery discharge.

Skin
- Face is red or may be pale.
- Palms are hot and sweaty.

Throat
- Irritation of larynx and of the trachea.
- Hoarseness.
- Congestion of the larynx with shortness of breath.

Tussilago farfara

This perennial herb is found growing in damp, heavy soil in Europe and Northern Asia. It is known as coltsfoot, because the leaf is somewhat shaped like a horse's hoof. The flower heads have yellow, ligulate rays in many rows; the florets of the disk are tubular and number about 20. The plant prefers clay, loam, marl and lime in the soil and is often considered an indicator of such soil.

To this day, *Tussilago farfara* is used in the form of a confection for coughs. The leaves are mucilaginous and were much used in scrofulous affections. Smoking the dried leaves relieves coughs. It is frequently used by itself or combined with other lung remedies as a medicine that relieves lung inflammation and has mucus-dissolving action in the respiratory organs. Cough, hoarseness, bronchitis and inflammations of the pharyngeal mucous membranes, as well as shortness of breath, bronchial asthma and pleurisy can be treated successfully with this remedy.

Below are proving symptoms by Dr. Irvin J. Lane. I chose this information, because it represents symptoms concerned with "flulike" symptoms.

Mental and Emotional State

- Dreamed about murder, burglars and so on most of the night, which would awake me and I would feel afraid for a short time.
- Feels quite cross.

Physical Symptoms
Abdomen
- Passage of a great deal of flatus, with rumbling of wind in the abdomen.
- Coliclike pains in hypogastric region that come in paroxysms, with flatulence in the abdomen and passage of a great deal of flatus.

Back
- Bruised, aching pain in lumbar region, aggravated by sitting up straight or leaning back; ameliorated by leaning forward or passing flatus.

Bladder
- Pass a great deal of light, nearly colorless urine.
- Had to get up twice during the night to urinate. (Seldom have to get up at all.)

Extremities (Arms and Legs)
- Weakness of the extremities.
- Right knee gave out while walking, as if I had no power in the muscles.
- Aching of the muscles of the right arm, worse at the elbow.
- Extreme weakness of the right side.
- Puffy swelling of hands still continues.
- Arm felt numb as if asleep when it was extended above the head.

Eyes
- Black, oblong specks with white rings around them before my eyes.
- Sensation as of sand beneath the eyelids in the morning on first awaking.
- Get the lines crossed while driving.

General
- Got tired very easily this afternoon, restless and sleepless last night after going to bed.
- Constant yawning and very sleepy.

Head
- Dull feeling in the forehead; aching pain at times in left temple.
- After bathing had a hot sensation in the forehead.
- Felt sleepy, with dull aching in forehead.
- Alternation of paleness and flushing (redness) of face.

Nose
- Thoughts or smell of medicine causes nausea.
- Burning, irritating sensation in the nose; aggravated by a long inhale through the nose.
- Constant irritation in left side of the nose.
- Burning sensation, with a discharge of watery mucus from the nose.

Mouth
- Base of tongue coated white with red, raised papillae.
- Thirsty, drinking little and often.

Throat
- Dry sensation in pharynx with difficulty swallowing.
- Had an irritating sensation in the upper part of the throat about four o'clock in the morning that caused a dry, hacking cough, aggravated by lying down or taking a deep breath.
- Dry sensation in the pharynx and frequent sneezing.
- Burning sensation in the throat, with dry, constricted sensation of pharynx; great difficulty in swallowing.

Veratrum viride

This is a plant indigenous to the U.S., known by the common names of Indian poke and itchweed. A homeopathic pharmacy prepares a tincture from the root. The remedy is used to treat simple fever without local inflammation but accompanied by vertigo, headache, dimness of sight, nausea, weakness and restlessness; infantile remittent fever with drowsiness, throbbing of the temporal arteries, hard and quick pulse, vomiting of mucus and bile as well as constipation; the invasive stage of scarlatina; and other toxemic fevers with much involvement of the head, high fever and the symptoms mentioned above. In those cases where the circulatory excitement and gastric irritation are beyond the scope of *Aconitum napellus*, *Veratrum viride* is an excellent substitute, especially when there is no threat of the typhoid conditions calling for baptisia.

Particularly in dealing with the onset of pneumonia, the drug is often valuable. Some American experiments indicate that in small doses, it can increase the specific bodily resistance to the pneumococcus. The remedy has great power over the muscles and nerves of motion, particularly in controlling spasm. It has also a considerable power in some cases of chorea. In many points, the pathogenetic effects of *Veratrum viride* resemble those of *Veratrum album* and in others, those of *Aconitum napellus*. It differs, however, from the latter in various ways and especially in that *Aconitum napellus* seems to exert a special action on the sympathetic nervous system, whereas the power of *Veratrum viride* shows over the vagus nerve centers.

The provers have not given us many symptoms—and those they have given us are general rather than specific—but *Veratrum viride* has prevented and cured many cases of pneumonia, bronchitis and pulmonary congestion (aconite, *Ferrum phos.* and belladonna can also deal with these conditions). The full pulse, marked dyspnea, hot head, cold extremities, dry tongue and high temperature are prominent symptoms.

For treating pneumonia that involves more than one lobe of a lung(s), use *Veratrum viride*; use it for very intense cases setting in with violent chill, very active congestion and delirium, followed by high fever with full, hard, bounding pulse. This remedy can be given in one- or two-drop doses every one-half to one hour until arterial excitement subsides.

Pulmonary hyperemia is one of the indications for *Veratrum viride:*

- Violent congestion in athletic persons.
- Thirst, nausea, high fever with throbbing, bounding pulse and red face.
- Difficulty breathing with sensation of a heavy load on the chest.

Mental and Emotional State
- Quarrelsome and delirious.

Physical Symptoms
Cough
- Dry or scanty cough.
- Acute coughs, high fever, bronchial or lung invasion.
- Short, dry cough; congestion of chest; rapid breathing; nausea and vomiting; high fever; very scanty, bloody saliva; oppression of chest.
- Difficult cough, high fever, flushed face, labored breathing, blood-streaked saliva.
- Difficult, dry cough; high fever; rapid, painful breathing; bound-

ing pulse; great excitement and distress; croupy pneumonia; saliva thick, scanty and very difficult.

- Stitching pleuritic pains around lungs; dry cough; high fever; great distress and prostration; face bluish-purple; pulse very rapid, short and hard.
- Pleuro-pneumonia.

Eyes
- Dilated pupils.

Face
- Face flushed.

Mouth
- Dry mouth and lips, dry all day.

Pulse
- Sinking, regularly intermittent pulse.
- Pulse hard, strong, quick or slow, weak, intermittent, near collapse.
- Reduces fever and arterial excitement, lessens pain and promotes expectoration of inflammatory products.

Respiration
- Labored breathing almost to suffocation; cannot lie down; face covered with cold sweat.
- Sensation of heavy load on chest, great anxiety, pneumonia.
- Labored breathing, quick, painful; high fever and pulse; bloody, mucous saliva.
- Breathing heavy, difficult, slow, short, convulsive, almost to suffocation; constriction of chest.
- Expectoration of pus and florid blood.
- Heavy load on chest, with great anxiety.
- Labored breathing, with bloody saliva.
- Stitching, pleuritic pains, high fever and rapid, short, bounding pulse.

Stomach
- Stomach faints, nauseated; faint feeling in pit of stomach.
- Vomiting.

Tongue
- Red streak through the center of the tongue.
- Tongue somewhat red in center; coated yellow with red streak in center.
- Feels scalded.
- Tongue white or yellow, with red streak down middle, or dry or moist, with white or yellow coating or no coating on either side.

Viscum album

This is mistletoe, and the whole plant is used to make the homeopathic remedy.

Mental and Emotional State

- Sad, tired, feels worn out, is apathetic but restless at the same time. Oversensitive to noise.
- Has aversion to people, wants to be left alone, cannot react adequately to people.
- Tendency to go to extremes: overstimulation, intense, almost maniacal ability to react and, more often, a depressive oversensitivity.
- Keeps waking at night thinking the most horrible things imaginable. Gets to sleep again soon by changing thoughts.
- Inclined to be violent.
- Feels as if going to do something dreadful while the tremblings are occurring.
- Great sensitiveness to noise.
- Spectral illusions (sees things that aren't there).
- Stupor, succeeded by almost entire insensibility; lying motionless with her eyes closed as if in sound sleep, but easily roused by a loud noise and then would answer any question; but when she relapsed into her former condition, there was a slight disposition to stertorous breathing.

Physical Symptoms

Breathing

- Breathing slow and stertorous (labored breathing).
- Spasm of glottis, comes with dry sensation in throat, followed by efforts to swallow, then a sort of complete block, making swallowing an effort and causing eyes to fill with tears.
- Breathing slow and labored.

Chest

- Pain across sternal region, below breasts, coming and going; worse when taking a deep breath or lying on left side.
- Stitching pain at upper part of left breast.
- Stitch in chest below left breast, again above right knee.

- Stabs under left false ribs and constriction of upper part of left lung, worse when taking deep breath.
- Creepy, chilly feeling on left side of lower outer chest.

Cough

- Dyspnea; feeling of suffocation when lying on left side.
- Spasmodic cough.
- Whooping cough (it has cured whooping cough within two days).
- Asthma, especially if connected with rheumatism and gout.
- Bronchial.
- Trembling of the heart.
- Lowered blood pressure.

Face

- Lips red, face red.
- Countenance suffused.
- Lips livid.
- Face flushed after palpitation.
- Face hot and flushed.

Fever

- Chilly even near a stove; cold, chilly feeling creeps over him frequently.
- Skin warm and very moist.
- First cold and then hot feeling without actually being hot.
- On waking always very hot except on knees, legs and feet, which are very cold.
- Hot feeling at night, during urination.

General

- Great weakness, especially tiredness of legs.
- Legs are restless.
- Feet may be burning hot or cold.
- Suppresses menses.

Pulse

- Pulse small, quick and very irregular (second day).
- Pulse slow, full and bounding.

Skin

- Skin warm and moist.
- Skin felt dry and burning.
- Red spots on neck and chest.
- Left side of neck large papule or small blood boil.

Modalities

- *Worse:* In winter, cold and stormy weather; in motion; when lying on left side.

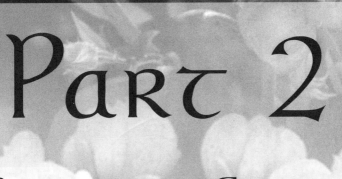

PART 2

Biological and Chemical Terrorism:

Homeopathic Strategy for Today's World

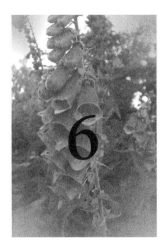

Modern-Day Epidemic Threats

Right now we're sitting on a powder keg of possibilities. Medical experts all agree that there is a flu epidemic coming that will wipe out people around the world. It's not even a question of if, but when. Keeping this in mind, we have many other epidemics that are quietly "blowing up" and moving through our population in a less dramatic fashion—but moving nonetheless. With that in mind, let's look at the possible culprits. (And, as always, seek help from your physician first, then call your homeopath to seek out secondary, backup support from this wonderful alternative medicine.)

The Hantavirus Epidemic

In 1993 there was an epidemic outbreak of the hantavirus. At first it was called the "Mystery Disease of the Four Corners Area." Then it was called the Navajo disease. The reservation was in pandemonium. The first victim was a teenage Navajo girl. Then her boyfriend died a few days later after contracting the same symptoms. A 13-year-old girl dancing at a party on the reservation in Shiprock, New Mexico, collapsed and died. By May of that year, 10 people had died in Albuquerque and Shiprock hospitals, all showing symptoms of this disease.

The symptoms were always the same: a raging pneumonia, with blood filling up the lungs in an explosive 48-hour period, causing the victims to die. No drug in the allopathic medical arsenal could stop it. Panic set in, but fortunately, a New Mexico biologist, Robert Parmenter, was able to trace the deadly dance of the events that lead up to the outbreak of the hemorrhagic fever back to its roots.

Parmenter had just completed a 10-year study of rodents. He noted that heavy rains had occurred from May 1992 through May 1993, leading to 10 times the normal population of rodents. Piñon trees grow throughout the deserts of the Southwest and rodents feed off these trees, which were numerous enough to keep the huge, multiplied rodent family alive and well. This population explosion among the rodents, which are carriers for the viruses of the bunyavirus family, meant that the hantavirus spread to many more in the human population than normal, and so the outbreak began. The epidemic subsided when the rains did not appear in 1994; Mother Nature herself intervened.

However, of 770 deer mice collected in Arizona, New Mexico and Colorado between June and August of 1993, 31 percent carried the virus. It was also found that 19 percent of the piñon mice, 7 percent of the brush mice, 15 percent of the chipmunks and 4 percent of the house mice carried this deadly virus.

The hantavirus is spread through inhaling the scent of the droppings from rodents. It is well known that rodents like to winter inside the walls of homes to avoid getting killed by the cold weather. They live there, they drop fecal matter, and even though it's dry, eventually the aerosol odor can travel to some unsuspecting human being nearby. For this reason, the Centers for Disease Control (CDC) have told us to avoid physical contact with mice or any other rodents and not to sweep or clean houses where rodent droppings are or were present without a respirator. One can catch the deadly disease simply by inhaling dried rodent droppings that become airborne.

Understanding the Hantavirus

One needs to step back in history to understand the hantavirus. It was originally seen during the Korean conflict when 2,000 soldiers were infected with this hemorrhagic fever. Until then it had been unknown to U.S. doctors. Many deaths occurred among the troops who became infected. Dr. Ho Wang Lee of Seoul, Korea, first isolated the hantavirus in 1978 in the lung tissues of the striped field mouse—a very common animal that is recognized as a major carrier of this virus. Dr. Lee named it the Hantaan virus, after the Hantaan River, which flows across the Korean demilitarized zone, in recognition of the troops there dying from the virus.

After collecting samples of the virus, scientists were able to identify that it was from the bunyavirus family. They found that the transmission of the virus from the rodent to the human population occurred via saliva, feces and especially urination for the duration of the rodent's life. It has since been conservatively estimated that there are over 100,000 cases of the disease annually in China alone.

Worse, virologists were able to trace this disease to the 1970s, when rats from Korea carrying the hantavirus were found in the port city of Osaka, Japan. Scientists panicked and ordered rats from shipping ports around the world, to test them for this virus. The results were chilling: Rats at every shipping port in the world carried the virus. In 1982 a new variety of hantavirus, known as the Prospect Hill strain, was found in wild voles outside the city limits of Washington, D.C.

A few years after that discovery, scientists found Baltimore rats carrying antibodies of another Seoul-type virus, which they named Baltimore rat virus (BRV). What was even more upsetting to the virologists was the fact that this rat didn't inhabit just the port area of Baltimore but could be found everywhere in the city, particularly in the inner-city trash and litter areas.

Symptoms of the Hantavirus

The major symptoms of this virus as reported by the World Health Organization (WHO) occur in the following order: a high fever; shock to the entire body; kidney and bladder impairment; loss of life-giving fluids from the body, chiefly through vomiting and loss of electrolytes; facial flushing or redness, especially on the neck where a red rash is usually seen, though it is sometimes limited to the armpit region; bruising, usually black/blue, purple/red or even yellow/green, all over the body; bloodshot eyes. The bottom line is that this deadly virus, which kills 60 percent of its victims, attacks the kidneys and they stop functioning. As a result, all the toxic body fluids, urine in particular, become impossible to release from the body and they continue to float around in the bloodstream.

The lungs become overburdened with too much liquid; the kidneys stop working and a person can no longer release fluid through urination. The lungs rapidly fill up and the victims literally drown in their own fluids and blood—a horrible form of self-suffocation or drowning from the inside out.

If a person is able to survive the virus—and numbers show 40 percent do—a marked pattern emerges: Survivors repeatedly show kidney damage, kidney-related infections and a higher probability of strokes as well as high blood pressure. Johns Hopkins Hospital identified 15 patients who had BRV antibodies in their bloodstreams, which meant they had contracted the Baltimore rat virus (the hantavirus showed up in Baltimore rats in 1985). Many of these patients had gone to the hospital and been diagnosed with one of these offshoot symptoms of the virus just mentioned.

So there is the possibility that many people out there have had a milder version of the hantavirus that got passed off as a deadly "flu" strain and recovered but later began to show a cycle of kidney-related problems (such as kidney infections, lower kidney function in general or possibly something as chronic as Bright's disease), had experienced mild to severe strokes (no matter what their age) or had high blood pressure come on for "no known reason." If you fall into this group, it wouldn't be a bad idea to have your blood tested for the hantavirus. If antibodies do show up, you had the hantavirus and survived it. Your next step should be to go to a classically trained homeopath for constitutional treatment, and hopefully, some of the damage can be reversed or minimized.

Dr. Gail Derin, Doctor of Oriental Medicine and trained classical homeopath from Cottonwood, Arizona, and I tried to find the symptoms of the hantavirus in September of 1993. We were going to open a clinic on the Navajo Reservation and help fight this virus homeopathically. Unfortunately, we were never able to interview the Navajo survivors of this disease, because among the Navajo you never talk about anything bad or evil; they believe that if you do, you draw it back to yourself and it will happen again.

So all we have are newspaper, magazine and television reports on the symptoms, which aren't very specific. However, they are specific enough that if someone came down with the hantavirus symptoms, that person could take the appropriate remedy on the way to the hospital to get antibiotic help. Between the two, you could very well save your life.

We want to list these symptoms as they appear in "rubric" (symptom) form from J. T. Kent's repertory. If you have these symptoms, you need to act very quickly and check out the homeopathic remedies, which you should keep on hand in the medicine cabinet or with you when you travel.

- Inflammatory fever, swift and sudden with high temperature.
- Complete debilitation from the fever.
- Fever with intense heat and high temperature.
- "Puerperal" fever: blood poisoning or septicemia and, as a result, high fever.
- Typhus/typhoid continued fever. Typhus symptoms are similar to those of hantavirus: sudden onset, high fever, body rash, face darkens and swells; this is followed by delirium and a stupor. In many cases, the rash leads to gangrene that destroys victims, literally rotting them alive.
- Fever with nervous-system involvement, which can cause the mental symptom of "floating in the air" that is part of the delusions that set in with the virus.
- Fever with typhus/typhoid muscular soreness. Many of the victims report that their muscles ache so badly that it feels as if their bones are going to break. Those who have had a flu virus that has hit them in the muscles and joints know this symptom well.
- Fever with typhus/typhoid bronchial pneumonia. This condition moves swiftly and is the one that will kill due to the lungs filling up with vast amounts of liquid and/or blood.
- Fever with typhus/typhoid toxemia. This condition, known as toxemia, results because the kidneys or renal system have shut down and the urine and other toxic/poisonous matter can't be expelled via urination. The victim's bloodstream becomes septic, and the body's fever rises swiftly and very high to try to combat this condition.
- A dry cough with fever; victims report coughing constantly.

- The victims appear as if they were drunk from too much alcohol—confused, speech badly slurred and barely able to walk. When they do walk, it is as if they were drunk.
- Aching bones, the kind of aching that makes one feel as if one will break if one moves or walks.
- Pain in the muscles, an intense pain that never lets up or goes away.
- Pain appears suddenly. Another symptom of the hantavirus profile is its sudden onset. It hits so violently that within hours of the virus awakening in the body to wreak its damage, the person is "felled like an ox with a sledgehammer."
- A severe sore throat.

Homeopathic Remedies

Based upon the above symptoms, which Gail and I could cull from our limited sources, we began to track down the homeopathic remedies that best fit the hantavirus symptom picture. In homeopathy, like cures like; therefore, we wanted a remedy with close-fitting symptoms, meaning that if a healthy person took the remedy, it would reproduce nearly the exact symptoms that the hantavirus wreaked on an individual. We found the following remedies, listed in the order of how closely they mirror the symptoms of hantavirus infection:

- *Pyrogenium*
- *Baptisia tinctoria*
- *Rhus toxicodendron*
- *Arsenicum album*
- *Echinacea angustifolia*
- *Belladonna atropa*
- *Bryonia alba*
- *Gelsemium sempervirens*
- *Lachesis muta*
- *Aconitum napellus*
- *Arnica montana*

Please go to the epidemic *materia medica* starting on page 202 and look up these remedies to get a fuller picture of the symptoms. If you think you've contracted the virus, match your symptoms with those of the above remedies while you're on your way to the hospital

emergency room and take the appropriate remedy. Thankfully, antibiotics *can* intervene on the hantavirus right now, but that may not
always be so in the future; then, possibly only these homeopathic
remedies stand between you and death from hantavirus.

It would be a wise idea to have the top five homeopathic remedies on hand in your medicine chest; if you travel, particularly into a
foreign country or into any "backwoods" kind of country in the
world, you should always have these remedies with you, just in case.

Locate your nearest homeopathic practitioner and show her
or him this information on the hantavirus. You can then have the
homeopath order these remedies for you in whatever potency
s/he feels you need, and all you need to do is keep them handy.

Lyme Disease

Lyme disease is carried by ticks. Many of us who go out into
the wilderness to hike, camp, fish or hunt are susceptible to tick
bites. Anyone who has ever been bitten by a tick knows that the
little creatures are hard to notice even after they've sunk their
teeth into our skin. Ticks will often hide in our hair, beneath a
shirt or in socks to remain invisible from prying eyes. Ticks also
like the folds of skin, particularly inside the knees and elbows.
Their favorite place is the hair on the scalp.

The tick carries an infection that is known as *spirochete borrelia
burgdorferai*. It was first found less than a decade ago in Lyme,
Connecticut, where it got its name. Lyme disease seems to be
found in a tight local area and does not occur everywhere in the
U.S., so not every tick carries this disease.

How the tick is removed can decide whether or not you're going to have complications. If you accidentally leave the "fangs" of
the tick in the skin when you try to pull it out, then you're a candidate for Rocky Mountain spotted fever, which is deadly too. My
father nearly died of it when I was a child of five. To this day I still
remember how they had to hospitalize him and how he almost
didn't survive.

My father was a great hunter and fisherman and I spent my
growing-up years in the forests of the West. As a result, one thing
I was taught at an early age was that if I found a tick on me, I
shouldn't try and pull it out with my fingers. My father was of

Kentucky hill people, wise in the ways of such things, and he would light a match, blow it out and place the hot end of it on the tick's body. There is enough heat left in the match head to force the tick to react and pull its fangs out of the skin. Then it can be removed in its entirety, assuring you that Rocky Mountain spotted fever won't get you and that Lyme disease doesn't have the best chances either.

Another, less popular, way is to heat up a sewing needle until the tip is glowing red (my mother always wore a kitchen glove to protect her fingers from the heat traveling up the needle) and then lay it against the back of the tick. The heat, again, forces the tick to remove its fangs from beneath the skin. Don't try to remove a tick with tweezers either, for fear of not getting all of it.

The above ways can protect you from spotted fever, but in a case in which the tick is carrying Lyme disease, even if you remove all of it, you can still be infected if the saliva juices of the tick have mingled with your blood and the disease is already circulating through your entire body. Go to your doctor immediately.

Symptoms of Lyme Disease

The signs and symptoms of Lyme disease usually appear 3 to 12 weeks after being bitten by the tick. The first sign is usually a large, red spot of skin that continues to grow in diameter. The spot, or lesion, is usually hot to the touch. Soon after that, many people experience multiple, smaller lesions without centers. This stage usually lasts several weeks.

The next stage of this disease (and you don't need to have all these symptoms), which might occur days after this or years afterward, is tiredness and exhaustion, chills, fever, headache and a stiff neck. Other, less common, symptoms include nausea, sore throat, lymph gland swelling, spleen enlargement, tenderness or pain in muscles or muscular rheumatism. Many times people think they have arthritis during the period of between two weeks and two months after the bite. There might be problems in all joints, but the knees seem to be the main target of this disease. There can be wandering pain moving from joint to joint, which is often misdiagnosed as polyarthritis.

The nerves may take a beating in this disease, and ailments such as the following can occur: meningitis (moderate irregular fever, loss of appetite, constipation, intense headaches, intolerance to light and sound, contracted pupils, delirium, convulsions and, finally, coma); chorea (a condition in which there are tics, tremors or muscle spasms that are involuntary and sometimes violent movements as if shocked with an electric current); Bell's palsy (the inflammation of a nerve in the face that renders the muscles slack and unable to move); adriculoneuritis (inflammation of the roots of the spinal nerves); or myelitis (inflammation of the spinal cord).

Another area of contention is the heart region. Myocardial abnormalities in the heart muscle itself might occur in one out of every 10 patients. This can result in atrioventricular blocks and an enlarged heart.

The synovial membranes around each joint can swell and fill with excess fluid, causing great pain and stiffness upon movement. Often, if this occurs, it is misdiagnosed as rheumatoid arthritis. One way to make the distinction is that Lyme disease usually does not include morning stiffness, nodules, mucosal lesions, rheumatoid factors or antinuclear antibodies, the last being more common in people with connective tissue diseases. Lyme disease can be misdiagnosed as juvenile rheumatoid arthritis, rheumatic fever or spondyloarthropathies, another form of arthritis.

Homeopathic Remedies

Homeopathically, there are a number of remedies that can help this condition. I strongly recommend going to a homeopathic practitioner to have your case taken for constitutional treatment, because Lyme disease is pervasive and affects so many different systems of the body. The following remedies are only some that can address this condition. They should not be taken without the consent of a homeopath.

Arsenicum album

This remedy is used when the skin eruption resembles a fleabite: The skin is red and bumpy and it burns and itches intolerably, particularly if it is scratched. The eruption might also look like a nettle rash. Eruptions of the pimples are small and they sometimes tickle. Pain results from scratching in the affected area.

Peripheral neuritis and fever with restlessness are also within this remedy's domain. Another keynote of this remedy is that it mimics—and hence treats—the burning sensation that is experienced in the joints, muscles or nerve endings, as well as the weakness that might occur, including the inability to walk or aggravation with movement of any kind, particularly when walking any distance.

Mentally, patients who are candidates for *Arsenicum album* have a sense of dread that something is wrong, but because of the usual comings and goings of Lyme disease's symptoms, some people might consider them little more than hypochondriacs. But this is not the case. Constant restlessness characterizes candidates for this remedy, along with inner anxiety that they are going to die. The heart might have violent palpitations and irregular beats that create anguish in the patient. There can be heat, burning or itching to the chest region.

Antipyrinum

Candidates for this remedy have a very scarlet rash along with swelling of that area. There is fever, accompanied by heavy sweating.

Belladonna

Patients who benefit from this remedy have a red rash that is hot to the touch and has a bright scarlet color. There can be fever spikes with the face becoming a bright red. The pupils are enlarged and very black-looking. There can be shifting, rheumatic types of pains, and the joints swell swiftly, are hot to the touch and have a bright red color that extends up or down from the central point in streaks. These patients also have a headache that is throbbing and intense and comes on suddenly.

Mercurius vivus

Candidates for this remedy have a red rash from which a thin, clear fluid leaks. The rash's bumps break easily and dry up quickly, but the redness lasts for one to two weeks. There is fever with heavy perspiration that is smelly, and there is a creeping chilliness. There might be swelling of the hands and feet and at joint sites. The skin may take on a greasy, shiny quality.

Rhus toxicodendron

Sufferers who benefit from this remedy have a red rash resembling the one you get from poison oak or ivy that progresses rapidly to the leaky stage. The rash is accompanied by swelling, heat and itching in those regions with formation of pus and scabs. There is a fever, accompanied by chills. Arthritic symptoms are better with movement and motion. There is swelling at the joint sites. The skin is a bright, shiny red color. There is stiffness when sitting or lying still, especially in the lower back region; upon sitting up or standing, the pain increases until full movement is accomplished, when the pain recedes and may go away almost completely. Headaches usually occur in the back of the skull, and there is stiffness in the neck.

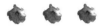

Lyme disease is often misdiagnosed, because few people remember being bitten by a tick. Sometimes chronic fatigue syndrome and general fatigue of no known origin are really Lyme disease. Get the blood test to find out.

Whooping Cough Epidemic

Eight years ago, in my homeopathic practice, a mother called me up in a frantic state. She and her baby had been diagnosed with whooping cough, also known as pertussis. She had shunned any vaccinations for herself and her child because she felt they were ultimately dangerous to the immune system. She was right: Vaccinations are dangerous. As I listened to their symptoms, *Drosera rotundifolia* (drosera), a very well-known whooping cough remedy, came to mind. I took their cases and, sure enough, drosera's symptoms matched theirs. The only problem was that I had only drosera 30C. Judging from the condition of the infant, which was worse than the mother's, I didn't feel 30C was strong enough. They both took the remedy. The baby improved about 50 percent, but I wasn't willing to let the situation go on and persuaded the mother to take her child to the emergency room and get a shot of antibiotics to finish off the bacterial infection (which it did). In the meantime, the mother's whooping cough was cured with three doses of drosera 30C and she didn't require any drugs.

Although most children get the DPT (diphtheria, pertussis and tetanus) shot when they are born, it has caused a lot of problems medically for some infants who received it. At one time, 16 pharmaceutical companies made this triple vaccine, but now, because of lawsuits, only one is continuing to produce it. Parents are becoming more educated, and many refuse to have their infants or children inoculated with this vaccine. (I recommend *A Shot in the Dark* by H. L. Coulter and B. L. Fisher for a real eye-opener concerning why *not* to rely on vaccinations.) DPT is a deadly combination to give children and can create terrible and life-long problems.

Whooping cough symptoms vary, and there are a number of homeopathic remedies that respond to this acute illness. I'm going to list some of the more frequently used remedies based upon the symptoms listed below, but you should see your homeopath for treatment, as this disease can be a killer if it's let go or is not monitored properly. The good news is that antibiotics can still stop it; someday, with the mutations occurring among the bacteria and viruses, they won't, and then all that will remain to prevent us potentially dying from whooping cough will be homeopathic remedies.

Symptoms of Whooping Cough

- An incubation period of between 7 and 14 days. There is rarely a fever with this illness.
- The upper respiratory tract, the lungs, begin to secrete or try to secrete a lot of mucus. At first it's rather runny and loose, or what is medically known as serous. Later, as the illness grows, the mucus becomes thick and sometimes nearly impossible to cough up; this is when the rales and repeated coughing begin to occur. (The body's defense against anything collecting in the lungs is to cough it up and out.) With whooping cough, this thick, sticky mucoid matter can become gelatinous, or even so tough or stringy that a person will cough for many minutes, gag and even vomit before throwing up some small mucoid matter from the lungs.
- Usually, this coughing begins at night and will appear like a simple upper respiratory ailment. Many might think it's just a chest cold at first, but it's not.

• As the illness takes its course, the first 10 to 14 days present the catarrhal, or flowing-mucus, stage. The cough then sets in and continues until the fourth week. The convalescent stage ends in about the sixth week for most people.

Whooping cough bacteria are very transmissible, infecting others through coughing or sneezing. In other words, they are airborne bacteria. Sometimes people are fooled initially into thinking they might have the flu, a viral chest cold, bronchitis or pneumonia. You should consult with a doctor and get a diagnosis—don't guess on this one.

Homeopathic Remedies

Here is a list of some of the major homeopathic remedies that cured whooping cough long before antibiotics were around. Remember, this is only a partial list and you should consult with a homeopath and have your case studied to determine which remedy you need—it may or may not be on this list. The remedies listed below are the ones I stock in my homeopathic kit at home, just in case.

• *Drosera rotundifolia*
• Pertussis nosode (Only your homeopath can order this one.)
• *Antimonium tart.*
• *Hepar sulphuris*
• *Aconitum napellus*
• *Carbo vegetabilis*
• *Cuprum metallicum*
• Ipecacuanha
• *Belladonna atropa*

Go to the epidemic *materia medica* starting on page 201 and look up the symptoms for these remedies. (You won't find the pertussis nosode there, since you can only get this through your homeopath.) If you find a match for your symptoms, then that is the remedy for you. Consult with your homeopath first to verify this, and s/he will tell you how much of it to take, at what potency and when.

Strep A—Flesh-Eating Bacteria

We are currently experiencing a wavelike surge of strepto-coccus A bacteria. For a time, this wave retreated, but it has now become stronger and more powerful and is reemerging around the world.

In January 1994, in Gloucester, England, a nurse went into the hospital for a hysterectomy. Ten days later she felt a jolting pain down her left leg and noticed some mild bruising on it. When she awoke the next morning, she saw bruises through her skin, her abdomen was black and the color extended down the left side of her body and deep into her leg. Fortunately, she made it in time: The hospital surgeon had to cut off her leg and put her on powerful antibiotics, but her life was saved. A plumber from Cardiff, Wales, came down with a sore throat and for two weeks afterward felt pain in his legs. He went to the hospital, thinking he'd strained some muscles, and died 18 hours later—of strep A. A third British victim was making breakfast for his children one morning when his leg began to swell up. His symptoms included a "firestorm of pain sweeping through his body." His wife said, "It got hold of him so fast. In the end I don't think he really knew who I was. He was just staring at me, looking really frightened."

More than a few scientists and doctors are frightened too. The Gloucester epidemic (seven cases) of necrotizing (flesh-eating) bacteria—*Streptococcus myositis* and *fasciitis*—is unsettling to the entire world community. Before this outbreak, there had been 10 cases a year in England and Wales. At first this strain was said to be "new." However, after further research, scientists said it wasn't a new strain.

The "cluster cases" in Gloucester are alarming because the odds against this type of outbreak are a thousand to one. Not all of the seven victims had been in the hospital, where it's easier to catch this bacteria. Those who caught it in the hospital had been in completely different hospitals—not the same one! As a result, scientists suggest that there could not have been only one carrier.

On one hand, it could mean, in scientific terms, that the cluster of cases was a "random occurrence." On the other, there is speculation that this is the result of a virus creating deadly, mutating strains of strep A. Scientists discovered four different strains of group A strep in this cluster of cases, which makes it even more alarming and worrisome.

It's estimated that 10 percent of the world population carry group A strep in their bodies, which might cause nothing more than a case of strep throat. Most strep bacteria are spread through breathing or airborne respiratory droplets (sneezing and coughing). Some bacteria can be spread through the contamination of food or milk or soiled hands, or by unsterilized instruments (as in a hospital surgery) being introduced into an open wound.

Strep A is known in medical terms as group A, and its clinical symptoms are fever, headache, sore throat and abdominal discomfort. It can also cause impetigo (a skin condition), cellulitis (inflammation of the cells and connective tissue of the body) or erysipelas (a life-threatening and rapidly progressing soft-tissue infection). Erysipelas produces fever and local redness on the skin; usually, the skin becomes shiny red, swollen and very tender. It is often accompanied by high fever, chills and malaise. Many times, these symptoms occur without obvious injury. Unchecked, this infection goes deep into the body to produce necrosis (dying flesh), pneumonia, nephritis (kidney inflammation) and meningitis.

The strep A variety that eats away the flesh, at a rate of as much as one inch an hour, began its deadly attack in 1986. Scientists recognized then that a more virulent strain had appeared and treated toxic shock syndrome with symptoms such as a dramatic drop in blood pressure, failure of multiple organs and a raging fever.

In the U.S., 20 to 30 million people have strep infections every year. The Centers for Disease Control estimate that 15,000 of these cases are invasive strep A and that between 5 and 10 percent are of the necrotizing, or flesh-eating, variety. The CDC don't have a clue as to whether this strain is on the rise, although many scientists think it is increasing around the world. According to Patrick Schlievert of the University of Minnesota, "There was an increase in the late '80s. Then, it [the invasive strep A] took a dip, and now it's gone back up above what it was before" (Rachel Novak, Flesh-Eating Bacteria: Not New, but Still Worrisome," *Science* 264 [June 17,1994]: 1665). Again we're seeing the wave theory in action. Schlievert notes that in 1991 and 1992, his lab would see two samples of invasive strep A in a week. As of June 1994, the rate had become two samples a day!

Strep A, the necrotizing variety, was first seen in 1924 in China. It was a less aggressive variety at that time, killing only 20 percent of its victims—and that was without antibiotic treatment available. The recent British epidemic stood in startling contrast: 70 percent of those who contracted invasive strep A died, even with antibiotic treatment. The bacteria are back—bigger, stronger and more lethal than decades before.

What is disturbing is that no one is keeping tabs on this silent stalker. The World Health Organization says that surveillance of this invasive strain of strep is "grossly inadequate." Thomas Prentice, spokesperson for WHO, has pointed out that he includes the U.S. in this statement and that the CDC has abandoned active surveillance of this type of bacteria!

What's so different about this strain? What makes it a killer instead of just causing a sore throat? Scientists have analyzed invasive strep A and found that there are two culprits, both proteins. One is exotoxin A, which is known as a "superantigen." A superantigen can wreak havoc on the human immune system by overtriggering the T cells meant to protect us. Cytokines, the signal carriers between cells, are then overproduced in the bloodstream. This excess production of cytokines damages the cells lining our blood vessels and fluid leaks out, the blood flow reduces and the tissue, waiting for oxygen carried by cells in order to remain alive, begins to die. That is how necrotizing strep A reacts chemically within us.

Exotoxin A has a deadly partner, chemically speaking, in this invasive strep A form. A second chemical, exotoxin B, begins to destroy tissue by breaking down the protein. This powerful one-two punch will send any immune system reeling into a state of shock. The two chemicals make the invasive variety of strep A even more highly contagious than the other forms of streptococcus.

Jim Henson, the world-famous Muppeteer, died of a virulent strep A infection, which caused a drop in blood pressure (one of the symptoms of this variety). Another famous person, Lucien Bouchard, leader of the Bloc Quebecois of Canada, was struck down with necrotizing myositis, the invasive strep A. It cost him his left leg and almost his life. Luckily, he got to the hospital in time.

This deadly killer can be contracted not only in the hospital operating room, but also through something as simple as a slight cut on the finger or through any other open wound, such as a skinned knee or a slight abrasion to the skin.

Invasive strep A seems to like the lower part of the body, particularly the feet and legs, and also the hands and arms. The bacteria enter the bloodstream and find an area where there is poor blood flow, such as around a bruise. Here, the bacteria are protected from the soldier T cells of the immune system and begin churning out toxins A and B. Toxin B creates an even larger area of dead cells, giving the bacteria more room to grow; the more they grow, the more toxins are produced and the more cells die. Eventually, this dying skin, or tissue—which, as said before, can die at a rate of one inch an hour—must be amputated to halt the merciless destruction of this life-threatening infection.

Homeopathic Remedies

Using the *Merck Manual* to determine the symptoms for invasive strep A, the following homeopathic remedies, in order of importance, may mean the difference between life and death. If you suspect you have invasive strep A, get to the hospital immediately. Do not waste any time. On the way to the hospital, match your symptoms against those for the remedies below and take whichever remedy shows the closest match. Contact your homeopath after you've gotten antibiotic treatment at the hospital.

- *Crolatus horridus*
- *Lachesis muta*
- *Aconitum napellus*
- *Arsenicum album*
- *Rhus toxicodendron*
- *Pyrogenium*
- Sepsis nosode (Only a homeopath can order this.)

Go to the epidemic *materia medica* starting on page 201 and look up the symptoms for these remedies. (You won't find the sepsis nosode there, since you can only get this through your homeopath.) As always, consult your homeopath about these remedies beforehand and find out what potencies you should carry in your medicine cabinet should this life-threatening ailment arise.

Measles and Mumps

Unfortunately, traditional medicine is treating childhood diseases such as measles and mumps as horrendous, life-threatening problems; they are not. The pharmaceutical companies have created the MMR (measles, mumps, rubella) shot to halt illnesses that children have been coming down with for thousands of years. I meet many, many parents who have seen their children getting sicker and sicker after every vaccination, and they no longer want their children's immune systems compromised by such shots.

Vaccinations don't work forever as the general public was told. Just look at the recurrence of measles and mumps in our schools. Our children were inoculated years ago, and there are now epidemics of these diseases in schools. The good news is that once you've had measles and mumps the old-fashioned way—that is to say, you didn't get the vaccination but you got sick, then you got well—you are immune for life. You don't have to keep taking shots to keep it that way.

When a germ such as a measles or mumps germ gets passed on through hand-to-mouth or finger-to-mouth contact, the first place a germ goes is into the saliva. Then it moves down through the esophagus to the stomach and intestinal tract before it ever reaches the bloodstream. Because of this natural occurrence, the body has the time it needs to begin amassing help from the immune system, and by the time the germ finally reaches the bloodstream via osmosis through the intestinal tract, the immune system is ready to counteract the disease. As the germ's journey ends, the body has strengthened itself against ever again being overtaken by that particular disease. This is natural immunization at its finest. The body is set up to deal with such invaders.

Unfortunately, when a vaccination, which is filled with a lot of toxic materials, animal cells and embryo parts and pieces, is given, it is sent directly into the bloodstream. The normal, natural system the body has set up has been avoided so that the gastrointestinal system is never involved. It's no wonder, in my opinion, that vaccines can't and won't last in the body and that they cannot promise lifelong immunity.

I was born in the 1940s when, luckily, most of the vaccinations weren't available. I did have to take one polio shot and two sugar cubes later on, but basically, my immune system was not compromised. I got mumps and measles and chickenpox, as did every other kid. These childhood diseases are meant to come along when the immune system is still growing, stretching and learning how to become strong. Measles, mumps and chickenpox are rites of passage for the immune system. Everyone knows that adversity creates strength, and it's no less true for the body.

Homeopathic Treatment for Childhood Diseases

Homeopathically, there are three ways to deal with childhood diseases in lieu of taking a vaccination.

First, one can go to a homeopath's office and ask for nosodes (we use diseased material from a human and then succuss it with alcohol and water to the desired potency) to give to a child. For instance, we can make a nosode from the diphtheria germ, potentize it and put the resulting remedy on sucrose pellets. These are then given to the infant or child and they will stimulate the immune system to create antibodies.

Naturopathic doctors are trained to give homeopathic remedies in a prophylactic form, that is, to give a homeopathic remedy that parallels the symptoms of a disease. This is a much gentler form that goes via the mouth and digestive tract—unlike a vaccination, which skips this crucial phase—and then signals the body's immune forces to be alert and create more "soldiers," the antibodies.

Normally, I recommend taking the tetanus shot and not taking the nosode and so do many other knowledgeable homeopaths. With strep, it is best to see your homeopath directly and not try to immunize with homeopathy yourself. Let the practitioner take your child's case homeopathically so that s/he can determine what remedy should be used or if the child should have antibiotics instead. I would rather take my child to a homeopath, get a throat culture to verify whether it is strep or not, and then take the appropriate homeopathic remedy to get rid of it, if possible.

A second way to deal with these childhood diseases is this: If your child comes home from school and says, "Mommy, there's mumps going around school," you can give your child (with your homeopath's approval and direction) parotidinum 6C three times a day for five days. This will prevent the child from contracting the mumps or, at the very least, it will shorten and lighten the disease if the child gets it anyway.

A third way to use homeopathic remedies is indicated if your child already has the disease. Again with your homeopath's prior approval, you can give the correct remedy to shorten the duration of the disease as well as to limit the intensity of it. If your child comes down with the mumps, giving parotidinum 6C every four hours for four days helps limit the mumps cycle. There is less swelling, less fever and so forth, and the child has to deal only with a very mild case of the illness. Another remedy that is very useful in limiting the effects of mumps is called pilocarpus. It's a powerful glandular stimulant and creates a lot of sweat in the feverish individual.

Homeopathic Remedies for Mumps

Here are some remedies for mumps. I prefer to use a 6C potency or, secondarily, a 30C. If you have a 6C, you may give it to your sick child every four hours for up four days. If you have a 30C potency, give it twice daily for three days. Check with your homeopath prior to using any remedy.

Abrotanum artemisia

This remedy is used if the mumps affects the testes of a male or the breasts of a female. If there is swelling in either of these areas, consider this remedy if *Pulsatilla nigricans* (see page 130) fails to help.

Aconitum napellus

This is for fever with restlessness and anxiety. Note that this remedy will work only within the first 24 hours of the contraction of the mumps, with the first signs of onset. Don't use it if the mumps is more than 24 hours old.

The child who is a candidate for *Aconitum napellus* is extremely restless, cannot sit still or stay in one room or on one piece of furniture but will move from bed to couch to chair to another room to a rug on the floor—you get the idea; as sick as s/he may be, the child is in constant motion.

Belladonna atropa

This is a premier mumps remedy when the illness has a very swift onset, when it strikes out of nowhere and the child has a full-blown case within 12 hours of contracting the illness.

Belladonna is the remedy to use when the child's face is red, the pupils of the eyes are dilated (enlarged) and s/he is very sensitive to touch, noise, jarring and everything in general. A red face and enlarged pupils are keynotes to this remedy, but other symptoms include the swelling of the right parotid gland on the neck—not the left (or if the left is swollen, the swelling is less)—and violent, shooting pains from the swollen region that make the child wince and cry constantly or at the very least put her or him in a very angry or irritable frame of mind. The child is also extremely sensitive to cold, and the skin is very hot to the touch, almost as if s/he is a furnace burning out of control.

Bromium

This remedy is used when the left parotid gland is swollen (the right may be too, but to a lesser degree). There is swelling with hardness of the gland, and it is warm to the touch. There is slow inflammation of the glands; the onset may take three or four days (unlike the mumps you want to treat with belladonna, which will become a full-blown case within 12 hours). Children who are candidates for treatment with bromium are very sensitive to cold and drafts when the mumps finally arrives. They also feel worse in humid, hot weather.

Carbo vegetabilis

This remedy is utilized if there is swelling in the testes or breasts and if the child's face is pale and cold.

Lachesis muta

This remedy is used when the left parotid gland is the one that's most affected and when it is enormously swollen, sensitive to even the hint of someone touching that area. The child who is a candidate for *Lachesis muta* jerks away to avoid anyone touching the swollen region. There is severe pain associated with it and the child can hardly swallow liquids or food. The eyes can have a glassy, glazed or wild look to them, which is a keynote for this remedy. The face is bright red and swollen.

Lycopodium clavatum

Use this remedy when the mumps begins in the right parotid gland, then moves to the left, and when the child desires warm drinks.

Mercurius vivus

This remedy is usually for right-sided mumps, when only the right parotid gland is involved. The child who is a candidate for treatment with *Mercurius vivus* sweats heavily and has a foul or rotten odor to her or his breath. The sweat is very offensive, and there may be a greasy look to the skin.

Parotidinum

This might be used—even though it is a nosode—when a child has never been well since having had the mumps. Parotidinum forces the disease to complete its cycle in the child's body and finally leave. If the child exhibits exhaustion and listlessness or is disinterested in life in general after having had the mumps, this would be the remedy of choice. (You could also give *Gelsemium sempervirens* if parotidinum doesn't work).

Phytolacca decandra

For this to be the remedy of choice, it is the right parotid gland that is swollen, as is the region beneath the jaw (the submaxillary region). The glands are hard and feel stony. Pain shoots up into either ear, especially upon swallowing. The child is worse when the weather is cold and wet. There is also an abnormal amount of stiffness in the neck.

Pilocarpine

This remedy acts quickly and relieves pain. It is used for swelling of the testes or breasts. If swelling subsides due to a chill, this is the remedy of choice.

Pulsatilla nigricans

This is good for intense swelling of the glands, testes or breasts. Use it for the child who becomes cold easily and when there is pain in either ear or in both ears that is sharp and excruciating.

Rhus toxicodendron

Usually, the left parotid gland is involved and the swelling and enlargement are huge when this is the recommended remedy. The glands beneath the jaw can also become highly involved. *Rhus toxicodendron* is for the children who are worse in cold weather, chills and drafts. They may or may not have herpes on the lips at the same time. These children are highly restless, moving constantly; interestingly, as long as they are moving around, they feel better; only when they are stationary do the children feel worse, an important keynote symptom for this remedy.

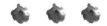

Homeopathic Remedies for Measles

A number of remedies can be used if a child has been exposed to measles, another childhood ailment. They will be mentioned as such, along with other remedies that, once your child has contracted measles, can be used to shorten and modify the course of the ailment. Dosage and potency are the same as for mumps; see page 128. As always, be sure to first check with your homeopath.

Aconitum napellus

This remedy is used when there is fever along with chill and both are very marked. There can be coldness alternating with heat. The child is always thirsty for juice or water and highly restless; s/he moves around but does not necessarily feel better because of it. The spots look like small red flea bites on the hands and body. This is also one of the remedies that may be given if the child has been exposed but does not have symptoms of the measles yet.

Arsenicum album

Use this remedy when the child is very cold, chills easily and is restless and anxious. This is another remedy that can be used if the child has been exposed to measles but hasn't developed symptoms yet.

Belladonna atropa

This is the remedy to use when measles comes on violently and suddenly—within 12 hours, the child has a full-blown case. The fever is high or spiking, the face is bright red, the pupils are enlarged. This child is sensitive to everything: touch, jarring, noise, temperature and so forth. There is a throbbing and burning sensation to the skin. Despite the high temperature, the child is thirstless and does not want water or juice. The eruptions are like a red rash spreading across the body. There may be a violent cough with the condition and an inclination to rub the nose.

Bryonia alba

This remedy is used when the child has a fever with a hard, full, bounding pulse that is tense and quick. There may be a dry cough and a chill that makes the child bundle up in a lot of blankets to stay warm. Children who are candidates for bryonia want to be left alone, not be fussed over in this condition and prefer the room quiet and dark. They won't move from wherever they choose to sit or lie down, as any motion make them feel worse. These children are worse in hot weather and may complain of a dryness in the throat.

Pulsatilla nigricans

The child who can be treated with *Pulsatilla nigricans* has a runny nose and runny eyes along with the measles. The cough may be loose during the day but becomes dry at night, with a tightness in the chest. There may be a fever, including a hot head and dry lips. The child is thirstless and despite fever or sweating does not want to drink any liquids. The eruptions, when fully out, often have a dark appearance to them. There is itching of the eyes, which is made worse by rubbing them.

Pulsatilla nigricans is another remedy that can be given to a child who has been exposed to measles but has not yet developed any measles symptoms.

West Nile Virus

When I wrote *Poisons That Heal* in 1995, I predicted a number of epidemics that would hit the shores of the U.S. shortly. One was Dengue fever, which is now a reality in Florida, Texas and Arizona and continues to slowly spread. I envisioned that unknown or little known viruses or bacteria would creep up on us, and this has become a reality with the West Nile virus, a form of encephalitis.

The bad news is: West Nile virus encephalitis (WNVE) is here to stay and will continue to spread. The good news is: Homeopathy may potentially help combat this virus concomitantly with standard medical treatment. And if you think you have the virus, it's imperative you get to your doctor to have the test run to confirm it. Sometimes, depending upon the individual, medical help may be used right alongside a homeopathic remedy.

What Is West Nile Virus Encephalitis?

An inflammation or infection of the brain can be caused by bacteria or a virus, and in the case of WVNE, it is a virus. WNVE is closely related to the St. Louis encephalitis virus, which was found in the U.S. before WNVE arrived here in 1999.

As of December 31, 2002, a total of 4,156 cases of WNVE in humans were reported in the U.S., with 284 fatalities. In the state of New York, 62 cases were reported in 1999, with 7 resulting deaths. In the New York City area, 21 cases were reported in 2000, with 2 deaths; in 2001 there were 66 cases and 9 deaths. You can see how this virus is gathering steam and becoming a consistent killer.

West Nile virus is a flavivirus. Other viruses that are associated with it are St. Louis encephalitis, Dengue fever, tick-borne encephalitis and yellow fever, among others. West Nile has its roots and origin in Uganda's West Nile Province, where it was first isolated in an adult woman and named in 1937. Since then, it has killed people in Israel (1957); France (early 1960s); South Africa, Algeria, Russia and Romania (1996); the outbreak in Romania also signaled that the West Nile virus had emerged as clinically important in Europe. In North America, the virus emerged from obscurity in New York in 1999.

Where Is the West Nile Virus in the U.S. as of 2004?

June 15, 2004

The CDC data table indicates avian or animal infection reported to CDC ArboNET for public distribution as of June 15, 2004, from the following states:

Alabama, Arizona, Arkansas, California, Florida, Georgia, Illinois, Indiana, Kentucky, Louisiana, Michigan, Mississippi, Missouri, New Jersey, New Mexico, New York, Ohio, Oklahoma, Pennsylvania, South Dakota, Texas, Virginia, Wisconsin and Wyoming.

Human cases have been reported in Arizona, California, New Mexico, South Dakota and Wyoming.

May 21, 2004

The CDC data table indicates cases reported to CDC ArboNET for public distribution of avian, animal or mosquito infection as of May 21, 2004:

Alabama, Arizona, Arkansas, California, Colorado, Connecticut, Delaware, District of Columbia, Florida, Georgia, Illinois, Indiana, Iowa, Kansas, Kentucky, Louisiana, Maine, Maryland, Massachusetts, Michigan, Minnesota, Mississippi, Missouri, Montana, Nebraska, New Hampshire, New Jersey, New Mexico, New York, North Carolina, North Dakota, Ohio, Oklahoma, Pennsylvania, Rhode Island, South Carolina, South Dakota, Tennessee, Texas, Utah, Vermont, Virginia, West Virginia, Wisconsin and Wyoming.

Human cases have been reported in Alabama, Arizona, Arkansas, California, Colorado, Connecticut, Delaware, District of Columbia, Florida, Georgia, Idaho, Illinois, Indiana, Iowa, Kansas, Kentucky, Louisiana, Maryland, Massachusetts, Michigan, Minnesota, Mississippi, Missouri, Montana, Nebraska, Nevada, New Hampshire, New Jersey, New Mexico, New York, North Carolina, North Dakota, Ohio, Oklahoma, Pennsylvania, Rhode Island, South Carolina, South Dakota, Tennessee, Texas, Utah, Vermont, Virginia, West Virginia, Wisconsin and Wyoming.

Worldwide Distribution

The West Nile virus is one of the most widely distributed of all flavaviruses and has reached Australia, South Asia and the Middle East as well as North America. Migratory birds are felt to be the reservoire host, which means they carry this pathogen and serve as a source of infection without detriment to themselves.

The virus is transmitted by a mosquito vector, and *Culex pipiens* has been proposed as the carrier. (Ticks were found to carry it in Russia.) In all, 40 different species of mosquitoes that carry the virus were found, in addition to ticks. Among these are the *Adedes japonicus* and *A. albopictus* (Asian tiger mosquito). It should be noted that *A. albopictus* is also the carrier for Dengue fever and Dengue hemorrhagic fever and has of late landed on the West Coast, particularly the Northwest, where it has been shown to be carrying Dengue on plants imported from Asia.

West Nile Virus and Animals

Amplifying Hosts

The wild birds of the world serve as amplifying hosts. To date there are 138 species of birds that have been hosts for this virus. Overseas, the bird population that carries this virus usually does not die. However, the virus has upped the ante and in its U.S. version, it does kill its host. An experiment by Russian scientists has found the virus to live in the Russian frog *Rana ridbunda*. This shows the adaptability of this particular virus to use many hosts in order to stay alive and spread.

Humans and some domestic animals such as horses, dogs and cats can be infected. Although neurologic disease has been prominent in some epidemics, infection with West Nile virus is usually asymptomatic in areas of the world where the virus is endemic.

Human and animal infection occurs when the person or animal is bitten by the offending species of mosquito. It should be noted that this mosquito flies only at *dusk* and *dawn*, so people need to take precautions (type of clothing they wear) at that time if they are going to be outdoors.

There is no evidence that handling a dead bird can transmit the virus to the person picking up the bird. Scientists say it is possible that an animal can become infected by eating a bird that has the disease, but this possibility has not been documented.

Dogs, Horses, Cats

Dogs have been tested in New York and shown to be frequently infected, but to date, no indication of them having the symptoms has been documented. The West Nile virus was isolated in a dead cat in 1999, but so far this has been the only one. Cats and dogs may get WNV, but it does not cause extensive illness for them. There is *no* evidence that you will get the virus from touching your infected dog or cat, nor is there any evidence that a dog or cat can transmit the West Nile virus to another animal.

Horses are a known target of the West Nile virus—they get bitten by the mosquito—but they do not need to be destroyed if they get the symptoms. Data suggests that most horses recover from the infection; 40 percent do die from it. A West Nile virus vaccine has been licensed, but its effectiveness remains to be seen.

Other Animals

Other animals that have been infected with West Nile virus are bats, a chipmunk, a skunk, a squirrel and a domestic rabbit.

Transmission and Susceptibility

An infected bird, dead or alive, is bit by a mosquito who draws the virus up in the blood it drinks. The insect then has an incubation period of 10 days before it can transmit the virus to the next host (human or animal).

People of any age or gender who have compromised immune systems are apt to be more reactive to the bite and virus, and this pertains especially to the elderly; from a homeopathic perspective, these are those who are "susceptible." From a practical standpoint, people at risk are those who do not take necessary precautions against mosquito bites.

The mortality rate of WNVE is very low. The majority of people are asymptomatic (meaning, no symptoms appear after they are bitten), and the fatality rate is less than 1 percent. The number of those who have been hospitalized with it may range from 3 to 15 percent, and the number is highest among the elderly.

Symptoms for West Nile Virus

Once a person is bitten, it takes 3 to 14 days for the symptoms to occur. The diagnosis can be confirmed by isolating the virus or by serologic (blood) testing. Many times, however, the symptoms (especially mild ones) may present as other potential acute diseases and a doctor is misled by them. Only lab testing can confirm the absence or presence of West Nile virus.

Depending upon the person (susceptibility), there are some who may have *no* symptoms after being bitten. In those who do, the symptoms are often mild or moderate and include fever, headache, bodyaches (often with a skin rash on chest and arms that generally lasts for less than one week), diarrhea, abdominal pain, loss of appetite and swollen lymph glands.

Those who have more severe symptoms may experience headache, high fever, neck stiffness, muscle weakness, stupor, disorientation, convulsions, paralysis, coma and, rarely, death. All these symptoms generally last one week and complete and rapid recovery usually follows (unless the person's immune system is compromised or s/he is elderly).

Central nervous system (CNS) manifestations may occur with more severe reactions, and these can be serious. The common manifestations of encephalitis are disorientation, altered consciousness and generalized motor weakness; 13 percent of patients developed coma.

Myocarditis and pancreatitis are other rare complications of West Nile virus infection. West Nile virus can cause hepatitis; a fatal case of hepatitis due to this virus resembling yellow fever was reported from the Central African Republic.

Mild Infection Symptoms

As of December, 2003, the Centers for Disease Control have put out the following information regarding clinical symptoms. Most West Nile virus infections are mild and often clinically unapparent. Approximately 20 percent of those infected develop a mild illness, West Nile fever. The incubation period is thought to range from three to fourteen days, and symptoms generally last three to six days.

Reports from earlier outbreaks describe the mild form of West Nile virus infection as a febrile illness of sudden onset often accompanied by:
• Malaise
• Anorexia
• Nausea
• Vomiting
• Eye pain
• Headache
• Myalgia
• Rash
• Lymphadenopathy

The full clinical spectrum of West Nile fever has not been determined in the United States.

Severe Infection Symptoms

Approximately 1 in 150 infections will result in severe neurological disease. The most significant risk factor for developing severe neurological disease is advanced age. Also, encephalitis is more commonly reported than meningitis.

In recent outbreaks, symptoms occurring among patients hospitalized with severe disease included:

- Fever
- Weakness
- Gastrointestinal symptoms
- Change in mental status

A minority of patients with severe disease developed a maculopapular or morbilliform rash involving the neck, trunk, arms or legs. Several patients experienced severe muscle weakness and flaccid paralysis.

Neurological presentations included:

- Ataxia and extrapyramidal signs
- Cranial nerve abnormalities
- Myelitis
- Optic neuritis
- Polyradiculitis
- Seizures

Although not observed in recent outbreaks, myocarditis, pancreatitis and fulminant hepatitis have been described.

Spread of West Nile Virus through Our Blood Supply

During the 2002 epidemic of West Nile virus in the U.S., a total of 23 persons were reported to have acquired West Nile virus infection after receipt of blood components from 16 West Nile virus-viremic blood donors, and an estimated 500 viremic donations might have been collected (B. Biggerstaff, PhD, CDC, personal communication, 2003). Because of the possibility of recurrent West Nile virus epidemics in the U.S., blood collection agencies (BCAs) recently implemented West Nile virus nucleic acid amplification tests (NATs) to screen all donations and quarantine and retrieve potentially infectious blood components.

Although nearly all human West Nile virus infections result from mosquito bites, transfusion-associated West Nile virus transmission resulted in a small number of West Nile virus infections in 2002. Implementation of national blood donor screening for West Nile virus in 2003 has reduced this risk substantially, by removing hundreds of units of potentially infectious blood donated by asymptomatic donors.

Preventing West Nile Virus

There are a number of preventive things you can do in your backyard:

- Make sure there is no standing water in containers such as buckets, old tires or pots; in clogged roof gutters; or anywhere else where water may sit and accumulate and stagnate, such as bird baths.
- Put a cover over your swimming pool when it is not being used.
- At dusk and dawn, wear a long-sleeved shirt or blouse when going outside; wear pants instead of shorts and wear socks to protect the ankle area.
- Make sure the screens on your windows are in good condition.
- Use an insect repellant as recommended by the CDC.

An experimental inactivated (making virus inactive) vaccine against this virus for humans is under investigation, but no vaccine has been licensed. Personal protection to avoid mosquito exposure and mosquito control programs are recommended during epidemics.

Treatment of WNVE by the Medical Establishment

Currently, treatment of West Nile virus infection is supportive, and there is no specific therapy. In severe cases, intensive supportive therapy is indicated through hospitalizing the person, IV (intravenous) fluids, airway management, respiratory support (ventilator) if needed and prevention of secondary infections such as pneumonia or urinary tract infections, as well as good nursing care.

Symptoms of WNVE

Keeping in mind the understanding that each person's case must be considered individually, there are central symptoms of WNVE. No one person will have all of these, and someone may have other symptoms mentioned here but not added to the list below. The items in the following list are my choices, and you may see other symptoms that are unique to an individual case.

- Headache (this is a form of encephalitis, an infection of the brain).
- Skin rash.
- Lymph glands are swollen.
- Body aches.
- Neck stiff.
- High fever.

Some of the more serious infection symptoms are:
- Person becomes disoriented.
- Coma.
- Paralysis.
  And in some cases, death can occur as the final outcome.

Homeopathic Remedies for WNVE

Remember, homeopathy is based upon the law of similars, like cures like. We can find certain remedies that parallel the symptoms of West Nile virus infection, and I've chosen the following symptoms from our *materia medica*:
- Cerebrospinal fever.
- Continued fever, typhus, typhoid, exanthemic.
- Exanthemata fevers.
- Zymotic fevers.
- Stiffness in back, cervical region.
- Swelling of back, glands of nape.
- Skin eruptions rash.
- Convulsions, exanthemata repelled or do not appear.
- Paralysis.

When these symptoms are entered into a homeopathic software program, certain remedies that cause them will show up, and these are the ones that should be considered. Only one of the remedies should be chosen, however—the one that fits most closely to a person's unique set of symptoms.

Belladonna atropa

Use this remedy if the infected person displays the following symptoms:

Abdomen
- Violent pain in abdomen that allows no rest.
- Pressure on abdomen, as if from a stone, chiefly in groin area.
- Cramplike, contractive and constrictive pains and pinching.

- Digging sensation in abdomen; cutting and shooting pains like from knives.
- Heat and rash across the abdomen.

Head
- Fullness, cloudiness and apparent intoxication, worse in the morning.
- Pressure is violent in the head, chiefly in the forehead, above the eyes and nose or on one side of the head.
- It feels as if head was going to burst open; there is a great and painful pressure inside.
- Sharp, tractive, shooting pains; strong pulsation of arteries in head.
- Congestion of blood in head, worse on stooping.
- Stunning headache that starts in neck and goes into head bringing heat and pulsation with it.
- Boring headache in right side of head, changes to stitches in the evening.

Neck
- Painful swelling and stiffness in the neck and at nape of neck.
- Painful swelling in neck glands and in glands of nape of neck.
- Red and purulent pimples on back and nape of neck.
- Veins in neck swollen.
- Sour sweat, only on the neck.

Skin
- Swelling with heat and scarlet redness of the whole body or several parts, chiefly the face, neck, chest and abdomen and the hands.
- Red, scaly eruption on lower part of body.
- Smooth, even shining, redness of the skin, with bloating, dryness, heat, burning and itching.

Bryonia alba
Use this remedy if the infected person displays the following symptoms:

Abdomen
- Pains in the liver, mostly shooting, tensive or burning.
- Shootings in the region of the spleen.

Head
- Bursting headache, left occiput to frontal to entire head.
- Bursting, splitting or heavy crushing headache, frontal occiput.

* Worse when moving eyes, coughing, straining a stool, stepping, stooping. It begins in the morning and gradually becomes worse.

Neck
* Painful stiffness in neck.
* Rheumatic stiffness and tension in nape of neck and in neck.
* Red spots on the sides of the neck.
* Red, miliary eruptions on neck with violent itching.

Skin
* Yellow color, moist and clammy.
* Burning and prickling all over body, as if from nettles after slight emotions; nettle rash.
* Miliary eruptions, especially in children.
* Hard knots and blotches.

Phosphorus

Use this remedy if the infected person displays the following symptoms:

Abdomen
* Feels cold.
* A very weak, empty, gone sensation in cavity.
* Pancreatic disease.
* Pressure above epigastrium.
* Sore spot in pit of stomach.
* Sharp, cutting pains.
* Rubbing abdomen brings relief.

Extremities
* Coldness in hands.
* Numbness in hands in the morning and upon waking.
* Numbness in feet upon crossing limbs.
* Ascending sensory and motor paralysis from ends of fingers and toes.
* Can hardly hold anything in hands.
* Tearing left shoulder at night.
* Arms and hands become numb.
* Burning sensation in feet, ice-cold feet.
* Toes cramp; formications (bug crawling sensation) of hands and feet.

Head
- Must be kept warm.
- Congestion in head and burning pains.
- Heavy feeling in head over one eye with hunger.
- Burning temples, vertex (top of head) throbs.
- Feels as if is pulled by hair; skin of forehead feels too tight.

Neck
- Rigidity of nape.
- Swelling of neck, engorgement of axillary glands, neck glands and those of nape of neck.

Skin
- Ecchymosis (purple bruising on skin), jaundice, brownish or blood red spots here and there.

Other Possible Remedies

Here is a list of possible remedies based upon all symptoms:
- *Rhus toxicodendron*
- Sulphur
- *Apis mellifica*
- *Carbo vegetabilis*
- *Zincum metallicum*
- *Hyoscyamus niger*

Other remedies to consider are:
- *Crolatus horridus*
- *Cuprum metallicum*
- *Ammonium carbonicum*

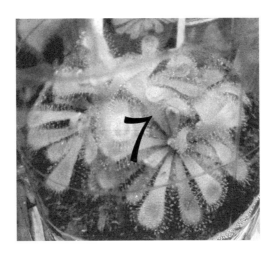

Smallpox

The History of Smallpox

Smallpox was a highly contagious disease. I say *was* because it was declared eradicated in 1980 by the World Health Organization (WHO). The last case of smallpox occurred in Somalia in 1977. Smallpox is caused by the virus *viriolae* and is available in two flavors: *Viriole major* (severe symptoms and a high mortality rate of about 20 to 40 percent) and *Viriole minor* (less severe symptoms with a low mortality rate of about 1 percent). This virus is known to have existed for at least 3,000 years and estimates have it killing up to 100 million people during its crusade. The 200 million people it didn't kill, it left blind and horribly scarred. Since smallpox is a virus, there is *no* allopathic cure for it, which is why a vaccine was eventually discovered and used to prevent many more deaths.

Was it really eradicated? Well, yes and no. No human being has contracted smallpox since 1977, but there are colonies of smallpox virus living comfortable, happy lives in labs. Two such labs are known: one is at the Centers for Disease Control (CDC) in Atlanta, Georgia in the U.S., and the other is at the Institute for Viral Preparations in Koltsovo in the Soviet Union. Is there more out there somewhere? Realistically, yes, there could be. There was talk of destroying the remaining virus samples in 1999, but from what I was able to determine, this did not happen. If anyone has proof to the contrary, perhaps you will consider taking a bold step and enlighten the rest of us.

Now comes the tricky part: the CDC confirm having 15 million vaccines available. They cannot, under any circumstances, release these vaccines for public use. I suspect that could change in the event of an outbreak, but that won't do any good to anyone who has actually contracted smallpox. In fact, in the grand scheme of things, by the time the vaccines are released and dispensed to 15 million people, it wouldn't amount to saving many lives, unless the epidemic was very small, which is unlikely. Immunity after living through smallpox is permanent; immunity after a vaccine most likely lasts up to 10 years.

Symptoms of Smallpox

Symptoms of smallpox include sudden onset of fever, headache, backache (the backache associated with smallpox is about the worst backache known to man), vomiting, marked prostration and delirium; it can end in blindness from scarring in the conjunctiva. The early stage may make you very ill. Also early in the illness (in about 10 percent of the cases), a fleeting rash in the form of a reddening of the skin may appear, not unlike the rash caused by German measles. There is nothing obvious about this rash to arouse suspicion of smallpox. The incubation period, from exposure to the onset of this feverish illness, is nearly always 12 days, with little variation, and you want to try to catch the illness at this stage, if possible.

About two to three days after the onset of illness, the true smallpox rash appears and the early rash fades. This true (focal) rash is normally diagnostic of smallpox, characterized by its evolution and distribution on the body. It begins as discrete, pink spots (macules), which enlarge and become slightly raised papules. Each of these spots progresses, and by the third day a tense blister (vesicle) about six millimeters in diameter has developed, set deep in the skin. After two more days, the fluid inside becomes thick and opaque. In the course of the following days, these vesicles shrink and dry up to become hard, lentil-like crusts in the skin. Eventually they separate, leaving a sunken scar. The hard crusts then detach, containing smallpox virus in their substance.

Diagnostic Information

The distribution of the focal rash is characteristic, affecting the head and extremities as well as, to a lesser degree, the trunk. These symptoms actually make smallpox easy to diagnose clinically once the thought of smallpox has entered the mind—which could take some time. There is some correlation between the severity of the illness and the extent of the focal rash. Toxemia may be so severe that death may occur before the rash is fully developed. However, it is more common for death to occur between the 11th and 15th day of the rash, if it is going to occur at all. In severe cases, the rash may cover the entire body and the individual lesions will run into one another.

The severe disease may also be hemorrhagic, which can further complicate diagnosis. Since the person is bleeding into the skin and from bodily orifices, it may be mistaken for another hemorrhagic disease. Yet another diagnostic difficulty arises from individuals who contract *variola sine eruptione,* in which no rash follows the onset of the illness. Very occasionally, even these individuals may be infectious, via droplets from the mouth.

Infection usually occurs through the respiratory tract and local lymph nodes. The virus then enters the blood (primary viremia), and internal organs are infected. Smallpox then reenters the blood (secondary viremia) and spreads to the skin. These events occur during the incubation period, when the patient is still well. The rash is the result of virus replication in the skin.

Homeopathic Treatment of Smallpox

Luckily for us, many great homeopaths lived through the onslaught of smallpox and we can use the knowledge and remedy information they have left behind. Some people are concerned that smallpox used in biological warfare would be mutated, rendering any treatment method ineffective. Granted, no one can tell for sure. However, I have spoken "unofficially" to a couple of MDs and even a vet. All agreed that they found this doubtful, that there is no need to mutate smallpox because of its high mortality rate and because it is unlikely that anyone is immune anymore. Unfortunately, by the time it would be realized that a smallpox outbreak was occurring, the only treatment option for those already infected would probably be outside allopathic medicine. Homeopathy can play a role in this.

Hahnemann taught us that it is okay to use nosodes as a preventive in the event that one finds oneself in an epidemic situation. That is one option. If you find yourself at ground zero, smallpox speaking, taking either variolinum, malandrinum or *Vaccininum* nosodes would be a great idea. (Do not take them all, though!) Failing that, you need to treat the symptoms, and that needs to be accomplished via the law of similars, or the *simillimum*. This requires repertorizing. However, since the symptoms follow a more or less specific pattern, the most likely remedy candidates can be determined ahead of time. So remedies to consider are *Antimonium tataricum*, baptisia, *Bryonia alba*, *Carbolicum acidum*, *Hepar sulphuris*, *Kali bichromicum*, *Mercurius sulphuricus*, *Rhus toxiocodendron* and thuja.

To recap: Variolinum, malandrinum and *Vaccininum* are *nosodes*, which means that they are made from diseased material—smallpox in the case of variolinum, grease of horses in the case of malandrinum and vaccine matter in the case of *Vaccininum*. It is sometimes argued that this treatment method takes the form of isopathy, which is using the exact remedy for a specific condition rather than a similar one. This is a debate that will continue to pop up. I believe that the current thinking follows that isopathy is, in fact, a nosode made from the individual, strictly for the individual's own use. These definitions are not important, however, to our mission at this time.

The Nosodes

In discussing nosodes, it is important to reiterate that you should *not* take any of them unless provided by a professional homeopath. Though it is true that they can be used as a preventive, they should only be taken if the threat of infection is real, for example, if a smallpox epidemic occurs. Vaccinia, smallpox and grease of horses are interrelated diseases, and the nosodes of each are available for the treatment or prevention of all three.

Malandrinum (Grease of Horses)

This is made from the grease from the skin of a horse and matches the following symptoms:

Mental and Emotional State
- Dullness, dizziness.

Physical Symptoms

Abdomen
- Pains around umbilicus.

Back
- Pain along back, as if beaten.

Ears
- Profuse, purulent, greenish yellow discharge mixed with blood.

Eyes
- Red stripes under eyes.
- Sensation of motion in the eye.
- Severe pain in the left eye as if a saw was drawn up and down vertically through the eyeball.

Extremities (Arms and Legs)
- Sore pains in limbs and joints.
- Run-around on nails of hands and feet.
- Impetiginous crusts on extensor sides of forearms.
- Pains, especially in left tibia with petechia-like patches on anterior aspect of left leg from knee to ankle. Petechia on both thighs, worse on the left.
- Toes felt as if scalded and itch terribly underneath.
- Sensation of a draft of air blowing on feet at night, must get up and tuck in the bedsheets, which relieves.

Face
- Scab on upper lip with stinging pain when torn off.

Head
- Aching in forehead.
- Frontal and occipital headache.
- Impetigo covering head from crown to neck and extending behind ears.
- Thick, greenish crusts with pale, reddish scabs, itching worse in the evening.

Mouth
- The tongue is coated yellow, with a red streak down middle (typhoid); cracked and ulcerating down middle, swollen.

Skin
- Impetigo covering back of head, extending over back to buttock and even into vagina, covering labia.
- Impetigo on extensors of forearms.
- Dry, scaly, itching cracks of hands and feet in cold weather and from washing.
- Boils; malignant pustules.
- Bad effects from a vaccination (dry, harsh skin).
- Small, dusky red spots on legs, not disappearing on pressure.
- Typhoid fever; petechial typhus.
- A sensation of rawness of the skin over the chest and shoulders after bathing, as if the skin had been scraped with burning acid, smarting by covering parts.
- Felt a creepy sensation in his skin, particularly in the face, as if ants were crawling over it.

Stomach
- Vomiting of bilious matter, nausea.

Stool
- Dark, cadaverous-smelling stool.
- Yellowish, foul-smelling diarrhea.

Comments

Indications according to Burnett (J. C. Burnett, *Curability of Cataracts with Medicines* [London: The Homeopathic Publishing Company, 1880]) are:
- Lower half of body, greasy skin and greasy eruption.
- Slow suppuration, never ending, as one heals another appears.
- Impetigo, pustular disease, fat, greasy-looking pustular eruptions are particularly acted on by this remedy.

A. L. Marcey relates a striking experience with malandrinum 30C. (R. Murphy, *Homeopathic Remedy Guide* [Colorado: The Hahneman Academy of North America, 2004], 530). In the presence of a smallpox epidemic, he vaccinated himself, taking at the same time malandrinum 30C night and morning. The vaccination did not take. It was twice repeated and still did not take, nor was smallpox contracted. Called to vaccinate four children in a family whose parents were recovering from smallpox, he vaccinated all and gave malandrinum 30C to three of them at the same time; the remaining child was the only one whose vaccination "took." This was so severe that malandrinum had to be given to modify its intensity, which it did effectively. The other three were revaccinated but none "took." Of five children from six to seventeen years of age, only the eldest had been vaccinated and he had a good scar. All except the eldest were given malandrinum and were vaccinated and none of the four "took." The eldest took smallpox. Malandrinum was then given and in a few days, he was convalescent.

In another case of smallpox, malandrinum was given and the disease lasted only a few days, the eruption drying up. In Straube's proving, the symptoms were worse in the evening. Burnett considers malandrinum a very deeply acting remedy and one not to be repeated more often than once a fortnight.

Homeopaths of yesteryear found it to be effective in the prevention of smallpox. As said before, A. L. Marcey vaccinated himself and also used malandrinum 30C morning and night during a smallpox epidemic. The vaccination never took, even after being repeated twice, but he remained free from smallpox with the nosode. He also used malandrinum to effectively cure smallpox in a very short period of time, in only a few days!

Vaccininum

Some documentation shows *Vaccininum* 6C, taken in water for one day and repeated after eight days, to have acted as a preventive in 600 cases.

Mental and Emotional State

- Crying, ill humor, restless sleep.
- Nervous, impatient, morbid fear of getting smallpox.

Physical Symptoms

Fever

- Fever with heat, thirst, tossing about, crying, aversion to food.
- Chill with shaking.

Head
- Frontal headache, forehead feels as if it would split in two from root of nose to top of head.
- Stitches in right temple, eruption looks like *crustea lacteal* (crusty, milklike).

Respiratory
- Shortness of breath with aching in pit of stomach.
- Pressure in region of heart.

Stomach
- Aching in pit of stomach, with shortness of breath.

Skin
- A general eruption, similar to cowpox.
- Red pimples or blotches in various parts, most evident when warm.
- Eruption of pustules with a dark red base, a roundish or oblong elevation filled with pus of a greenish yellow color; some as large as a pea; without depression in the center; coming with a round, hard feel in the skin; very itchy.
- Tingling and burning in skin over whole body.

Variolinum

The cardinal symptoms of smallpox are the keynote symptoms (matches) for variolinum.

Mental and Emotional State
- Delirium with initial fever.

Physical Symptoms
Head
- Vertigo, loss of consciousness when attempting to rise.
- Forehead very hot, face red and bloated, carotids pulsating violently.
- Headache with or right after a chill, all over head, particularly in forehead; severe in vertex, as if a band tightly encircled head.
- Intolerable pain in occiput.

Respiratory
- Oppressed respiration, troublesome cough, with serous and sometimes bloody sputa.
- Hawking up thick, viscid, bad-smelling slime.

Skin
- Exanthema (eruption) of sharp, pointed pimples that are usually small, suppurating, dry, resting on a small red areola and frequently interspersed with spots of red color; sometimes severe itching.

Stomach
- Soreness in pit of stomach and across epigastric region.
- Frequent vomiting of bilious and bloody matter.
- Vomits milk immediately after drinking it.

Other Homeopathic Remedies

Antimonium tartaricum, Baptisia tinctoria, belladonna, *Bryonia alba, Carbolicum acidum, Hepar sulphuris, Kali bichromicum, Mercurius sulphuricus, Rhus toxicodendron* and thuja are remedies made from various sources. Certain remedies have specific keynotes in their symptoms that can be of great value in determining the correct one. I will include mental symptoms too, although in the eventuality that we need to repertorize, the physical symptoms will probably be more important.

Antimonium tartaricum (Tartar Emetic)

Mental and Emotional State
- Vertigo alternating with drowsiness, great despondency, fears being alone.

Physical Symptoms
Back
- Violent pains in sacro-lumbar region.
- Slightest effort to move causes retching and cold, clammy sweat.
- Sensation of heavy weight at coccyx, dragging downward all the time.

Fever
- Coldness, trembling and chilliness.
- Intense heat, copious perspiration.
- Cold, clammy sweat with great faintness.

Head
- Bandlike feeling over forehead.
- Headache as from a band compressing.

Keynotes
- Rattling of mucus with little expectoration.
- Drowsiness, debility.
- Sweat, chills and pains in the muscles.

Respiratory
- Burning in chest, which ascends to throat.
- Breathing is rapid, short and difficult; sufferers feel like they are suffocating.
- Pulse rapid, week, trembling.

Skin
- Pustular eruption, leaving a bluish mark.
- Smallpox.

Stomach
- Difficulty swallowing fluids, vomiting in any position, except when lying on right side.
- Nausea, retching and vomiting, especially after food.
- Thirst for cold water, little and often; desire for apples, fruits and acids generally.

Modalities
- *Worse*: In evening, from lying down at night; from warmth, in damp weather; from all sour things and milk.
- *Better*: Sitting erect; from eructation (belching) and expectoration.

Baptisia tinctoria (Wild Indigo)

Mental and Emotional State
- Wild wandering feeling.
- Inability to think, mentally confused, thinks s/he is broken or double.
- Vertigo.

Physical Symptoms
Back
- Neck tired.
- Stiffness and pain, aching.
- A drawing on arms and legs.
- Pain in sacrum, around hips and legs.
- Sore and bruised.

Fever
- Chill, with pains and soreness all over body.
- Heat all over, with occasional chills.
- Chill about eleven o'clock in the morning.
- Adynamic (causing a lack of strength or function) fevers.

Head
- Pressure at root of nose.
- Skin of forehead feels too tight.
- Skin of forehead seems drawn to back of head.
- Soreness of eyeballs.

Keynotes
- Septic conditions of the blood.
- Indescribable sick feeling.
- Great muscular soreness and putrid phenomena.

Respiratory
- Lungs feel compressed, breathing difficult.
- Seeks open window.
- Fears going to sleep due to nightmares and sense of suffocation.

Skin
- Livid spots all over body and limbs.
- Burning and heat in skin.
- Putrid ulcers with stupor, delirium and prostration.

Stomach
- Can swallow only liquids.
- Vomiting from spasm of esophagus.
- Constant desire for water.
- Sinking feeling in stomach.
- Pain in epigastric region.
- All symptoms worse from beer.

Modalities
- *Worse:* Humid heat, fog, indoors.

Belladonna atropa (Deadly Nightshade)

Mental and Emotional State
- Vertigo, with falling to left side or backward.
- Sensitive to least contact.

Physical Symptoms

Fever

- A high feverish state with comparative absence of toxemia.
- Burning, pungent, steaming heat.
- Feet icy cold.
- Superficial blood vessels distended.
- Perspiration dry, only on head.
- No thirst with fever.

Head

- Much throbbing and heat in head.
- Pain and fullness, especially in forehead.
- Pain worse from light, noise, jarring, lying down and in the afternoon.
- Headache worse on right side.

Keynotes

- Sudden and violent onset of symptoms.
- Loss of consciousness, delirium, rage, oversensitive in all senses.
- Bleeding from inner parts, exanthemata (eruptive disease) of a scarlet color.

Respiratory

- Dryness; tickling, short, dry cough, worse at night.
- Larynx feels sore.
- Cough with pain in right hip.
- Barking cough, whooping cough with pain in stomach before attack and with expectoration of blood.
- High, piping voice.
- Moaning at every breath.

Skin

- Dry and hot.
- Swollen, sensitive.
- Burns scarlet, smooth.
- Eruption like scarlatina, suddenly spreading.
- Glands swollen, tender, red.
- Boils, suppurative wounds.
- Alternate redness and paleness of skin.
- Indurations after inflammations.

Stomach

- Loss of appetite.

- Averse to meat and milk.
- Constriction; pain runs to spine.
- Nausea and vomiting.
- Great thirst for cold water.
- Empty retching; dread of drinking.
- Uncontrollable vomiting.

Modalities
- *Worse*: Touch, jarring, noise, draft, afternoon, lying down.
- *Better*: Lying semierect.

Bryonia alba (Wild Hops)

Mental and Emotional State
- Exceedingly irritable, talk of business.
- Vertigo, faintness on rising.
- Confusion.

Physical Symptoms
Fever
- Pulse full, hard, tense and quick.
- Chill with external coldness.
- Internal heat.
- Sour sweat after slight exertion.
- Easy, profuse perspiration.

Head
- Bursting, splitting headache made worse from stooping, motion and opening eyes.
- Cannot sit up, gets faint and sick.
- Headache becomes seated in occiput.
- Frontal headache, with frontal sinuses involved.

Keynotes
- Grouchy (bryonia is *the* grouch remedy).
- Aggravation at 9 PM.

Respiratory
- Dry, hacking cough from irritation in upper trachea.
- Dry cough at night, must sit up. Worse after eating or drinking, with vomiting and stitches in chest.

Skin
- Yellow, pale, swollen.
- Hot and painful.

Stomach
- Nausea and faintness when rising up.
- Abnormal hunger, loss of taste.
- Great thirst.
- Vomiting of bile and liquid immediately after eating.
- Worse with warm drinks, which are vomited.
- Stomach sensitive to touch.

Modalities
- *Worse*: Warmth, any motion, morning, eating, hot weather, exertion, touch.
- *Better*: Lying on painful side; pressure, rest, cold things.

Carbolicum acidum (Carbolic Acid)

Physical Symptoms

Head
- Doesn't like mental work.
- Tight feeling, as if head was compressed by a rubber band.
- Orbital neuralgia over right eye.
- Headache is better from drinking green tea and while smoking.

Keynotes
- Very marked acuteness of smell.
- Terrible stomach pains that come and go suddenly.

Skin
- Itching vesicles (fluid-filled blister) with burning pain.
- Burns tend to ulcerate.

Stomach
- No appetite.
- Desire for stimulants and tobacco.
- Constant belching, nausea and vomiting; vomit is a dark olive green.
- Painful flatulence, often marked in one part of the bowel.

Hepar sulphuris (Calcium Sulphide)

Mental and Emotional State
- Anguish in the evening and at night, with thoughts of suicide.
- Irritable, dejected and sad.
- Vertigo.

Physical Symptoms

Fever
- Chilly in open air and from slightest draft, dry heat at night.
- Profuse sweat; sour, sticky, offensive.

Head
- Headache when shaking the head or riding; scalp sensitive and sore.
- Boring pain in right temple and in root of nose every morning.
- Cold sweat on head.

Keynotes
- When handling involved areas, pain is felt as if from subcutaneous ulceration; great sensitiveness of affected parts to touch.

Respiratory
- Dry, hoarse cough.
- Loose, rattling cough, worse in the morning.
- Cough excited whenever any part of the body gets cold or uncovered or from eating anything cold.
- Suffocative attacks, has to rise up and bend head backward.

Skin
- Abscess.
- Papules (a small, solid, usually conical elevation of the skin).
- Easy bleeding.
- Ulcers with bloody discharge, smelling like old cheese; ulcers are very sensitive to contact.
- Can't bear to be uncovered, wants to be wrapped up warmly.
- Putrid ulcers, surrounded by little pimples.
- Great sensitivity to slightest touch.
- Smallpox.

Stomach
- Longs for acids, wine and strong-tasting food.
- Aversion to fatty food.

- Frequent belching without taste or smell.
- Distention of stomach, compelling person to loosen clothing.
- Heaviness and pressure even after a slight meal.

Modalities

- *Worse*: From dry, cold winds; cool air; slightest draft. From touch and lying on the painful side.
- *Better*: In damp weather; from wrapping head up, from warmth; after eating.

Kali bichromicum (Bichromate of Potash)

Mental and Emotional State

- Vertigo with nausea when rising from seat.

Physical Symptoms

Head

- Headache over eyebrows, preceded by blurred vision.
- Aching and fullness in glabella (smooth area between the eyebrows).
- Semilateral headache in small spots.
- Frontal headache, usually over one eye.
- Bones and scalp feel sore.

Keynotes

- Symptoms worse in the morning.
- Pains migrate quickly.

Respiratory

- Voice hoarse, worse in the evening.
- Metallic, hacking cough.
- Profuse, yellow expectoration; very glutinous (gluelike) and sticky; coming out in a long, stringy and tenacious mass.
- Pain at bifurcation (branch) of trachea on coughing, from mid-sternum to back.

Skin

- Papular eruptions.
- Ulcer with punched-out edges, with tendency to penetrate and tenacious exudation (oozing).
- Pustular eruption, resembling smallpox, with burning pain.
- Itching with vesicular (blisterlike) eruption.

Stomach
- Feels as if digestion has stopped.
- Dilation of the stomach.
- Stitches in region of liver and spleen, through to spine.
- Gastritis.
- Dislikes water; cannot digest a meal; desire for beer and acids.
- Vomiting of bright yellow water.

Modalities
- *Worse*: From beer; in the morning, hot weather; when undressing.
- *Better*: From heat.

Mercurius sulphuricus (Yellow Sulphate of Mercury)

Mental and Emotional State
- Low-spirited, with chilliness and yawning.
- Ill humor after eating.
- Sensation of giddiness while standing, after headache.

Physical Symptoms

Fever
- Chilliness running up back, with yawning and depression, followed by a dull pain in the forehead, burning in the face and ears.
- Light fever.
- Chilliness, restlessness and heaviness in upper part of abdomen.
- Frequent yawning and diminished secretion of urine (afternoon).

Head
- Fullness in head, with occasional stitches.
- Soreness and heaviness through head (after breakfast and while walking about.)

Keynotes
- Worse in the afternoon, from 4 to 5 PM.

Respiratory
- Roughness and hoarseness in throat.
- Sensation of heat in larynx.
- Increased expectoration of mucus from larynx and trachea.

Skin
- Induration (hardness, inflammation) of the glands.

Stomach
- Violent, yellow vomit; stomach is so irritated that nothing will stay down.
- Pain and weight in stomach, tenderness.
- Vomiting and diarrhea.

Rhus toxicodendron (Poison Ivy)

Mental and Emotional State
- Listless, sad, suicidal thoughts.
- Extreme restlessness with constant change in position.
- Delirium with fear of being poisoned.
- Great apprehension at night, cannot remain in bed.
- Vertigo when rising.

Physical Symptoms

Head
- Feels as if board was strapped to forehead.
- Pain in forehead that proceeds backward.
- Heavy head.
- Brain feels "loose" as if it were struck against the skull on walking or rising.
- Headache in occiput, painful to the touch.
- Humid eruptions on scalp, itching greatly.

Keynotes
- Red, shiny swellings and vesicular (blisterlike) erysipelas (inflammation of the skin and subcutaneous tissue).
- Eczematous eruptions with great burning and itching; tendency to form scales.

Respiratory
- Tickling behind upper sternum.
- Dry, teasing cough from midnight until morning, during a chill or when sticking hands out from underneath covers.
- Oppression of the chest, cannot get breath with sticking pains.

Skin
- Red, swollen; itching intense.
- Glands swollen.

- Vesicles, herpes, urticaria (raised, swollen patches of skin), pemphigus (large blisters on skin or mucus membranes, often associated with itching and burning).
- Burning eruptions with tendency to scale formation.

Stomach
- No appetite, but unquenchable thirst, with dry mouth and throat.
- Bitter taste.
- Nausea, vertigo and bloated abdomen after eating.
- Desire for milk.
- Pressure in stomach as from a stone.
- Drowsy after eating.

Modalities

- *Worse*: During sleep; at night; during rest; when lying on back or right side. In cold, wet, rainy weather; after rain.
- *Better*: In warm, dry weather. When in motion, walking; changing position; from stretching out limb. Rubbing, warm applications.

Thuja occidentalis (Arbor vitae)

Mental and Emotional State

- Fixed ideas, as if a strange person was at her or his side, as if body and soul were separated, as if something were alive in the abdomen.
- Emotional sensitiveness; music causes weeping and trembling.

Physical Symptoms

Fever
- Chill, beginning in thighs.
- Sweat only on uncovered parts or all over, except head; when sleeping.
- Sweat profuse, sour, smells like honey.

Keynotes
- One-sided complaints (left side).
- Aggravation at 3 AM and 3 PM.

Respiratory
- Dry, hacking cough in afternoon, with pain in pit of stomach.
- Stitches in chest; worse with cold drinks.

Skin
- Perspiration sweetish and strong.
- Herpetic eruptions, tearing pains in glands, glandular enlargement, eruptions only on covered parts; worse after scratching.
- Very sensitive to touch, coldness of one side.

Stomach
- Complete loss of appetite; dislike for fresh meat and potatoes; cannot eat onions.
- Rancid belching after fatty foods; flatulence, pain after food.
- Sinking sensation in epigastrium before food.
- Indigestion from drinking tea.

Modalities
- *Worse*: At night, from heat of bed; at 3 AM and 3 PM; from cold, damp air. After breakfast, fat, coffee, vaccination.
- *Better*: Left side, from drawing up a limb.

Homeopathic Journal Proves Use of Homeopathy Against Smallpox

Another course of treatment for smallpox is stated in the *Homeopathic World*, 1909:

> 1rst stage- fever. Hit it high with Ferrum Phos
>
> 2nd stage-inflammation of serous membranes . . . exudation fibrinous in character- Kali Mur low.
>
> If it doesn't work you need to give Nat. Mur low as it is a KCl /NaCl thing going or visa versa in administration.
>
> If it doesn't stop exuding switch to Nat phos in alternation with Sil or if the pustules should run confluent use Nat Mur in place of Nat Phos.
>
> For Small Pox one thing I uncovered was Hempel's work with Acetic Acid in the form of VINEGAR!! Two Tbsp after breakfast and in the evening for two weeks. To half-grown and feeble persons he gave ½ this dose. Almost the whole village had been stricken and not one died even if they had been quite stricken. 8 out of 10 who were exposed didn't even catch it all. "A small number of the

sick was but little affected; pustules were few and sequela none."

(C. Sterling Saunder, L.R. C. P., "Kali mur. with Special Reference to Its Antidotal Power Against Small Pox and Vaccine Poisoning, Etc." *Homeopathic World* [1909]:75.)

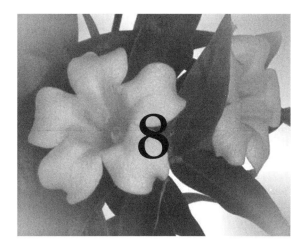

Anthrax and Homeopathic and Antibiotic Treatment Protocols

Anthrax Biological Warfare Information

Iraq, Russia and as many as 10 other nations have the capability to load spores of *B. anthracis* into weapons. The spores of *B. anthracis* can be produced and stored in a dry form and they remain viable for decades in storage or after release. When released, the spores are easily dispersed in air for inhalation by unprotected troops (or civilians downwind) and can remain in the soil for many years. Anthrax spores are apparently one of the top choices of weapons for biological warfare.

The following is an excerpt from the *U.S. Navy Manual on Operational Medicine and Fleet Support*, entitled "Biological Warfare Defense Information Sheet":

> The disease anthrax is caused by the bacteria *Bacillus anthracis*. Anthrax is normally found in sheep, cattle and horses but can be transmitted to humans who contact infected animals or their products. Usually, humans acquire the disease by skin contact with the bacteria or by inhaling the bacterial spores found in sheep wool.

As an agent of biological warfare (BW), it is expected that a cloud of anthrax spores would be released at a strategic location to be inhaled by the personnel under attack. As such, the symptoms of anthrax encountered in BW would follow those expected for inhalation of spores as opposed to those expected for skin contact or ingestion of the bacteria. These symptoms are discussed in the sections below.

Use Bleach and Water

If you suspect that you've been sprayed with anthrax, it will be all over everything. The only way to help protect yourself is with the use of *bleach* and *water* as stated in the "Biological Warfare Defense Information Sheet" in the *U.S. Navy Manual on Operational Medicine and Fleet Support*: "Disinfection of contaminated articles may be accomplished using a 0.05 percent hypochlorite solution (1 tbsp. bleach per gallon of water). Spore destruction requires steam sterilization."

Paths of Infection

There are three ways to become infected with anthrax bacteria: by inhalation (pulmonary anthrax), through the skin (cutaneous anthrax) and by ingestion (gastrointestinal anthrax).

Pulmonary Anthrax

Pulmonary anthrax, also called inhalational anthrax, is contracted by inhaling anthrax spores. The symptoms mimic those of a bad flu and, within a few days, pneumonia. This makes diagnosis difficult. Intravenous antibiotic treatment should begin immediately. The Centers for Disease Control (CDC) state that despite treatment, pulmonary anthrax is fatal in at least 80 percent of all cases. One should take into consideration that overall, our information on pulmonary anthrax is sparse. It is believed that there are a number of variables that can affect the outcome of the disease, including the virulence of the strain of anthrax (there are said to be 22 or 23 known strains, 50 percent of which are harmless), the number of spores inhaled and the speed with which the disease is diagnosed and treated.

Cutaneous Anthrax

Cutaneous anthrax (anthrax of the skin) is contracted by having anthrax spores come in contact with a scratch, cut and so forth. A rashlike inflammation of the skin, not unlike that caused by a spider bite, is the most obvious symptom of the first phase of the disease. During the second phase, a blackened ulcer forms and a fever is present. This manifestation of anthrax, though difficult to diagnose, responds rapidly to intravenous antibiotic treatment. Cutaneous anthrax is fatal in only 25 percent of untreated cases and in less than 1 percent of treated cases.

Gastrointestinal Anthrax

Gastrointestinal anthrax is most often contracted by consuming food that has been infected with anthrax spores. Infection is characterized initially by lack of appetite, nausea, vomiting and fever. Second-phase symptoms are abdominal pain, diarrhea and vomiting of blood. Diagnosis is difficult because of the initial flulike symptoms. Intravenous antibiotic treatment is given. Gastrointestinal anthrax can be fatal in 25 to 60 percent of treated cases.

Below are expanded descriptions of symptoms for all three paths of infection.

Symptoms of Pulmonary Anthrax

Disbursement of anthrax from an airplane could be harmful to a large number of people, depending on the weather conditions and wind patterns. Under the most favorable conditions, aerosolized anthrax spores sprayed from a plane can cover a path of about eight kilometers. This has the potential of affecting hundreds of thousands of people if dropped in a metropolitan area. Pulmonary anthrax symptoms have *two stages*.

Stage One—Flulike Symptoms

About one to six days after inhaling *Bacillus anthracis* spores, there is a gradual onset of vague symptoms of illness such as fatigue, fever, mild discomfort in the chest and possibly a dry cough.

One might think one has the flu. The symptoms improve for a few hours or for up to two to three days. This is followed by a sudden onset of difficulty in breathing, profuse sweating, cyanosis (blue-colored skin), shock and death within 24 to 36 hours.

These symptoms are essentially those of woolsorter's disease, which is caused by inhalation of bacterial spores (*Bacillus anthracis*) from contaminated wool or hair. Here is a list to summarize the first set of anthrax symptoms, which mirror nonspecific flulike symptoms:

- Progressive fatigue.
- Possible fever.
- Chills.
- General discomfort, uneasiness or ill feeling (malaise).
- Headache.
- Nausea and vomiting.
- Shortness of breath/breathing problems.
- Dry cough.
- Mild chest discomfort with a nonproductive cough.
- Joint stiffness.
- Joint pain.
- Possible sore throat (rare).
- Possible night sweats.
- Loss of appetite.

Homeopathic Symptoms for Pulmonary Anthrax at Stage One

Here are the symptoms to look for when considering homeopathic treatment of the first stage of pulmonary (inhalational) anthrax. Remember, though, that the first line of defense is your physician. Use homeopathy only as an adjunct to accepted medical practices.

- Heat in general, fever.
- Coldness in general, chill.
- Headache, general pain.
- Nausea, vomiting, diminished appetite.
- Dry cough.
- Suffocative (difficult) respiration.
- Congested nose.
- Sensation of fullness in throat.
- Chest catarrh.
- Stiffness, general pain, feeling of influenza in extremities.

- Mental and emotional state shows discomfort, discontentedness, restlessness.

Homeopathic Remedies
- Anthracinum (anthrax nosode)
- *Arsenicum album*
- *Lachesis muta*
- *Secale cornutum*
- *Bryonia alba*

The affected person experiences improvement; the symptoms seem to abate for one to three days, and the person feels better.

Stage Two Symptoms

The second phase will hit the person hard and usually within 24 to 36 hours. This phase is marked by high fever, dyspnea (shortness of breath), stridor (lungs filling with fluid), cyanosis (blue-colored skin; the victim is unable to get sufficient oxygen into the body due to breathing problems) and shock. Then the person dies. Here is a list to summarize the second set of anthrax symptoms:
- Breathing problems/pneumonia
- Shock
- Swollen lymph glands
- Profuse sweating
- Cyanosis (skin turns blue)

Homeopathic Symptoms for Pulmonary Anthrax at Stage Two

These are the symptoms to look for when considering homeopathic treatment of the second stage of pulmonary (inhalational) anthrax. However, the first line of defense is your physician. Use homeopathy only as an adjunct to accepted medical practices.
- Fever, heat in general, perspiration
- Coldness in general, chill
- Headache, general pain
- Nausea, vomiting, diminished appetite
- Dry cough
- Suffocative (difficult) respiration, pneumonia
- Congested nose
- Sensation of fullness in throat

- Chest catarrh
- Stiffness, general pain, feeling of influenza in extremities
- Swelling of cervical region
- Mental and emotional state shows discomfort, discontentedness, restlessness
- Cyanosis, asphyxia

Homeopathic Remedies
1. *Arsenicum album*
2. Phosphorus
3. *Lachesis muta*
4. *Carbo vegetabilis*
5. *Baptisia tinctoria*
6. *Pyrogenium*

Symptoms for Cutaneous Anthrax

Contact through the skin is the most common "naturally" occurring form of anthrax and is characterized by swelling and boils on the skin. Skin infection begins as a raised, itchy bump that resembles an insect bite but develops into a vesicle (fluid-filled blister) within one to two days and then into a pain-less ulcer, usually one to three centimeters in diameter and with a characteristic black, necrotic (dying) area in the center. A reddish brown sore develops, which breaks open and forms a scab. Usually, one finds a typical painless lesion (ulcer) at the site of infection with a black, necrotic eschar (scab). Lymph glands in the adjacent area may swell.

About 20 percent of untreated cases of cutaneous anthrax will result in death, but deaths are rare with appropriate antimicrobial therapy. Here is a list to summarize the symptoms of cutaneous anthrax:

- Skin infection, begins as a raised, itchy bump that resembles an insect bite; develops into a vesicle within one to two days and then into a painless ulcer with a characteristic black, necrotic area in the center.
- Reddish brown sore develops, breaks open and forms a scab.
- Lymph glands in the adjacent area may swell.
- Local swelling is often prominent.
- Possible fatigue.
- Possible chills.

Homeopathic Symptoms for Cutaneous Anthrax

These are the symptoms to look for when considering homeopathic treatment of cutaneous (skin) anthrax. However, the first line of defense is your physician. Use homeopathy only as an adjunct to accepted medical practices.

- Vesicular eruptions of skin, swelling of affected part, blackish discoloration, itching.

Homeopathic Remedies

1. *Arsenicum album*
2. *Lachesis muta*
3. Nitric acidum
4. *Secale cornutum*
5. *Carbo vegetabilis*

Symptoms for Gastrointestinal Anthrax

The intestinal disease form of anthrax may follow the consumption of contaminated meat and is characterized by an acute inflammation of the intestinal tract. Initial signs of nausea, loss of appetite, vomiting and fever are followed by abdominal pain, vomiting of blood and severe diarrhea. Intestinal anthrax can result in death in 25 to 60 percent of treated cases. Here is a list of symptoms indicating gastrointestinal anthrax:

- Inflammation of the intestinal tract
- Nausea, loss of appetite
- Fever
- Abdominal pain, vomiting of blood
- Severe diarrhea

Homeopathic Symptoms for Gastrointestinal Anthrax

These are the symptoms to look for when considering homeopathic treatment of gastrointestinal anthrax. Again, remember that the first line of defense is your physician. Use homeopathy only as an adjunct to accepted medical practices.

- Appetite wanting
- Vomiting in general, vomiting blood
- Nausea
- General pain in abdomen
- Diarrhea, frequent stool

Homeopathic Remedies
1. *Arsenicum album*
2. Ipecac (*Cephaelis ipecacuanha*)
3. Phosphorus
4. *China officinalis*
5. *Veratrum album*

What Else Can I Do?

If you find yourself under attack, we suggest Rescue Remedy every 10 to 15 minutes (4 drops beneath the tongue) to help with your anxiety and panic reactions. Once you settle down, then you can take Rescue Remedy on an "as needed" basis.

We can't stress enough the importance of the communication between you and your medical doctor. If things get bad, there is going to be panic, so you need to have your own house in order; you need to have your homeopathic kit, your remedies and your instructions as well as phone numbers of your homeopath (if you have one) and your medical doctor. Panic serves no one.

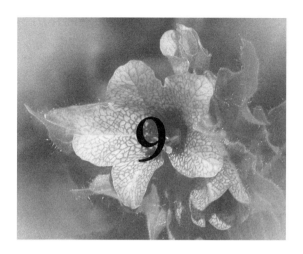

A Terrorist Attack
Releasing Plague

A weapon designed to aerosolize the plague bacterium could cause a rapidly severe and fatal disease in exposed persons. The *Yersinia pestis*, the causative agent of plague, is found in rodents and their fleas in many areas around the world. It can be grown in large quantities and disseminated by aerosol. The result could be an epidemic of the pneumonic (lung form, from breathing it in) form with the potential for a secondary spread of cases.

A bioterrorism attack would be characterized by pneumonic cases occurring simultaneously in persons one to six days following a common exposure and in a secondary wave as a result of unprotected contacts. There are no effective environmental warning systems to detect an aerosol of plague bacilli.

Although pneumonic plague is an uncommon form of the disease, large outbreaks of pneumonic plague have occurred. Most people who get the plague are those who handle dead rodents, especially gophers. However, bioterrorism is different. It uses the least known and most virulent form of plague, the type that hits our lungs after we breathe in the bacteria.

What Is Plague?

Plague is a disease of rodents that can be spread to humans and other animals by infected fleas. In people, plague has three forms: bubonic plague (infection of the lymph glands), septicemic plague (infection of the blood) and pneumonic plague (infection of the lungs). Pneumonic plague is the most contagious form because it can spread from person to person in airborne droplets.

Use the information presented in this chapter to determine whether you or someone you know may have the plague. There are three types of plague:

Bubonic plague: Bubonic plague is the most common form of plague. It occurs when an infected flea bites a person or when materials contaminated with *Y. pestis* enter through a break in a person's skin. Patients develop swollen, tender lymph glands (called buboes) and fever, headache, chills and weakness. Bubonic plague does not spread from person to person.

This strain is extraordinarily virulent and can last up to two months. Death usually occurs within two days. Symptoms include ugly black sores, mass hemorrhaging and strong propensity for eating away lung tissue.

Pneumonic plague: Pneumonic plague occurs when *Y. pestis* infects the lungs. This type of plague can spread from person to person through the air. Transmission can take place if someone breathes in aerosolized bacteria, which could happen in a bioterrorist attack. Pneumonic plague is also spread by breathing in *Y. pestis* suspended in respiratory droplets from a person (or animal) with pneumonic plague. Becoming infected this way usually requires direct and close contact with the ill person or animal. Pneumonic plague may also occur if a person with bubonic or septicemic plague is untreated and the bacteria spread to the lungs.

This strain affects the lymphatic system. Common symptoms include swollen glands, constant fever and external buboes under the arm or in the groin area. This disease usually runs its course within three days.

Septicemic plague: Septicemic plague occurs when plague bacteria multiply in the blood. It can be a complication of pneumonic or bubonic plague or it can occur by itself. When it occurs alone, it is caused in the same ways as bubonic plague; however, buboes do not develop. Patients have fever, chills, prostration, abdominal pain, shock and bleeding into the skin and other organs. Septicemic plague does not spread from person to person.

This strain races through the body within a matter of hours, saturating blood with bacteria, which causes immediate death. Common symptoms of this strain include a high fever and grotesque boils.

Where Is Plague Found?

Plague is found in some semiarid areas in Asia, Eastern Europe, Africa, South America and North America. In the U.S., most cases in humans occur in two regions: (1) northern New Mexico, northern Arizona and southern Colorado; and (2) California, southern Oregon and far western Nevada. In the southwestern U.S., rock squirrel fleas are the most common source of infection in people, and in the Pacific states, California ground squirrel fleas are the most common source. Many other types of rodents—including other ground squirrels, prairie dogs, chipmunks, woodrats, wild mice and voles—suffer plague outbreaks and are occasional sources of human infection. Domestic cats can be infected by fleas or by eating infected wild rodents and can be a direct source of infection to people. Dogs rarely suffer severe illness and have yet to be shown to be sources of infection for humans.

Is Plague a New or Emerging Infectious Disease?

Plague is an ancient disease that occurs in irregular cycles and remains a public health hazard in parts of Asia, the Middle East, Eastern Europe, Africa and South America, as well as the United States. Epidemics of plague in humans usually involve house rats and their fleas. Rat-borne epidemics continue to occur in some developing countries, particularly in rural areas.

Highly publicized outbreaks of bubonic and pneumonic plague occurred in 1994 in India, leading to a heightened international reaction. The last rat-borne epidemic in the U.S. occurred in Los Angeles in 1924-1925. Since then all human plague cases in the U.S. have been associated with plague outbreaks in wild rodents and their fleas.

What Is the Infectious Agent That Causes Plague?

Plague is caused by *Yersinia pestis*, a bacterium that is spread from rodent to rodent by infected fleas. Periodic outbreaks of plague kill large numbers of rodents (called a "die-off"). The risk of infection to humans and other animals in the area increases when the rodent hosts die and infected fleas look for other sources of blood.

Plague Is Aerosol-Transmissible to Other People

Primary pneumonic plague results from the inhalation of plague bacilli. Person-to-person transmission of pneumonic plague occurs through respiratory droplets, which can infect only those who have direct and close (within six feet) exposure to the ill patient.

Yersinia pestis is very sensitive to the action of sunlight and does not survive long outside the host. Research suggests it may survive in the exposed environment for up to one hour. This is good news compared with anthrax, which doesn't die for 50 years or more and makes plague as a biological warfare item less interesting to terrorists, although it still is on the "A" list of possible biological weapons that can be used against us.

If You Suspect You Have It, You Should . . .

Before antibiotic treatment, nearly 100 percent of cases were reported to be fatal. A pneumonic plague outbreak would initially resemble an outbreak of other severe respiratory illnesses but would quickly be distinguished by the rapid development of life-threatening respiratory failure, sepsis and shock.

Important medical information: Antibiotics need to be given within 24 hours of first symptoms to prevent a high chance of mortality.

The fatality rate of patients when treatment is delayed more than 24 hours after symptom onset is extremely high. This means, if you *think* you have plague, get to the emergency room of your nearest hospital and get tested. Don't feel stupid or dumb about this—this is one time you cannot afford to wait around and think about it. You have one day after contracting the inhalant plague to

get antibiotics or . . . you will more than likely die. Don't guess. Go!
Immediate notification of suspected plague to local or state health
departments is essential for rapid investigation and control activities and for definitive tests through a state reference laboratory or
the Centers for Disease Control (CDC).

What Traditional Medicine Will Do

Confirmatory testing for *Yersinia pestis* usually takes from 24 to
48 hours; presumptive identification by fluorescent antibody testing takes less than 2 hours. The only problem is that few physicians in the U.S. have ever seen a case of pneumonic plague. They
are simply not trained to see it or test for it, so you may have to de-
mand the test that can confirm whether or not you have plague.

Vaccine against plague does not prevent the development of
primary pneumonic plague and is not presently available in the
United States. Early treatment and prophylaxis with streptomycin
or gentamicin antibiotics or with the tetracycline or fluoroquinolone
classes of antimicrobials is advised. In a community experiencing a pneumonic plague epidemic, all persons who develop a fever or new cough should promptly begin antibiotic treatment.

Those in close contact with persons with untreated pneumonic plague in the household, the hospital or at other venues
should receive postexposure antibiotic treatment for seven days.
(Close contact is defined as contact with a patient at a distance of
less than two meters, or about six feet.) The use of disposable surgical masks is recommended to prevent the transmission of pneumonic plague to persons in close contact with cases.

Preventing Plague

How can you prevent plague? There are many precautions
and preventive measures you can take to minimize your risk.

If You Are in an Area with Active Plague Infection . . .

People who live, work or play in areas with active plague infection in wild rodents should take these precautions:
- Allow health authorities to use appropriate and licensed insecti-
  cides to kill fleas during plague outbreaks in wild animals.
- Treat pets (cats and dogs) for flea control regularly.

- Eliminate food and shelter for rodents around homes, work places and certain recreation areas, such as picnic sites or camp-grounds where people congregate. Remove brush, rock piles, junk and food sources, including pet food.
- Avoid sick or dead animals and report such animals to the health department. Hunters and trappers should wear rubber gloves when skinning animals.
- Use insect repellents when outdoors in areas where there is a risk of flea exposure.

Preventive Treatment with Antibiotics

Preventive treatment with antibiotics is recommended for the following groups:
- People who are bitten by fleas during a local outbreak or who are exposed to tissues or fluids from a plague-infected animal.
- People living in a household with a bubonic plague patient, since they may also be exposed to infected fleas.
- People in close contact with a person or pet with suspected plague pneumonia. Close contact is defined as face-to-face con-tact (within six feet) or being in the same closed space, such as a room or vehicle.

If You Travel . . .

People who travel to countries where plague occurs should take these additional precautions:
- Avoid exposure to fleas from diseased rats. The risk of being bitten by infected fleas is especially high after large numbers of plague-infected rats have died. Therefore, avoid places that are infested with rats or where large numbers of rats have reportedly died.
- If travel to such areas is essential, apply insect repellent contain-ing DEET to legs and ankles. Also apply repellents and insecti-cides to clothes and outer bedding according to manufacturers' instructions.
- Take preventive antibiotics if the risk of exposure is high.

For Whom Is Plague Vaccine Available?

Plague vaccine is available for the following groups:
- Persons who work with the plague bacterium in the laboratory or in the field; and

- Persons who work in areas where human plague outbreaks occur or who handle potentially infected animals.

Symptoms of Pneumonic Plague

The person typically experiences fever, prostration and rapidly developing shortness of breath, chest pain and cough. This is often accompanied by gastrointestinal symptoms such as nausea, vomiting, abdominal pain and diarrhea.

The first signs of illness, one to six days after exposure, would be fever, shortness of breath, chest pain, headache, weakness and cough with bloody, sometimes watery sputum. In two to four days, the illness leads to septic shock and has a high mortality rate if left untreated.

Homeopathic Treatment for Pneumonic Plague

Homeopathic Symptoms

These are the symptoms to look for when considering homeopathic treatment of pneumonic plague. However, the first line of defense is your physician. Use homeopathy only as an adjunct to accepted medical practices.

- Weariness, flabby feeling, heaviness, lassitude, lie down, relaxation, weakness; septicemia, blood poisoning, pyemia; shock; swelling glands.
- Respiration is difficult (asthmatic, impeded).
- Heat in general, fever.
- Coldness in general, chill.
- General pain in chest.
- Headache, general pain.
- Bloody saliva.
- Chronic cough.
- Nausea, vomiting in general.
- General pain in abdomen.
- Diarrhea, frequent stool.

Homeopathic Remedies for Pneumonic Plague

- Pestinum (This is a nosode.)
- *Arsenicum album*
- *Crolatus horridus*

- *Lachesis muta*
- *Naja tripudians*
- Phosphorus
- *Mercurius vivus*
- *Nitricum acidum*

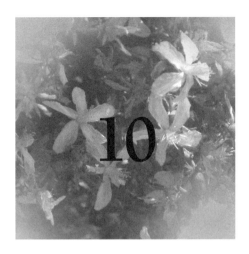

Botulism and Bioterrorism Attack

Botulism toxin is the most potent lethal substance known to humankind (lethal dose is 1ng/kg). It is made by the bacterium *Clostridium botulinum*. Botulinum toxin was developed as an aerosol weapon by several countries. No human data exist on the effects of inhaling botulinum toxin, but the symptoms may resemble those of the food-borne illness. Breathing in the toxin or ingesting the toxin via contaminated food or water—for example, in a bioterrorist attack—are the most likely routes of exposure that might lead to a serious illness (food-borne botulism).

Spores of *C. botulinum* are found in soil worldwide. Terrorists with the technical capacity to grow cultures of the bacterium and harvest and purify the toxin could therefore use it as a bioterrorism agent. Contaminating food with botulism toxin could create a devastating event. About 25 cases of food-borne botulism already occur each year, usually due to improperly prepared home-canned or Native Alaskan foods. Outbreaks from commercial products and foods improperly prepared in restaurants have also occurred.

What Is Botulism?

Botulism is a muscle-paralyzing disease caused by a nerve toxin that is made by a bacterium called *Clostridium botulinum*.

The toxin types most commonly associated with human disease are types A, B, E.

Three Kinds of Botulism

There are three main kinds of botulism: food-borne botulism, infant botulism and wound botulism.

Food-borne botulism occurs when a person ingests *preformed* toxin that leads to illness within a period of a few hours to several days. Only food-borne botulism is a public health emergency, because it could indicate that a food is still available to other persons (besides the patient).

Infant botulism is a condition that occurs in a small number of susceptible infants each year. For unknown reasons, the botulism bacteria is able to grow in their intestines. Infant botulism is not a public health emergency, because the infants are not consuming food with toxin; rather, they are consuming *C. botulinum* spores (which are everywhere in the environment) and, for unknown reasons, are susceptible to gut colonization.

Wound botulism is caused by the growth of living botulism bacteria in a wound, with ongoing secretion of toxin that causes the paralytic illness. In the U.S., this syndrome is seen almost exclusively in injecting drug users.

Symptoms of Botulism

Symptoms of botulism include double vision, blurred vision, drooping eyelids, slurred speech, difficulty swallowing, dry mouth and muscle weakness, which always descends the body: first shoulders, then upper arms, lower arms, thighs, calves and so forth. Paralysis of breathing muscles can cause a person to stop breathing and die, unless s/he is assisted by a ventilator.

Clinical Information

How Soon Do the Symptoms Manifest?

For food-borne botulism, symptoms begin from 6 hours up to 2 weeks after eating toxin-containing food; most commonly, the delay is about 12 to 36 hours. Infants with botulism appear lethargic, feed poorly, are constipated and have a weak cry and muscle tone.

The clinical syndrome of botulism—whether food-borne, infant or wound botulism—is dominated by neurologic symptoms and signs.

Incubation Periods

For food-borne botulism, incubation periods are reported to be as short as 6 hours or as long as 10 days. However, the time between toxin ingestion and onset of symptoms generally ranges from 18 to 36 hours. The ingestion of other bacteria or their toxins in the improperly preserved food or changes in bowel motility are likely to account for the abdominal pain, nausea and vomiting as well as diarrhea that often precede or accompany the neurologic symptoms of food-borne botulism. Dryness of the mouth, inability to focus to a near point (prompting the patient to complain of "blurred vision") and diplopia are usually the earliest neurologic complaints. If the disease is mild, no other symptoms may develop and the initial symptoms will gradually resolve. The person with mild botulism may not come to medical attention.

In more severe cases, however, these initial symptoms may be followed by hoarseness, dysarthria (difficulty speaking), dysphagia (difficulty swallowing) and peripheral muscle weakness. If the illness is severe, respiratory muscles are involved, leading to ventilatory failure and death unless supportive care is provided. Recovery follows the regeneration of neuromuscular connections. A two- to eight-week duration of ventilatory support is common, although patients have required ventilatory support for up to seven to twelve months before the full return of muscular function.

Death occurs in 5 to 10 percent of cases of food-borne botulism. Early deaths result from a failure to recognize the severity of the disease or from secondary pulmonary (lung) or systemic (blood) infections, whereas deaths after two weeks usually result from the complications of long-term mechanical ventilatory management.

Perhaps because infants are not able to complain about the early effects of botulinum intoxication, the neurologic dysfunction associated with infant botulism often seems to develop suddenly. The major manifestations are poor feeding, diminished suckling and crying ability, neck and peripheral weakness (the infants are often admitted as "floppy babies") and ventilatory failure.

Constipation is also often seen in infants with botulism; in some this precedes the onset of neurologic abnormalities by many days.

Loss of facial expression, extraocular muscle paralysis, dilated pupils and depression of deep tendon reflexes have been reported more frequently with type B than with type A infant botulism.

Treatment with aminoglycoside (medical doctors' prescription drug of choice when indicated) antimicrobial agents may promote neuromuscular weakness in infant botulism and has been associated with an increased likelihood of the requirement for mechanical ventilation. Fewer than 2 percent of reported cases of infant botulism result in death.

Diagnosis

Botulism is probably substantially underdiagnosed. The diagnosis is not difficult when it is strongly suspected, as in the setting of a large outbreak, but since cases of botulism most often occur singularly, the diagnosis may pose a more perplexing problem. Findings from many outbreaks have suggested that early cases are commonly misdiagnosed. They may be diagnosed only retrospectively, after death, when the subsequent clustering of cases of botulism-like illnesses finally alerts public health personnel to an outbreak of botulism.

Botulism should be suspected in any adult with a history of acute onset of gastrointestinal, autonomic (for example, dry mouth, difficulty focusing) and cranial nerve (diplopia, dysarthria, dysphagia) dysfunction, or in any infant with poor feeding, diminished suckling and crying ability, neck and peripheral muscle weakness and/or ventilatory distress.

Medical Treatment

The mainstays of treatment of food-borne and wound botulism are as follows:

1. Administration of botulinum antitoxin in an attempt to prevent neurologic progression of a moderate, slowly progressive illness, or to shorten the duration of ventilatory failure in those with a severe, rapidly progressive illness.

2. Careful monitoring of respiratory vital capacity and aggressive respiratory care for those with ventilatory insufficiency (monitoring of respiratory vital). Except for antitoxin administration instructions, other information included in the antitoxin package insert is accurate.

The Centers for Disease Control (CDC) maintain the national botulism antitoxin supply. Physicians diagnosing cases of botulism and wishing to treat their patients with antitoxin must contact the CDC through their state health departments. This way public health officials are alerted immediately about potential cases of botulism. The CDC provide clinical consultation on botulism cases for physicians 24 hours a day and ship botulism antitoxin when needed.

If symptoms occur, individuals should seek treatment. Botulism can be fatal and should be considered a medical emergency.

The paralysis and respiratory failure that occur with botulism may require a patient to be on a breathing machine (ventilator) for weeks, in addition to intensive medical and nursing care. The paralysis slowly improves, usually over several weeks. If diagnosed early, food-borne and wound botulism can be treated with an antitoxin from horse serum, which blocks the action of toxin circulating in the blood. This can prevent patients from worsening, but recovery still may take many weeks.

If You Suspect Botulism . . .

State public health officials should immediately contact CDC if botulism is suspected. If a commercial food product is a suspected vehicle for botulism, the United States Department of Agriculture (USDA) or the U.S. Food and Drug Administration (FDA) should also be notified. Investigation of a suspected case of botulism includes an immediate search for other possible cases and identification of suspected food exposures, as well as confirming the diagnosis. If a number of people are affected, a rapid and detailed epidemiologic investigation is launched to assure that the source is identified and controlled. Diagnostic testing of both case specimens and foods should be performed as needed.

Homeopathic Treatment

Homeopathic Symptoms

- Diplopia, blurred vision (dim, foggy).
- Falling of eyelids.
- Swallowing difficult, impeded, impossible; food lodges; obstruction when swallowing.

- Dryness in mouth.
- Weakness in extremities.
- Paralysis; paralytic weakness.

Homeopathic Remedies

- Botulinum (nosode)
- *Gelsemium sempervirens*
- *Arsenicum album*
- *Carbolicum acidum*
- *Nux vomica*
- Phosphorus

If you feel you have been exposed to a chemical release by terrorists where you live, here's what you must do:

1. Get to the emergency room of your local hospital as soon as humanly possible.
2. Call your homeopath immediately after you've gotten medical help.

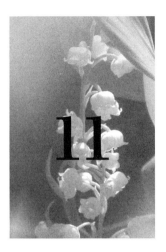

Nerve and Chemical Agent Attack

The following information comes from the Centers for Disease Control (CDC). I am providing the homeopathic information to help you deal with such a situation. If you feel you have been exposed by terrorists to a nerve/chemical release where you live, here's what you must do:

1. Get to the emergency room of your local hospital as soon as humanly possible or call your medical doctor immediately.
2. Check the following information for your symptoms. Call your homeopath immediately and take the homeopathic remedy s/he recommends because it most closely parallels your symptoms.

Types of Nerve Agents

Nerve agents listed by the CDC include those listed below. These are the types of gas that could be dispensed both on the ground and through the air. You can inhale them or come into skin contact with them.

- Tabun (GA)
- Sarin (GB)
- Soman (GD)
- VX gas

Note that all these have the same symptom picture and you may not know which one you've inhaled or come into contact with, but it doesn't matter. What matters is your symptoms.

Plain Talk on the Symptoms

Nerve agents acquired their name because they affect the transmission of nerve impulses in the nervous system. All nerve agents belong chemically to the group of organo-phosphorus compounds. They are stable and easily dispersed, highly toxic and have rapid effects both when absorbed through the skin and via respiration. Nerve agents can be manufactured by means of fairly simple chemical techniques. The raw materials are inexpensive and generally readily available.

Manifestations of nerve agent exposure include rhinorrhea (thin, watery discharge from the nose); chest tightness; pinpoint pupils (the pupils of your eyes contract and look like a small, black pinhead in size; they will *not* dilate when light is flashed into them but remain small and pinpoint); shortness of breath; excessive salivation (a lot of saliva coming out of your mouth) and sweating (skin perspiration); nausea, vomiting, abdominal cramps; involuntary defecation and urination (loss of control of your bladder and bowels; you pee and poop without control); muscle twitching; confusion (this is a mental symptom and you can have changing levels of consciousness; you can come in and out of it and will most likely behave like a drunk); seizures; flaccid paralysis (weakness of muscles; they won't respond and are too weak to lift); coma; respiratory failure; and death.

Nerve agents alter cholinergic synaptic transmission at neuro-effector junctions (muscarinic effects), at skeletal myoneural junctions and autonomic ganglia (nicotinic effects), and in the central nervous system (CNS). Initial symptoms depend on the dose and route of exposure (inhaling it or having skin contact with it).

Types of Homeopathic Symptoms

Homeopathic symptoms can be grouped into muscarinic effects, relating to the smooth muscles of the body, and nicotinic effects, relating to the skeletal muscles.

Muscarinic Effects

"Muscarinic" refers to the smooth muscles of our body, and the effects include pinpoint pupils; blurred or dim vision; conjunctivitis; eye and head pain; hypersecretion by salivary (a lot of saliva coming out of the mouth), lachrymal (tears watering from the eyes), sweat (perspiration on skin) and bronchial (coughing up a lot of mucus) glands; narrowing of the bronchi (like an asthma attack; we have trouble breathing); nausea, vomiting, diarrhea and crampy abdominal pains; urinary and fecal incontinence (we lose control of our bowels); and slow heart rate (heart beats very slowly, thuds along).

Homeopathic Symptoms

Abdomen
- Pain.
- Cramping, griping.

Bladder
- Involuntary urination.

Expectoration
- Copious expectoration.

Eyes
- Pupils contracted.
- Vision blurred, dim, foggy.
- Loss of vision; weak vision.
- Inflammation; conjunctivae.
- General pain.
- Profuse lachrymation.

Head
- General pain.

General
- Hypertension

Mouth
- Copious saliva.

Perspiration
- Perspiration in general.

Rectum
- Diarrhea.
- Frequent stool.
- Open, relaxed anus.

Respiration
- Asthmatic, difficult, impeded.
- Asthmatic cough.
- Feeling of oppression in chest.

Stomach
- Nausea, vomiting.

Homeopathic Remedies

- *Arsenicum album*
- *Belladonna atropa* (contains atropine)
- *Gelsemium sempervirens*
- *Mercurius vivus*
- *Digitalis purpurea*
- Phosphorus
- *Pulsatilla nigricans*

Nicotinic Effects

"Nicotinic" refers to our skeletal muscles, that is, the muscles attached to our bones. Nicotinic effects include skeletal muscle twitching, cramping and weakness. Nicotinic stimulation can obscure certain muscarinic effects and produce rapid heart rate and high blood pressure.

Homeopathic Symptoms

Chest
- Affections of the heart.

Extremities
- Twitching, weakness, cramps.

General
- Hypertension.

Homeopathic Remedies

- *Belladonna atropa*
- *Cuprum metallicum*
- Phosphorus
- *Arsenicum album*
- Sulphur

Small to Moderate Vapor Exposure

Relatively small to moderate vapor exposure causes pinpoint pupils, rhinorrhea (thin, watery discharge from the nose), broncho-constriction (like an asthma attack; you either cannot breathe or breathing feels restricted), excessive bronchial secretions (coughing up large or small quantities of phlegm/mucus from lungs) and slight to moderate dyspnea (shortness of breath).

Mild to Moderate Dermal (Skin) Exposure

Mild to moderate dermal exposure results in sweating and muscular fasciculations at the site of contact, nausea, vomiting, diarrhea and weakness. The onset of these mild to moderate signs and symptoms following dermal exposure may be delayed for as long as 18 hours.

Higher exposures (any route) cause loss of consciousness, seizures, muscle fasciculations, flaccid paralysis, copious secretions (from any orifice of the body; could be mucus, urine or fecal matter—loss of control over bowels), apnea (stops breathing for periods of time) and death.

Behavioral and Psychological Changes

Central nervous system agents cause behavioral and psychological changes in humans. CNS symptoms include irritability, nervousness, fatigue, insomnia, memory loss, impaired judgment, slurred speech and depression. High exposures may produce loss of consciousness, seizures and apnea (breathing stops).

Homeopathic Symptoms

Mental and Emotional State

- Irritability, anger, disposition to contradict, discontent; discouraged, quarrelsome, sensitive, unfriendly.
- Restless, nervous; restless activity; anguish, driving from place to place, delirium, excitement, fear, impatience, desire to wander.
- Weak memory, loss of memory, concentration is difficult, dementia, dullness.

- Has fancies, is confused and forgetful, has deficient ideas, makes mistakes.
- Does not recognize relatives, vanishing thoughts.
- Foolish behavior, behavior as if drunk.
- Sadness, despondency, dejection, mental depression, gloom, melancholy, brooding, delirium, despair, discouraged, dwells on things, grief, hypochondriasis; is inconsolable, sighing, weeping.
- Unconsciousness, coma.
- Stupor, stupefaction.

Physical Symptoms

General
- Weariness, flabby feeling, heaviness, lassitude; wants to lie down, relax, feels weak.
- Convulsions, convulsive movements.

Speech and Voice
- Disconnected speech.
- Foolish speech, talks as if drunk.

Extremities
- Convulsion, convulsive motions.

Respiration
- Intermittent Cheyne stokes respiration (sounds like snoring).

Homeopathic Remedies
- *Belladonna atropa* (contains atropine)
- *Hyoscyamus niger*
- Stramonium, datura
- *Opium* (can only be obtained through a homeopathic MD)
- *Mercurius vivus*
- *Atropinum purum* (this is homeopathic atropine)
- Phosphorus

Respiratory Inhalation

Respiratory inhalation (breathing in) of nerve agent vapors causes respiratory tract effects within a short time, from seconds to minutes. Symptoms include excessive rhinorrhea (thin, watery discharge from nose) and bronchial secretions (coughing up or hawking up large or small amounts of mucus), chest tightness and difficulty breathing due to constriction of bronchial muscles and mucous secretions. Respiratory failure may occur due to CNS depression.

Homeopathic Symptoms

Chest
• Tightness around chest, constriction.
Expectoration
• Copious.
Nose
• Thin discharge.
Respiration
• Difficult, asthmatic, impeded.
• Asthmatic cough, oppression in chest.

Homeopathic Remedies

• *Carbo vegetabilis*
• *Hepar sulphuris*
• *Iodium purum*
• *Laurocerasus*
• *Coccus cacti*

Cardiovascular Symptoms

Vagal stimulation may produce bradycardia (slow heartbeat, slow heart rate of beating), but pulse rate may be increased due to ganglionic stimulation. Pulse may be racing or feel faster than it should be (80 to 100 beats per minute is "normal"). The person may also experience hypoxia (oxygen starvation; the lungs cannot bring enough oxygen into your body). Bradyarrhythmias (slow beat of heart, but it will come and go) and hypertension (high blood pressure) may also occur.

Homeopathic Symptoms

Mental and Emotional State
• Stupefaction as if intoxicated, dullness, weak memory, labors with mental tasks, protration of mind (inability to think).

- Dullness of senses, torpor.
- Unconsciousness, as if in a dream.
- Unobserving.

Physical Symptoms
Chest
- Hypertrophy of heart.
- Arrhythmia.

General
- Hypertension.
- Pulse is frequent, accelerated, elevated, exalted, fast, innumerable, rapid.

Respiration
- Arrested, impeded, interrupted.

Homeopathic Remedies

- *Digitalis purpurea* (bradycardia)
- *Veratrum album*
- Phosphorus
- *Aconitum napellus* (bradycardia)
- *Crataegus oxyacantha*

Gastrointestinal Symptoms

Gastrointestinal symptoms (digestive symptoms) such as abdominal pain, nausea and vomiting are common manifestations of exposure by any route but may be the first systemic effects from liquid exposure on skin. If these symptoms occur within an hour of dermal exposure (this means you came into physical contact with it and it is on your skin somewhere), severe intoxication is indicated; you will appear "drunk". Diarrhea and fecal incontinence (loss of bowel control) may also occur.

Homeopathic Symptoms

Mental and Emotional State
- Stupefaction as if intoxicated, dullness, weak memory.
- Dullness of senses, torpor, unconsciousness as if in a dream, unobserving.
- Labors for mental tasks, prostration of mind.

Physical Symptoms

Abdomen
• General pain.

Rectum
• Diarrhea, frequent stool.
• Relaxed anus, open anus.

Stomach
• Nausea, vomiting in general.

Homeopathic Remedies

• Phosphorus
• *Apis mellifica*
• *Arsenicum album*
• *Veratrum album*
• *Nux vomica*

Ocular (Eye) Symptoms

Ocular symptoms (those referring to your eyes) may occur from local effects of vapor exposure and from systemic absorption. Pinpoint pupils and spasm of the muscle of visual accommodation (that is, ciliary muscle) lead to blurred and dim vision, aching pain in the eye and conjunctivitis.

Homeopathic Symptoms

Eye
• Pupils contracted.
• General pain, aching pain.
• Inflammation, conjunctivae.

Vision
• Blurred, dim, foggy.
• Weak vision, loss of vision.

Homeopathic Remedies

• *Belladonna atropa*
• *Aconitum napellus*
• *Pulsatilla nigricans*

- *Arsenicum album*
- *Rhus toxicodendron*

After-Exposure Symptoms

When you survive exposure to a nerve or chemical agent, you can expect potential sequela, that is, a potential condition following and resulting from the disease. Central nervous system effects such as fatigue, irritability, nervousness and impairment of memory may persist for as long as six weeks after recovery from acute effects. Although exposure to some organo-phosphate compounds may cause a delayed mixed sensory-motor peripheral neuropathy, there are no reports of this condition among humans exposed to nerve agents.

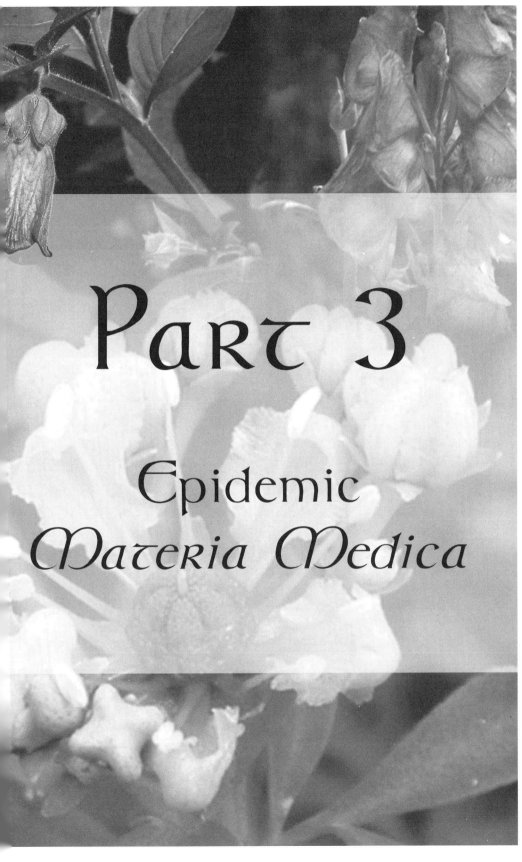

Part 3

Epidemic Materia Medica

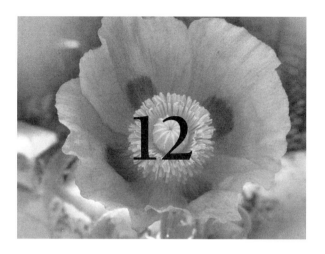

Homeopathic Epidemic
Materia Medica

All homeopathic *materia medicas* are composed of parts of the body—the mind, head, mouth, extremities and so on. The homeopathic remedies and the symptoms they will help are then listed.

The homeopathic remedies below do not present a complete picture but were especially chosen for their strength in combating acute and chronic ailments and also in fighting against the epidemics discussed in this book. There are many more remedies than are listed here, but you would have to purchase a complete *materia medica*, such as Boericke's (see Bibliography) for 450 of the 2000 remedies in our pharmacopoeia, to get even larger and more complete symptom pictures than those presented here.

I've chosen symptoms that correlate with epidemics, flu and other acute ailments most people deal with on a regular basis; the lists don't include all the symptoms under a particular remedy. Match your symptoms to the ones presented. If they fit, call your nearest homeopathic practitioner (if you don't have one, go to Appendix B and call the National Center for Homeopathy [NCH], since they have directories of homeopaths in the U.S.) and confer with him or her about your complete symptom picture. If the homeopath gives you permission to take the remedy, do so. If s/he doesn't, you should not take the remedy because there will be one that fits your symptoms more closely — but your homeopath can determine that. *It's important to work with a professional homeopath, especially if an epidemic occurs.* Find out about your local homeopaths and become a patient.

Aconitum napellus

The "personality" of aconite is one of suddenness, surprise, shock and trauma. This remedy, made from the herb bearing the same name, is of immense help to people who have suffered a heart attack or stroke. It is also used as a shock remedy if someone has had an accident and is in shock. This is one of the minor remedies for the hantavirus. It can also be used for those who experience any kind of shock, including bad news, a divorce, separation, getting fired from a job, move to another city or state and so forth.

Mentally, the person is restless and nervous. There might be an overriding fear of death or dying. It is one of the great remedies for panic attacks or anxiety attacks and also for posttraumatic stress disorder (see also arsenicum on page 209, *Mercurius vivus* on page 248, *Nux vomica* on page 254 and sulphur on page 266).

Aconite works especially well on any illness that comes on suddenly, without warning, or from a change in the weather. It is useful for severe hypotension, or loss of blood pressure, which is seen with invasive strep A, the flesh-eating bacteria, and is a secondary remedy for that condition when the symptom of loss of blood pressure is present with it. Whooping cough will respond to this remedy *if* it is caught *early* in the prognosis, within a few days of being infected and while the bacteria are still at the incubation stage and have not developed symptoms. It will not help in the latter stages.

Mental and Emotional State
Anxiety attacks; anxiety in general.
Dentist, fear of (give one hour before).
Earthquake remedy.
Fainting from fear.
Insomnia caused by fear or panic or after a shock/trauma; restless.
Panic caused by bleeding.
Panic attacks.

Shock from fear of any sort (or any kind of trauma that produces fear).
Surgery, fear of (give one hour before).

Physical Symptoms

Cold or fever, sudden onset of first stage.

Convulsions.

Cough: A croupy type, hoarse and dry with loud, labored breathing. Child grasps at throat every time she coughs; very sensitive to air breathed in, especially if it's cold air, then cough will
start again. Hot feeling in the lungs; blood may come up with
hawking or coughing.

Croup: If it does not work within two hours, try *Hepar sulphuris*
(page 236)—both are croup remedies.

Diarrhea due to hot weather or change in weather.

Disk that has slipped in back all of a sudden, with onset of severe
pains.

Earache: External ear will look bright red, painful and swollen. If
pain persists after an hour, check out hypericum (page 237)
symptoms.

Epileptic seizures if brought on by fright.

Eye inflammation or pain; excellent for any eye injury.

Headache that comes on suddenly and is violent, throbbing in
temples with a burning or bursting pain.

Hypotension, a sudden drop in blood pressure.

Larynx in throat very sensitive during any cough.

Lungs: Constant pressure feeling in chest, particularly the left side,
oppressed breathing with even the smallest motion. Shortness
of breath, worse after midnight.

Septicemia conditions (see *Crolatus horridus* on page 226, *Lachesis
muta* on page 244, *Pyrogenium* on page 262); get antibiotic treatment at the first sign of this condition.

Shock, postoperative.

Stroke aftermath (to calm patient).

Throat: A burning sensation or a dry, constricted sensation, with
prickling or stinging. Tonsils will be swollen and dry.

Vomiting from shock/trauma/fear of some sort.

Modalities

Better: In open air.

Worse: In a warm room, lying on the injured or affected side, from music, from tobacco smoke, dry/cold winds or drafts, in the evening and night.

Ammonium carbonicum

Carbonate of ammonia is formed during the putrefaction, or destructive distillation, of those organic substances that contain nitrogen. The anhydrous neutral carbonate can only be obtained by bringing together dry carbonic-acid and ammoniacal gases.

Ammonium carbonicum is for those who lead a sedentary life, have a slow reaction generally and are disposed to frequent use of the smelling bottle. *Ammonium carbonicum* is adapted to stout women who are always tired and weary, take cold easily in winter and suffer from cholera-like symptoms before menses and who lead a sedentary life. Dr. Gallavardin has cured uncleanness in bodily habits with *Ammonium carbonicum*.

Guernsey, a great 19th-century homeopath, said that this remedy was very useful in "delicate" women who fainted easily. Constitutionally, the *Ammonium carbonicum* woman is weak, with deficient reaction and of the lymphatic type (think of a woman who carries a lot of edema or water weight in her flesh). So this remedy is for a woman who does not exercise much, for example—a couch-potato type of woman. In Guernsey's experience, patients like this want stimulants; in his practice, they requested ammonia, camphor, musk and alcohol. At the onset of cerebro-spinal meningitis, Guernsey found, *Ammonium carbonicum* is an excellent choice of remedy for this type of person. It is definitely a stimulant; there's no question about that. By taking it, the vital force of the individual is "excited" into action and places her (or him) in a condition where the next remedy can be chosen as indicated by the symptoms.

Mental and Emotional State

Aggravation in evening and during wet weather.

Mental depression, anxiety, malaise. Cries a lot; hypersensitive. Sad, anxious, especially in the morning when the weather is damp, stormy; better at night. Weakening of the intellect, mainly the memory.

Talking and hearing others talk affects him greatly.

Temperament: Stout type, flabby, fatty, lymphatic, indolent, sedentary, weak and delicate although looking robust.

Another type, that of the woman fainting easily, needing camphor and music.

Physical Symptoms

Circulation: Affects the heart, circulation and blood; heart becomes weak; collapse. Circulation becomes sluggish; under-oxygenation of blood produces lividity, weakness and drowsiness. Vitality becomes low and there is lack of reaction.

It is adapted to fat patients with a weak heart, with wheezing and suffocative feeling; to stout women who are always tired and weary, take cold easily and suffer from cholera-like symptoms before menses and who lead a sedentary life.

Cough: Dry cough as from dust in the throat; cough either only at night or only in daytime.

General: The right side of the body is mostly affected; reappearance and aggravation of some symptoms from washing (bleeding of the nose, swelling of the veins of the hands, blue hands). Excoriation (burning) of the mucous membranes.

Limbs: Stinging and tearing pains. Tearing in the joints, relieved by the heat of the bed. Drawing and tension as from the shortening of the muscles. Inclination to stretch the limbs. Pain as of dislocation in the joints. Pains as from subcutaneous ulceration.

Debility that permits only to lie down. Disinclination to walk in the open air and from that aggravation of many complaints. Restlessness of the body in the evening.

Skin: Eruptions of a scarlet color. Itching eruptions, desquamation of the skin. Great sensitiveness to the cold.

Soreness: Very sensitive to cold air. Great aversion to water, cannot bear to touch it. Heaviness in all organs. Uncleanliness in bodily habits. Pains are bruised and sore. There is internal, raw burning.

Discharges are hot, acrid, adherent. Hemorrhages dark, thin. Prostration from trifles. Old age. Lies down because of debility or soreness of whole body.

Modalities

Worse: Right side; at night, from 3 to 4 AM; from cold, wet applications, washing, during menses.
Better: In dry weather; lying on the abdomen or on the painful side.

Antimonium tartaricum

This remedy is made from double tartrate of antimony and potassium. It is for anyone who experiences great exhaustion, drowsiness or debility when ill. *Antimonium tartaricum* is a premier lung and respiratory disease remedy—especially if there are a lot of rattling sounds in the chest with little expectoration (mucus) being coughed up, such as in whooping cough, or pertussis. It is especially useful at the stage of this disease when there's a lot of mucus and coughing. The greater the prostration of the person, especially from viral or bacterial complaints, the more this remedy should be considered in those situations—providing the symptom picture fits.

Physical Symptoms

Asthma: "Dry" type with above symptoms.
Dizziness brought on by coughing.
Lungs: Great rattling sounds due to loose mucus though very little is coughed up. Burning sensation in chest that rises into the throat. Coughing and gasping. Edema, or water in the lungs. Useful for bronchitis, pneumonia and emphysema.
Person is usually pale and tired looking.
Pulse is rapid, weak and trembling.
Shortness of breath.

Modalities

Better: From sitting up, from coughing up mucus/phlegm.
Worse: In the evening; from lying down at night; from warmth or from damp, cold weather; from sour liquids and milk.

Apis mellifica

One of the great allergy reaction remedies, apis is made from the venom of the honeybee. Where there is sudden, violent swelling of body tissue, apis should be considered. For anaphylactic reaction to any kind of allergy, apis can be used to save a life, if necessary.

Physical Symptoms

Allergic reaction: Bee sting allergic reaction; insect bite allergic reaction. Drug allergic reaction; food allergic reaction.

Extremities: Hands and feet swell; knees swollen/shiny looking; sensation of sore, stinging, burning pains.

Eyes: Lids swell and become red, inflamed; they burn and sting. A lot of watering from eyes, which might swell closed.

Face: Red, swollen with sticking pains; flushed red with burning heat and pain.

General: Bowel movement involuntary with any motion; feels as if anus is open and raw. Milk, craving for.

Head: Head or neck swelling; lips swollen; tongue swollen, fiery red, with scalding sensation in mouth and throat.

Herpes zoster with large blebs and stinging/burning; cool cloth helps.Incision, swelling of after surgery.

Lungs: Difficulty breathing, breathing hurried and labored; a feeling of suffocation and not being able to draw in another breath of air.

Pain, of a stinging or burning nature.

Skin: Swelling after bites, sore and sensitive; stinging sensation; red skin with burning sensation; puffing up of skin anywhere on body. Anaphylactic or allergy reaction, hives with intolerable itching. Sunburn.

Throat: Swollen; uvula swollen, tonsils swollen; entire area is red, swollen and puffy with a sensation as if a fishbone were stuck in throat. Everything is fiery red with a varnished, shiny look to the membranes.

Modalities

Better: In open air, with cold cloth/bath/shower.

Worse: Heat in any form (temperature/bath/cloth/shower), touch, pressure, after sleeping, in a closed or heated room, lying on right side. Symptoms always worsen in the afternoon.

Arnica montana

Made from a plant bearing the same name, there is probably no broader-based remedy than this one. Arnica's sphere is usually muscle injuries, but it also works particularly well on injured tendons, ligaments and inflammation around joints/bones. It is a premier remedy to halt hemorrhages, from acute nosebleeds to hemophilia.

Arnica ointment can be spread on the skin. If there is an open wound, place the ointment around the outer edges and it will instantly reduce swelling/bruising. *Never put arnica tincture or any arnica product into an open wound or laceration!* It is wonderful for fingers crushed in a car door or smashed by a hammer or for any other, similar type of blow to any part of the body (I would also use some hypericum to stop the pain). For a black eye, smear ointment around affected area, but never in the eye itself.

Physical Symptoms

Abscess with bluish color to it, deep inflammation and pain.
Black eye (use hypericum, page 237, if there is pain).
Concussion.
Dental operation (after root canals or any sort of surgery or extraction of a tooth; use hypericum if pain persists afterward).
Eyes bloodshot.
Fractures: Ledum (page 248) followed by symphytum will also aid in quick recovery and knitting of bone).
Injury: Improves and speeds healing.
Pain: Swelling or soreness associated with sprains, bruises, muscles, falls, fractures (use symphytum to mend the break itself) or any kind of blow resulting from an accident.
Shock, especially when there has been blood loss.
Spinal injuries (use hypericum if pain persists).
Stroke (belladonna, see page 212, may prove useful in tandem with arnica).
Tennis elbow or similar injury.
Wasp stings (if this does not work, see apis on page 206).

Modalities

Better: Lying down or having head lower than rest of body.
Worse: From touch, any motion, from resting, from damp cold, from drinking wine.

Arsenicum album

Arsenicum is made from arsenic poison. In the small doses utilized in homeopathy, it poses no threat to the individual taking it. This is one of the Ebola virus remedies. Invasive strep A, the flesh-eating bacteria, may also respond to this remedy, provided the symptoms match — get to the hospital immediately if this condition is suspected and take this remedy on the way there. *Arsenicum album* is also a noted posttraumatic stress disorder remedy. (See also *Mercurius vivus* on page 248, *Nux vomica* on page 254, sulphur on page 266.) People who need this remedy are often very restless in nature, a type A personality, hurried workaholics who get very short-tempered and impatient with others who don't move at the speed of light as they do.

Mental and Emotional State

Exhaustion brought on by nervous strain or stress.
Irritability.
Panic attacks, with great anxiousness about health state; insomnia after midnight, restless with anxiety.

Physical Symptoms

Asthma, wet or dry (worsens after midnight).
Chilly in the extreme; can't get warm enough.
Colds, later stages of.
Diarrhea, acute, from food poisoning.
Eyes swell, with tearing and burning sensation.
Flu with watering eyes/nose, chilled and extremely weak.
Hay fever with violent sneezing; not relieved by sneezing (if it doesn't stop within an hour, try *Allium cepa* or sabadilla).
Head pain of a bursting nature.
Hemorrhaging.
Herpes zoster eruptions.
Hiccough brought on by swallowing cold drinks or rise in temperature.
Septicemia conditions: Get to the hospital immediately if this condition is suspected and take this remedy on the way there.
Skin: Turns blackish color; red with heat or burning sensation or rash that is sudden and improves with heat application. Eruptions, scaly eruptions that burn and/or itch; bruising, ecchymoses.

Thirsty all the time for cold drinks despite sipping them often.
Vomiting black; vomiting blood.

Modalities

Better: Heat of any kind (cloth/blankets/bath/shower/tempera-
ture), from having head elevated and warm drinks.

Worse: Cold (cloth/bath/shower/temperature), cold food or cold
drinks; lying on the right side or being at the seashore; midnight, 1 AM or 2 AM.

Atropinum

Synonyms are atropia and atropine; the formula is $C_{17} H_{23} NO_3$.
Atropinum is an alkaloid obtained from belladonna, especially
from the root.

Mental and Emotional State

Appears profoundly intoxicated.
Complete unconsciousness of all preceding events.
Delirium alternating with stupor.
Epilepsy.
Frenzied with excitement and frantic in her appeals.
Great fear and anxiety.
Hallucinations: Of hearing and vision; spectral illusions (sees ghosts).
Incoherent in observations, although thoroughly wakeful.
Insisted repeatedly that her blood did not circulate and that her
feet must be put into warm water or she should die.
Langour (sluggishness) of body and mind, rendering person inca-
pable of active bodily or mental exertion.
Laughed in an idiotic manner.
Mind confused; commenced a sentence and forgot what she wished
to say.
Mirthful humor.
Muttering and smiling.
Quarrel; began to quarrel incoherently with his supporters.
Rambling speech.
Sad and morose, preferring solitude and a dark room to company
of friends.
Slight delirium, picking and other motions of hands and fingers in
air, as if they came in contact with real objects.
Wakeful and partially delirious all day.

Physical Symptoms

Albuminuria

Arms: Could not hold a vessel of fluid in his hands nor carry it to his mouth two weeks after; gouty affection of right wrist, with stiffness and want of feeling of fingers; hands cold after two hours; bending in of thumbs.

Back: Burning in back under sternum and in region of stomach. Spinal irritation, pressure causes pallor, nausea, belching and retching. Constant burning pains in back, under sternum and in region of stomach. A large portion of the spine was so sensitive that she cried out on pressure, turned pale and was as seized with nausea, belching and retching. Painful affections from spinal irritation. Locomotor ataxia (muscle incoordination).

Chills alternating with flushes of heat.

Diseased pancreas.

Exaltation of brain and spine, followed by prostration.

Gastric disorder.

Great desire for open air (faintness), very weak in the open air, giddiness and staggering; better from motion.

Head: Feeling as if the head was screwed up, walking causes the most severe sticking pains. Fine, drawing, very sensitive stitches across the forehead and temples. Dull pain in the temples, coming on at intervals of perhaps a quarter of an hour; very sensitive sticking in the left temporal region on walking in the morning; spasmodic winking.

Hyperesthesia of some nerves: Ophthalmic, auditory, olfactory, vaginal, spinal, solar-plexus, nerves of uterus and bladder.

Legs: Continual dragging of legs when assisted, or rather held up, in walking; stiffness in left knee and lower leg, in right great toe.

She said, her limbs "feel like sticks" and thought she could not use them to walk across the room to the sofa, but with aid she did so with considerable difficulty; edema of legs.

Limbs: Numbness, heaviness, paralysis of limbs. Numbness and heaviness in her limbs so great that she feared the results of going to sleep lest she should never awaken. Hands and feet cold and covered with cold sweat. From sleeping in a damp bed acute rheumatism, pain in all his limbs, which are swollen and red; no sleep, generally feverish and profuse sweat.

Ovarian neuralgia.

Skin: Dark red or mottled, efflorescent redness of the skin; numbness of the skin.

Violent stitches in base of brain, above eyes and in temples.

Baptisia tinctoria

Made from the herb wild indigo, this remedy played a vital part in the 1918 Spanish influenza. It is also one of the major remedies for the hantavirus.

Mental and Emotional State

Confused: Might appear drunken; stupor, coma, inability to think; delirium, wandering, muttering, indifference to others; unhappy or sad during stupor condition.

Physical Symptoms

Bowel movements bloody.

Diarrhea with blood.

Face: Has a stupid or slack expression to it; flushed and red looking.

Fever: High, with chills and soreness over body; heat all over with chills.

Flu symptoms with sore, bruised feeling; aching muscles; no position is comfortable.

Liver sore and swollen.

Lungs: Breathing difficult and a sense of suffocation.

Mouth odor fetid or with a rotting smell to it.

Septic, blood-poisoning states.

Skin burning and heat to it, liver spots all over body, ulcers.

Thirst, constant.

Throat sore with difficulty swallowing anything, liquid or food.

Tongue swollen and speech slurred.

Vomiting due to spasms in stomach.

Modalities

Worse: Humid weather and heat, fog; being kept indoors.

Belladonna atropa

Belladonna is made from the herb by the same name. It is for people who have a highly sensitized nervous system, who start if jarred, who are like barometers reacting instantly to any kind of change. This is another Ebola virus remedy, although not one of the major ones. Anyone who experiences a sudden onset of symptoms, no matter what they are, should think of belladonna and/or aconite (see page 202). This is also a whooping cough remedy. Belladonna people are like highly strung thoroughbreds and just as mettlesome at times.

Mental and Emotional State

Light, sensitivity to.
Noise, sensitivity to.

Physical Symptoms

Earaches: Chronic and continual (usually right ear), but can help prevent possible shunt surgery.
Eyes, bleeding from.
Fever high and sudden; spike fevers, especially in a child; use *Ferrum phosphoricum* (page 234) if belladonna does not cure this symptom.
Headache, pain of a bursting nature.
Hemorrhaging, rapid and bright red.
Insomnia; sleepy, yet unable to sleep.
Lactation: Milk flows too freely; breasts red, swollen, hot and might be stonelike.
Lungs: Cough is ticking, short, dry and worse at night. The larynx becomes very sore and feels as if something was lodged in it every time one coughs. Voice might become high and piping. Stitches in chest when coughing. Cough might become barking or whooping, with pain in stomach before the attack. Breathing is oppressed, rapid and unequal. Moaning with every breath.
Premenstrual tension: Spasm and pain of a sudden, violent nature in uterus; flushed face or burning/heat sensation. Acuteness of all senses, causing an emotional roller coaster at this time of month.
Sunstroke.
Teething in infants (also see *Chamomilla* on page 219).
Throat sore with congested head, high temperature and sweating.
Tongue swollen and fiery red.
Vomiting blood.

Modalities

Better: Sitting semierect.

Worse: Being touched, jarred; noise or sound; from draft; in the afternoon and when lying down. Symptoms worse usually around 11 AM or 3 PM, or they begin to worsen at 11 AM and grow worse through 3 PM and then begin to alleviate and get somewhat better.

Bellis perennis

Follows arnica (page 208) well, especially if arnica does not take care of swelling or bruising a week after the surgery or injury.

Bothrops

This is the venom of the yellow viper, or fer-de-lance, from the island of Martinique. It is one of the secondary remedies for the Ebola virus epidemic and can mean the difference between surviving or dying; it ranks fourth behind *Crolatus horridus* (page 226), phosphorus (page 257) and *Lachesis muta* (page 244).

Physical Symptoms

Eyes: Blindness during the day; sunlight is too intense to cope with so dark glasses must be worn all day; even more severely blinded by sunlight, vision is badly impaired; photophobia; loss of vision when there is no pathological condition for losing one's sight.

Pulmonary embolus.

Retinal hemorrhage.

Modalities:

Better: Right side.

Bryonia alba

Made from wild hops, this is a minor remedy for the hantavirus. It is known as the "grump" remedy, and when ill, these people want to be left alone; untouched; in a dark, quiet room. They will lie still beneath a pile of covers. Bryonia is one of the great migraine remedies of all time, along with *Gelsemium sempervirens* (page 235).

Mental and Emotional State

Angry and rebuffs efforts of people trying to help. Wants absolute quiet without interruption.

Any sound is irritating.

Irritable, wants to be left alone in a dark room, unmoving.

Physical Symptoms

Abdomen is swollen.

Asthma of the dry variety; dry, hard, painful cough so that he has to hold his chest.

Constipation: Stool is dry, hard and black.

Cough: Hard and dry, shakes whole body.

Eyes: Sore to touch and when moving them, a pressing, crushing or aching pain is felt.

Flu and cold: Flu symptoms with fever, thirst, exhaustion and aches all over, made worse by movement. Colds if onset is slow to develop.

Headache: Migraine-type start on forehead that moves to the rear of the skull, with vertigo, nausea, faintness on rising and confusion. Headache begins in occiput, the rear of the skull, and is worse on any motion; even moving the eyes increases the pain; migraines with dizziness, nausea and/or vomiting.

Indigestion: With headache that intensifies if one tries to sit up; vomiting of bile and water immediately after eating. Colic from ingesting rich or fatty foods; possible vomiting.

Liver is enlarged and sore, burning pain with stitches.

Lungs: Breathing is difficult, with quick breathing or panting; desire to take a long breath to try and expand lungs. Mucus in lungs is tough and hard and can barely be coughed up; cough worsens in warm room or temperatures, must press hand against sternum when coughing; bloody mucus coughed up.

Mouth, bitter taste in.

Stomach is sensitive to touch; pressure sensation in the stomach, as if there's a stone sitting in it.

Thirst: Excessive; will drink cold drinks during a fever chill, but warm drinks make patient feel generally better.

Throat: Dry, sticking pain on swallowing; scraped sensation to it.

Modalities

Better: Lying on painful side, rest with no movement whatsoever; dark room, quiet; cold things.

Worse: Warmth (cloth/bath/shower/temperature), any movement, in the morning, eating, hot weather, exerting oneself, sounds of any kind, company when sick, sitting up (they get faint-feeling and nauseated); symptoms are always worse around nine o'clock in the evening.

Cantharis

Made from Spanish fly, this remedy is utilized for bladder problems. It also works in the reproductive and sexual area. If there is violent inflammation in any of these regions, then cantharis should be considered.

Physical Symptoms

Bladder: Infections, cystitis, frequent and intolerable urge to urinate accompanied with burning sensation; painful urging to urinate. Bloody urine, by drops; tremendous straining to urinate. Urine has scalding, burning sensation when it does come out; constant desire to urinate.

Burns, minor or first degree, that are relieved by cool cloth being applied.

Diarrhea, bloody stools with straining and burning sensation.

Feet, burning in soles.

Modalities

Better: Rubbing the affected area.

Worse: From touch, or approach; urinating, drinking cold water or coffee.

Carbo vegetabilis

This remedy is made from charcoal from vegetables. It is one of the premier suffocation and coma remedies. Whooping cough, at the early stage, will respond to this remedy. It is one of the few remedies that can help those who have "never been well since" their flu or cold or any other ailment to fully recover (also see *Gelsemium sempervirens* on page 235).

Physical Symptoms

Asphyxia, or suffocation, face blue mottle and cold sweat, puffy (use this after airway has been unobstructed). Particularly good for those who have a near-drowning experience, to be given on way to hospital.

Bleeding: Steady seep of dark-colored blood.

Cough: With rattle and itching sensation in throat; possible gagging or choking up of mucus. Itching sensation in larynx while coughing. Hoarseness, especially in the evening. Cough worsens at night.

Heartburn, sour belching or vomiting of food.

Hoarseness, worse in evening.

Indigestion: Burping, swollen abdomen, gas — especially after eating fatty foods or drinking wine.

Lungs: Gasping for air/breath; feels oppression in chest with a sore, raw feeling. Burning sensation in chest when coughing.

Salty foods, desire for.

Sweets, desire for.

Modalities

Better: From belching, from fanning oneself with something; cold temperature, wind, shower/bath/cloth.

Worse: In open air; from eating/drinking fat, butter, coffee, milk; warm or damp weather; symptoms always get worse in the evening and at night.

Carbolicum acidum

Also called carb-ac, phenolum, carbolic acid, phenol, monoxy benzine, phenic acid or phenyl alcohol, this is a solution in rectified spirit; trituration.

Physical Symptoms

Abdomen: Flatulence (bloated), frequent occurrence of coliclike pains, sinking feeling all over abdomen. Jolting during driving the car unpleasantly affects the abdominal organs, which feel hot and sore. Constant belching up of wind from stomach;

acid eructations and formation of gas, feels better by pressing hand on stomach. Rumbling and rolling in abdomen with sense of distension; dependent on imperfect digestion; smelly farts and stool.

Bladder: Passes mucus from rectum while urinating.

Face: Dusky (red-colored) face; pale about nose and mouth.

Head: Disinclined to mental work. Muddled and confused feeling in head. Tight feeling as if compressed by a rubber band, better with green tea and smoking. Orbital neuralgia over right eye; headache better with green tea, while smoking. Headaches appear at the time of menses; pain as if a hot ball was in forehead; scalp tender. Dull, heavy pain running from forehead to occiput. General mental and physical lassitude. Dull, heavy pain through temples, with bandlike constriction over forehead; the whole head feels hot. Brain appears compressed as in a tight bandage. Worse by noise, walking across room; better in fresh air. Monthly headache before, during or soon after menses.

Rectum: Constipation with retraction of abdomen. Shreddy stools; diarrhea like rice water, terrible odor. Constipation with very offensive breath. Bloodylike scrapings from the intestines; straining; diarrhea; stools thin, black, putrid.

Stomach: Fermentative indigestion with bad taste and breath; constant belching, nausea; vomiting, dark olive green. Heat rises up esophagus. Flatulent distension of stomach and abdomen; painful bloating, often marked in one part of the bowel. Nausea and vomiting, sea sickness, dark, olive green. Heartburn, sore stomach with bad breath and taste. Chronic vomiting, sarcinae (type of bacteria) in vomit; vomiting of everything taken into stomach, often with great restlessness, nervous vomiting.

Total loss of appetite, but desire for stimulants. Constant belching up of wind; regurgitation from stomach. Intense nausea and heartburn after raising a sort of sweetish-sour liquid. Sensation of warmth in pit of the stomach region; heavy weight in the pit of the stomach with constant inclination to relieve himself by fruitless efforts at eructations or by pressing the hand into the pit of the stomach. Incarceration of gas in abdomen; rumbling and rolling in abdomen; insufficient, sluggish stool.

Throat: Spasmodic and painful contraction of esophagus with inability to swallow; soreness of throat on empty deglutition; choking feeling in throat with disposition to hawk up phlegm.

Chamomilla

Made from German chamomile, a daisy, this remedy is a boon to all mothers who have children going through the "teething" stage. Colic is another area of expertise for *Chamomilla*—it has helped many a parent with a cranky, inconsolable child through this stage.

Mental and Emotional State

Nerves in turmoil; nothing is tolerable.

Physical Symptoms

Colic: Draws legs up and in great pain; stomach badly swollen.
Diarrhea: In infants, associated with teething; with slimy, green stools.
Earache with severe pain, made worse with application of heat.
Insomnia: Sleepless or restless first part of night.
Pain-sensitive.
Teething: Painful; irritable and/or feverish; convulsive fit in anger.

Modalities

Better: From being carried, warm, wet weather.
Worse: By heat of any kind, anger, open air, wind or draft; all symptoms are worse at night.

China officinalis

Also known as cinchona, this remedy is made from the bark of the Peruvian tree in South America and was used extensively in the 1800s for the malaria epidemics that ravaged Europe.

Physical Symptoms

Diarrhea: Acute, frequent, painless bowel movements that tire individual; can result from eating too much fruit.
Ears have a ringing noise.
Fainting caused from loss of blood.

Fever: A three-phase type with chills, severe shaking, fever; followed by sweating, thirst and exhaustion.

Hemorrhage, postpartum.

Menses: Dark clots with abdominal swelling, profuse and with pain.

Nosebleed: If it doesn't stop within 10 minutes, switch to *Ferrum phosphoricum* (see page 234).

Modalities

Better: Bending over, hard pressure to the affected area; open air; warmth (cloth/blanket/shower/bath).

Worse: Slightest touch, draft of air; periodicity of every other day; bending over; loss of vital fluids (electrolytes or dehydration); after eating; all symptoms are worse at night.

Coccus cacti

This remedy is made from the dried female insect, *Coccus cacti*, or cochineal. The insect, N. O. *hemiptera*, is native to Mexico, Peru, Central America, Spain and the West Indies. The remedy comes in form of a tincture and triturations.

Mental and Emotional State

Depressed, apprehensive and anxious.

Fit of unconsciousness and absence of mind.

Great indolence.

Ill-humored, fretful.

Lively, talkative mood.

Physical Symptoms

Breathing: Respiration somewhat laborious, with fatigue of vocal organs; difficult breathing, labored; shortness of breath.

Chest: With the chest troubles, there is much labored breathing. Bruised pain in left clavicle region, worse from motion; stretching-like pain in upper part of left chest, near clavicle; feeling as if a plug of mucus was moving in chest. Sensation of burning, soreness or pressure beneath sternum; stitches in upper part of chest. Soreness and pain of whole chest, worse at superior portion; oppression of lower part of chest, difficult breathing. Pressure upon chest, with hoarseness. Spasmodic difficulties of chest, with renal (kidney) pains; transient, very painful stitches, at times in left, at times in right side of chest. Sudden pulmonary (lung) congestion, with profuse mucous secretion and spasmodic suffocative cough. Accumulation of mucus in chest, difficult to raise, nearly causing strangulation and vomiting of food.

Cough: Cough with expectoration of much viscid albuminous mucus, draws out in long strings. Has expectoration of large quantities of viscid, stringy or albuminous mucus at the end of each spell of coughing.

He cannot walk without bringing on difficult breathing; he cannot ascend a height without suffocation. After the quantities of mucus are cleared out, the cough is better and he goes on for two, three or four hours before another one of these awful attacks comes on. Attacks are apt to be worse at night when he becomes warm in bed; if he can lie in a cool room without much covering, he will go longer without coughing.

The whooping cough is of a similar character. You will see the child lying in bed with the covers off. He wants the room cold, and the mother will tell you that if she can get to him quickly enough with a drink of cold water, she can ward off the paroxysm. The chest fills up with mucus until respiration cannot be carried on any longer and it must be cleared out, yet the child will resist and hold his breath to prevent coughing. You will be astonished to see how speedily *Coccus cacti* will change the character of that cough.

One of the earliest signs of improvement will be observed in the easier respiration. The cough becomes less violent; the retching passes away; and in a week or ten days, the cough will go too. Cough worse after eating, worse on waking, worse in a warm room.

Throat: Fatigue of vocal organs; even after speaking without exertion, the voice becomes rough and hoarse, respiration somewhat laborious; hoarseness.

Sensation as though a lump as large as a walnut was sticking behind larynx obliged him to swallow constantly; rawness of air passages, which frequently compels him to cough; tickling in larynx, very violent, waking him at 11:30 PM, causing cough with expectoration of much tenacious mucus for 10 minutes.

Scraping sensation in larynx, causing some paroxysms of cough, with expectoration of little balls of mucus. Scraping and dry feeling in larynx, worse toward evening, with hacking cough and hawking. Laryngeal irritation; feeling as of mucus ascending and descending trachea, causing tickling and cough, worse in a warm room, better in open air. Constant tickling in bronchi, caused by a feeling as if a plug of mucus was moving in chest, in spite of the profuse expectoration. Inflammation of the mucous membranes of larynx and air passages; chronic bronchitis; protracted bronchial inflammation of the mucous membranes remaining after whooping cough.
Urine turbid.

Coffea cruda

Made from the coffee bean, this remedy is well known for helping people who have a very low tolerance to *any* kind of pain. This remedy works primarily on the nervous system.

Physical Symptoms

Fainting from excitement; insomnia due to exhaustion or too much excitement.

Toothache aggravated by heat/hot fluids; could be an abscessed tooth; go to the dentist and find out.

Modalities

Better: Warmth of any kind (blanket/shower/bath/cloth/temperature), from lying down, holding ice cube in the mouth.

Worse: Excessive emotions (even joy; it doesn't have to be bad news), narcotics, strong odors, noise, open air, cold of any kind (shower/bath/cloth/temperature); all symptoms become worse at night.

Colocynthis

This remedy is made from the bitter cucumber and has a marked sphere of action involving spasms anywhere in the body. The person becomes extremely irritable and crabby due to the pain, which is a good symptom to indicate use of this remedy.

Physical Symptoms

Colic: Writhes or twists in pain; can't lie still.

Diarrhea: Colicky pains.

Menses: Cramplike pains that can double one over in order to relieve.

Modalities

Better: Doubling over, hard pressure on affected area; warmth of any kind; lying with head bent forward.

Worse: From anger, from humiliation or indignation; all symptoms worsen at 6 AM or from 4 PM to 5 PM.

Conium maculatum

The common name for *Conium maculatum*, N. O. *Umbelliferae*, is poison hemlock. The remedy is a tincture made from the fresh plant in bloom.

Mental and Emotional State

Delirium.

Derangement of ideas and mania; confusion of ideas as from drowsiness.

Hypochondriacal indifference.

Hysterical anguish, with sadness and great inclination to weep, from suppression of or from too free an indulgence in the sexual instinct.

Ill humor and moroseness.

Inaptitude for labor.

Irritability and disposition to be angry.

Superstitious ideas.

Timidity of character (fear of robbers); disposition to be frightened.

Want of mental energy; slowness of conception.

Wants to be alone and yet is afraid of solitude.

Weakness of the intellectual faculties and of the memory; ready forgetfulness, excessive difficulty of recollecting things.

Physical Symptoms

Arms: Shoulders painful, as if they had been bruised and excoriated. Humid, scabby and burning tetters in the forearms.

Back: Backache; weakness and lameness in small of back and general lassitude, worse on bending backward or after a short walk, with nausea and weakness. Ill effects of bruises and shocks of the spine, worse when laughing, sneezing to taking a quick breath. Staggering gait; coldness of limbs.

Bones: Sensation as if bones of upper and lower extremities were surrounded by tight bands. Periostitis, with throbbing and burning pain, as if from an ulceration; worse in morning and at night, also when standing, lying or lifting the part; better when letting limbs hang down and from notion, right side or left upper and right lower.

Hands: Weary, heavy, trembling, unsteady; numbness of the hands and especially of the palms of the hands. Cracking in the wrist joint. Sweat in the palms of the hands. Inactivity of the fingers; itching in the back of the fingers; yellow spots on the fingers and yellowish nails.

Heels: As if bone would push through them; shooting pain in heels.

Legs: Drawing pains in the hips. Arthritic pains in the knee, tearing and tensive; aggravated on beginning to walk after sitting down, with a sensation as if the tendons were too short. Restlessness and heaviness in the legs; weakness in the knees; cracking of the knee joints; painful swelling of the legs and of the feet; red spots on the calves of the legs, sometimes painful, becoming subsequently green or yellow as after a blow or bruise and impeding the movement of the foot, which is drawn back as if the tendons were contracted; cramps in the calves of the legs. Coldness and strong disposition to take cold in the feet (even from a slight exposure of the feet).

Limbs in general: Weak lower limbs, as if paralyzed; cracking in knee joint. Can walk straight and steadily with eyes closed, but staggers, becomes giddy; is nauseated when walking with open eyes. Heaviness and sense of weariness in all limbs; limbs feel bruised; paralyzed feeling in all limbs. Difficulty in using limbs, unable to walk; unpainful lameness, trembling of limbs; weakness and debility, especially of arms and legs. Shooting pains through arms and legs. Paralysis of lower, afterward of upper extremities, or the reverse; numbness of fingers and toes, the former looking as if they were dead. All the joints pain as if beaten; piercing and tearing pains through extremities and in joints, particularly in elbows and hip joints. Coldness of hands and feet.

Paralysis from periphery upward to spinal cord; general paralysis of involuntary muscles, weakness of legs and tottering gait; painless lameness; muscular palsy without spasms. Vision of fixed objects good, but accommodation sluggish. Acute ascending spinal paralysis (case of Socrates).

Shoulder: Shoulders feel bruised; clothes lie like a weight on them; axillary (armpit area) glands enlarged.

Crataegus oxyacantha

The common name for *Crataegus oxyacantha*, N. O. *Rosacea*, is Hawthorn. The remedy is a tincture made from the ripe fruit.

Mental and Emotional State

An unusual rush of blood to the head with confused feeling, followed by a feeling of quiet and calmness mentally.

Confused feeling, followed by a feeling of quiet and calmness mentally.

Despair, feels weak and fragile.

Hurried feeling with rapid action of heat.

Irritability, crossness, melancholy.

Mental dullness.

Physical Symptoms

Chest: Painful sensation of pressure in left side of chest below the clavicle.

Fingers and toes blue.

General: Cardiac neuralgia, palpitation, vertigo; irregular and intermittent pulse, with increased rate. Despondency and anxiety. Extremely labored breathing on slight exertion, usually accompanied with pain in the region of the heart. Mitral regurgitant murmur. Nervous indigestion with constipation from a weakened condition of the lower bowel. Great exhaustion from slight mental or physical exertion. Albumen and excess of phosphates in the urine. Swelling of hands and feet, with a feeling of prostration. Affections of the heart following attack of inflammatory rheumatism; valvular deficiency with or without enlargement.

Head: Rush of blood to the head, with confused feeling and followed later by a feeling as of quietness and calmness mentally.

Heart: Faintness and collapse; heart failure in hypertrophy and valvular disease. Palpitation and rapid action of heart; angina pectoris. Pain above and to left of stomach. Pulse strong and forcible, indications of hypertrophy. Very tender spot left side of spine. Hypertrophy from overexertion, from alcoholic, venereal and other excesses. Heart dropsy.

Skin: Excessive perspiration. Skin eruptions; burning, smarting eruptions on back of neck, axillae and chin; worse with heat and sweating and better with washing.

Stomach: Sensation as of fullness and weight in the stomach.

Throat: Sensation as of dryness and burning in the throat, accompanied by a slight, dry spasmodic cough caused by a tickling.

Modalities

Worse: Excitement, exertion, warm room.
Better: Fresh air, quietness, rest.

Crolatus horridus

This is the venom of the rattlesnake; it is the number-one remedy for the Ebola virus (Zaire, Sudan and Marburg) epidemic. (See also phosphorus on page 257, *Lachesis muta* on page 244 and bothrops on page 214; all are secondary but very important remedies to back up *Crolatus horridus*.) Interestingly, during the Spanish influenza, or the Great Flu, of 1918, which killed 22 million people globally and 500,000 people in the U.S., this was the major remedy that saved lives from this killing flu virus. Now we can use it again *if* the Ebola viruses, which are from the filovirus family, become epidemic and sweep across the U.S. or any other country. *Crolatus horridus* is also the leading remedy for invasive strep A, the flesh-eating bacteria, and in the 1900s, it was used with great success against deadly yellow fever, the plague, cholera and scarlet fever. Match your symptoms against those listed below on your way to the hospital—get help immediately if you suspect you have this condition and take the remedy on the way there!

Mental and Emotional State

Delirium that ranges from weeping mood, agony and despair to irritation; might cycle rapidly over a matter of hours.

Irritability; greatly emotional, with weeping; perception and memory clouded. Very impatient. Sadness predominates, might turn very talkative with a desire to escape.

Physical Symptoms

Bleeding: Without the ability to clot; from the abdomen, rectum or urinary tract; internal, anywhere in body.

Blood: Decomposing rapidly; bright red and won't clot. Coughing up blood.

Bowel movement: Stools bloody, bright red (bleeding from rectum); dysentery (diarrhea).

Face: Has masklike look, without any emotion or expression; zombielike, with puffiness apparent. Lips swollen and numb feeling. Leaden color and yellow face. Bleeding from eyes, bleeding from ears and "stopped up" feeling in right ear.

Fever: With flushes of heat all over body, sweaty and then chilled/cold.

Fingernails: Blood oozing from beneath.

General: Collapsed states in general; convulsions; delirium tremens; epilepsy seizures, *grand mal* and *petit mal*. Gangrene anywhere on body. Hemorrhage from every orifice in the body, including eyes, nose, ears, mouth, via urination or bowel movements; skin breaks open and bleeds without reason. Liver disorders, phlebitis, septicemia of all types. Spasms, jerking, convulsing of arms and legs. Swallows only with great difficulty.

Headache: At back of skull, throbbing; may extend over eyes; with pain and heat.

Heart: Palpitations with fever.

Mouth: Salivary glands bloody or frothy, large amounts of saliva in mouth; odor moldy smelling.

Nosebleeds: Uncontrolled, with black and stringy blood emerging.

Skin: Bruising appears on skin for no apparent reason. Has purple spots on it; eccymoses. Red-colored skin, yellow color to skin, blackish. Tender or sore feeling to it, tears and bleeds easily, has red pimples or eruptions/spots.

Throat: Sore, dry, swollen and dark red, with a feeling of tightness or constriction. Gangrenous with massive swelling. Cannot swallow any food but can swallow water; spasms of the esophagus.

Tongue: Enormously swollen, bright red, bleeding, swollen. Speaking difficult.

Vomiting: Black, bloody red or green.

Modalities

Better: Rest; head and stomach symptoms better in open air.

Worse: In morning upon waking or waking up in the night; eye pains in evening, from motion or exertion of any kind; cold air on throat; all symptoms are worse in the evening and in the morning.

Cuprum metallicum

Made from copper, this remedy sees action in spasmodic kinds of symptoms, including the rales of coughing with whooping cough. It is one of our great epilepsy remedies.

Physical Symptoms

Asthma, worse at 3 AM, with spasms and constriction alternating with spasmodic vomiting.

Convulsions.

Cough: Has a gurgling sound to it and is made better by drinking cold water. Whooping cough is better by sipping water.

Epilepsy.

Hands: Cold with cramps in the palms.

Legs: Cramps in calves of legs and soles of feet.

Lungs: Spasm and constriction in chest, with asthma and alternating with spasmodic vomiting. Spasms at the back of the tongue.

Muscular jerking and twitching.

Stomach: Cramping, preceded by hiccoughs.

Thirst for cold drinks, but a gurgling sound when swallowing liquid.

Modalities

Better: During perspiration or sweating, drinking cold water.

Worse: Before menses, from vomiting, physical contact; all symptoms worsen at night, particularly around three o'clock in the
morning.

Datura stramonium

The common names for *Datura stramonium*, N. O.
Solanaceae, are thorn apple, Jamestown weed or stinkweed. The
latter name stems from the plant's growing in the vicinity of cul-
tivation on rank soil where refuse is deposited, in all parts of the
world. The remedy is a tincture made from the fresh plant in
flower and fruit.

Mental and Emotional State

Delusions: Are present; hears voices during sleep; believes herself
all alone, abandoned; child jumps up with a start, believes he
is going to fall and clings desperately to his mother. Imagines
all sorts of things, that she is double, lying crosswise; in delirium desire to escape.

Rages reach the point of loss of control. Delirium is particularly wild and often associated with terror. The subject
wants to clutch hold of companions, uttering frantic cries;
holds out the arms as if seeking solace; adopts a kneeling posture; makes constant chewing movements.

Terrifying hallucinations obtrude; sees snakes, cats, bugs,
dogs and so forth at his side, coming out of the ground. Sees
"double," where he seems to have two bodies or an extra limb.

Desire for light and company.

Mania: Disposed to talk continuously; talks incessantly and ab-
surdly. Child is very cross and strikes or bites.

Sadness: Is a prominent feature associated with the desire for
company and sunshine. It may afflict especially in the evening
in bed and be accompanied by thoughts of death and copious
weeping. The subject is very adversely affected by darkness
and solitude, but curiously enough manifests a fear of brightly
glistening objects, such as light reflected from a mirror or anything suggesting water.

Sleep: Deep, stupid sleep.

Physical Symptoms

Arms: Convulsive movements of arms above head; convulsive movements of arms and hands. Contractile pain in arm, with acute lancinating in forearm. Distortion of hands, clenched fists, cramps in hands, trembling of hands, numbness of fingers.

Back: Liability to undue sensitivity of the spine, especially in the cervical region; drawing pains occur in the spine and also in the thighs.

Cold: General coldness of the whole body; chills, with great sensitiveness to uncovering. Skin icy cold and covered with cold sweat. Hands and feet livid; face, hands and feet blue and cold; limbs cold.

Extremities: Twitching of hands and feet, of tendons; trembling of limbs, they fall asleep; jerking in legs, as from a shock, with retraction. Violent, distracting pain in left hip when abscesses form; pain in muscle of outer side of right hip. Drawing pains in thighs; legs bend when walking (falls over own legs). Feet tremble; contractile cramps in feet.

General: Painless with most complaints. Twitching of single muscles or groups of muscles, especially of upper part of body. Spasms of the esophagus

Sweat: With thirst. Cold sweats over whole body; oily sweat.

Modalities

Worse: During perspiration, after sleep; when first awakens from sleep will shrink away as if in fear; in the dark, in solitude.

Better: In company.

Digitalis purpurea

Digitalis purpurea, N. O. *Scrofulariaceae*, comes in form of a tincture prepared from the leaves of a second-year plant known as foxglove.

Physical Symptoms

Arms: Paralytic pullings (tension in arms) and tearings (pain) in the arms; heaviness or paralytic weakness of the left arm.

Sharp pain in left shoulder and arm, tingling in arm and fingers, with heart affection.

Chest: Sensation of soreness in the chest. Respiration painfully restricted, especially at night, when lying down; or in the day, when walking or seated; in the morning. Suffocating constriction of the chest, forcing the patient to rise up in the bed. Pressure on the chest from keeping the body bent. Tension in the chest, with necessity to breathe deeply; contractile pain in the chest, when sitting with the body bent; smarting in the chest. Sensation of weakness in the chest, proceeding from the stomach; congestion in the chest. Shuddering or trembling of the breasts.

Face: Pale, deathlike appearance and bluish-red. Blueness of skin, eyelids, lips, tongue; cyanosis (oxygen starvation). Distended veins on lids, ears, lips and tongue.

General: There are three main symptoms in the digitalis pathogenesis that should be borne in mind: (1) slow, weak, irregular and intermittent pulse; (2) enlarged, sore, painful liver; (3) white, pasty stools.

Prostration from slight exertion; sensation as if the heart would stand still if he moved; must hold the breath and keep still. Sensation as if the brain were loose, as if something fell forward in the head on stooping, as if the brain were made of fine glass and shattered at a blow; as if something were running out of urethra; as of a weight attached to stomach; as if the internal parts were grown together; as if the lungs were constricted and tied up in bundles; as if heart stood still, as if heart had torn itself loose and were swaying to and fro by a thin thread; as if the stomach would sink into abdomen.

Terrible pain at root of nose after vomiting; discharged blood coagulates slowly or not at all.

Hands: Nocturnal swelling of the right hand and of the fingers. Coldness of the hands. Tearings in the joints of the fingers. Sudden and paralytic stiffness in the fingers; torpor and disposition to numbness of the fingers.

Legs: Pain in the hip joint. Great stiffness in the legs after being seated, which abates when walking. Want of energy and paralytic weakness in the legs. Swelling in the knee, like a sebaceous cyst is present.

Incisive pain in the thigh and burning sensation in the calf of the leg on crossing the legs. Tension in the hamstring muscles of the thigh. Coldness of the feet; swelling in the feet, by day only (diminished at night).

Pulse: Full, irregular, very slow and weak; intermittent every third, fifth or seventh beat.

Respiratory: Hoarseness in the morning after a night sweat. Hollow, spasmodic cough from roughness and scraping in the throat. Expectoration (only in the evening) of yellow, jellylike mucus, tasting sweet.

Hoarseness and a runny nose in the morning. Much phlegm in the larynx, which is detached by a slight cough.

Cough after a meal, with vomiting of food; dry cough, with pains in the shoulders and arms; cough with expectoration of matter resembling starch.

Smarting in the chest on coughing. Cough worse at midnight and during the morning hours.

Cough caused by talking, walking, drinking anything cold, when bending the body forward. Troublesome choking sensation with cough, mostly at night and on physical exertion.

Dry, cramplike cough, excited by prolonged conversation. Sanguineous expectoration on coughing (small quantities of dark blood).

Drosera rotundifolia

This remedy is made from the sundew plant; it acts primarily on the respiratory tract. One of the leading whooping cough remedies, it saved many lives before the use of antibiotics was introduced.

Physical Symptoms

Asthma: When talking, followed by contraction of the throat with every word. Voice might become deep, toneless, cracked; it might require a great deal of effort to speak.

Cough: Spasmodic; one cough follows the next without relief or reprieve so can hardly catch breath between attacks. Cough is deep and hoarse sounding. Harassing cough in children as soon as they lie down to go to bed at night. Sensation as if there were dry bread crumbs in the throat or as if a feather was tickling there. Yellow mucus with blood from the nose and mouth. Retching while coughing. Rough, scraping feeling in the upper mouth and back of throat.

Fever: With cold feeling inside of body; might shiver with hot face, but hands are cold. There is no thirst. Always cold, even in bed.

Lungs: Can hardly get a breath in or out due to rapid-fire coughing.

Modalities

Worse: Lying down, on getting into a warm bed, drinking, singing or laughing; all symptoms are worse after midnight.

Echinacea angustifolia

Made from the herb purple cone flower, this is a hantavirus remedy. It is also a flu remedy par excellence, especially when there is considerable muscleache. This remedy is powerful in addressing septic states of any type of blood poisoning (also see *Pyrogenium* on page 262), gangrene or even venom infections.

Mental and Emotional State

Confused and depressed, along with dizziness and profound tiredness.

Physical Symptoms

Chest: Muscles are painful; pain beneath sternum.

Face: Aches that are accompanied by a flushing in the face. Nosebleeds, particularly from right nostril; foul-smelling discharge from nostrils in general.

Fever: Spikes, come and go with great chilliness accompanied by nausea. Cold chills all over back.

Extremities: Arms and legs ache with great fatigue.

Mouth: Gums bleed easily; salivation is heavy and constant. Tongue dry and swollen, white coating of tongue with red edges.

Skin: Has boils, ulcers or gangrene.

Stomach: Has sour belching along with heartburn and nausea. These symptoms are better if lying down.

Throat: Sore and ulcerated. Tonsils might be purple or black looking.

Urination: Scanty, infrequent and involuntary.

Modalities:

Better: By lying down, by bending double.
Worse: After eating, from exposure to cold air.

Eupatorium perfoliatum

Made from the herb thoroughwort, *Eup. perfoliatum* is a wonderful flu remedy, particularly for a full-blown case of the flu with all the accompanying aches and pains.

Physical Symptoms

Cough: Chronic and loose; associated with flu.
Eyes: Eyeballs painful when pressure is applied.
Fever: Associated with the flu; with chills, thirst, sweating. Is highest at 7 to 9 AM. Flu symptoms of bone/joint pain, stiffness, restless with thirst.

Modalities

Better: By talking with someone, by getting on hands and knees.
Worse: From motion; all symptoms worsen between 7 AM and 9 AM.

Ferrum phosphoricum

Made from iron, *Ferrum phosphoricum* should be considered immediately when getting a cold or flu. If none of the symptoms have set in yet, this remedy can stop a cold or flu from developing! But it is important to take it *before* symptoms manifest. Also, it is an excellent remedy to take if a cold or flu has dragged on a long time. Anemia responds to this remedy. It is a great cure for fever.

Physical Symptoms

Abscesses, early inflammation of.
Bleeding: Bleeding from menses bright red and clots readily, same with bleeding from a knife or razor cut. Nosebleed, especially in children but also in adults.
Cough: Hard, dry with a tickle; chest aches from it.
Earache, early stages of.
Fever: With slow onset; pale but with red cheeks.

Flu, early stages of.
Head: Early stages of head cold. Throbbing headache that feels better with cool cloth.

Modalities

Better: Application of a cold cloth.
Worse: Touch, jarring, motion, right side; all symptoms worsen at night, particularly between 4 AM and 6 AM.

Gelsemium sempervirens

Made from the yellow jasmine shrub, *Gelsemium sempervirens* is known as the "relapse remedy"—any kind of relapse, whether it is acute or chronic. For instance, reappearance of a cold, flu, bronchitis or pneumonia can be prevented with this remedy. Chronic fatigue syndrome is often helped by this remedy, which is known to stop a relapse from occurring. *Gelsemium sempervirens* was one of the major remedies that saved lives during the Spanish influenza in 1918 in our country.

This is the premier remedy to consider when any kind of paralysis is involved, whether acute or chronic, no matter what the disease. It acts upon the central nervous system and is particularly helpful with polio and chronic fatigue syndrome, after strokes when there is paralysis or for any other type of injury to the spinal nerves. *Gelsemium sempervirens* is a hantavirus remedy.

Mental and Emotional State

Depression after the flu, pneumonia or any other debilitating ailment.
Listless or anxiety over forthcoming ordeal/stress.
Fear, paralyzed with it.

Physical Symptoms

Chronic fatigue syndrome.
Cold: Of summer variety from change in weather; might have chills up and down spine.
Eyes: Eyestrain, eyeballs sore. Lids droop and feel heavy. Vision dims.
Face: Hot, flushed and dull-looking or droopy. Lower jaw may be dropped, the mouth open and hanging. Tongue is numb, thick, coated yellow and will tremble or be paralyzed.

Fever: With chills up and down the back. Heat and sweating stage is long and exhausting; wants to be held because shaking so much; shivering. No thirst, will not want liquids in any form but must drink fluids or risk dehydration or electrolyte imbalance. Head is very hot with headache, wants it dark and quiet.

Hay fever: Eyes hot and heavy. Sneezing, throat tickling and dry. Pain in ear(s) if swallowing.

Head: Headache as if band around the head; hammering at back of head. Heaviness and droopy quality of eyelids. Migraines with vertigo, with dull ache; pain in temples extending into the ear or beginning at the base of the skull and involving the neck and shoulder region.

Heart: Sensation that they must move around or it will stop beating.

Limbs: Arms and legs have excessive trembling, shaking or a feeling of dragging weights. Incredibly heavy sensation to the limbs; stiffness.

Measles: With very high fever or delirium.

Menopause: When periods are late and scanty, heaviness in womb as if being crushed or squeezed. Neck is stiff, tight with a bruised sensation; shoulders drawn upward and can't relax.

Shivering.

Skin: Hot, dry, itchy with measleslike eruptions.

Throat: Sore, swollen, difficulty in swallowing with pain shooting from throat to ear when swallowing; no thirst. There may be a sensation of a lump in the throat that cannot be swallowed away.

Modalities

Better: From urinating, fresh air, bending forward, moving around and drinking stimulants such as coffee or tea.

Worse: During damp, rainy or humid weather; before a thunderstorm or front coming through. From receiving bad news or receiving news that excites them too much or thinking of their ailment; symptoms worsen around ten o'clock in the morning.

Hepar sulphuris

Made from calcareum sulphide, this remedy should be considered for people who, like the plaster of paris the remedy is made from, build walls to hide behind to protect themselves from the pain of the world around them. In the event of any kind of thick, yellow mucus discharge, this remedy should be used. It is an excellent whooping cough remedy in the latter stages, where mucus is thick and won't be coughed up.

Physical Symptoms

Cough: Suffocating-type of cough, croupy; mucus is thick, ropy, yellow or yellow-green in color; worse upon walking. Dry, hoarse cough that starts up if patient is uncovered or gets cold or chilled; might start up if something cold is eaten. Choking cough, mucous refuses to come up. Croup (if it doesn't work within an hour, try aconite [page 202]).

Ears: Earache, stitching-type pains. Sore throat, desire for heat. Nothing pleases.

General: Cold sores. Gums bleed easily, teeth sensitive to touch. Raynaud's phenomenon.

Lungs: Breathing is anxious, with wheezing sounds. Worse in dry, cold air and better in damp or humid air.

Nose: Ulcerated or sore.

Skin: Any kind of lingering skin condition that may have eruptions or boils, festers easily.

Modalities

Better: In damp weather, from wrapping head up, from warmth of any kind (shower/bath/cloth/temperature).

Worse: Dry, cold winds; cool air (air conditioning); slightest draft. Touch, lying on painful side.

Hypericum perforatum

Made from the herb Saint-John's-wort, this remedy's sphere of influence is primarily the body's nervous system. Dental pain is especially helped. *Hypericum perforatum* is an excellent remedy for crushed fingers or toes, after operations or for any injury involving the central nervous system or the motor nerves of the body.

Physical Symptoms

Bell's palsy (seventh facial nerve in face).

Burns: Relieves pain; one can use ointment form or take tablets.

Concussions of brain or spine.

Earache.

Eye injury.

Fractures: Takes away pain. Use arnica (page 208) to reduce swelling and finish up with *Bellis perennis* (page 214).

Hemorrhoids.

Insect bites/stings if there is pain shooting upward from bite/sting; if not, use apis (page 206).

Pain: Any nervelike pain associated with any type of trauma such as crushed toe or finger, skin abrasion, postoperative pain.

Teeth: Dental surgery of any kind; use before and after surgery. Kills pain after tooth extraction.

Wounds: Puncture, incised or lacerated.

Modalities

Better: Bending head backward.

Worse: In cold weather, dampness, fog; in a closed room. Least exposure to touch.

Hyoscyamus niger

A tincture is made of the whole fresh plant of *Hyoscyamus niger, L.* The action of hyoscyamus is often intermittent, whereas that of stramonium (page 229) continues; hyoscyamus has angular motions, whereas stramonium has graceful motions.

Mental and Emotional State

Delirium: Without consciousness, does not know anybody and has no wants (expect thirst). Loss of consciousness with eyes closed and raving about business. Delirium, sometimes with trembling; fits of epileptic convulsions. Delirium, sees ghosts, demons and so on. Wandering thoughts. Perversion of every action.

Hysteria: It is called for when the mental condition of the patient exhibits marked jealousy; she is talkative, nervous, full of suspicion, troublesome, but not maniacal. Well-marked, sudden twitchings and jerkings of groups of muscles; one arm will twitch, then the other. The motions are all angular. The head falls from side to side. There is a great deal of frothing at the mouth. The patient seems to be wild. She laughs at everything in a silly manner. She is sleepless or sobs or cries during sleep.

Mania: With loss of consciousness or with buffoonery and ridiculous gestures. Lascivious mania and occasional mutterings, uncovers his whole body.

Melancholy (depressed): Melancholy from unfortunate love, with rage, or inclination to laugh at everything. Fear of society (anthropophobia); suspicious; anguish and fear. Fright followed by convulsions and starts from sleep. Desire to run away from the house at night. Fear of being betrayed or poisoned.

Disposition to make a jest of everything. Loquacity (is talkative); talks more than usual, more animatedly and hurriedly. Jealousy with rage and delirium. Unfortunate love with jealousy, rage and incoherent speech. Peevish and quarrelsome humor. Rage, with desire to strike and to kill. Unconscious, with plaintive cries, especially on the slightest touch, and complete apathy. Loss of memory.

Physical Symptoms

Epilepsy: It is one of the most reliable remedies we have for epileptic convulsions, that is, if there is no other remedy indicated.

Suddenly starting jerking and twitching of single groups of muscles; one arm will twitch, then the other. The motions are all angular. During the paroxysm, the face is distorted and is apt to be of a deep red color, almost purple. Hunger appears before the attack, especially the children wake up from sleep hungry. There is a great deal of frothing at the mouth and biting of the tongue. The patient seems to be wild.

General: Chorea (twitching muscles); it is indicated in patients who are very weak, with tottering gait. Clutching motions of the hands and numerous incoherent muscular movements. Paralysis with constant tremor of muscles. They seem to have abnormal impressions of distances. They reach for something that seems to be within their grasp, when in reality it is on the other side of the room. It has well-marked local jerkings and twitchings of groups of muscles. In children convulsions from fright.

Extraordinary sinking of strength. Inflammation of internal parts, spasms and convulsions. Convulsive twitching, with thrashing about of hands and feet. Effects of taking cold and cold air. Epileptic attacks, terminating in deep, snoring sleep. Complaints are intensified in the evening and after eating and drinking.

Head: Confusion and heaviness of the head. Vertigo as from intoxication or with obscuration of the sight. Attacks of cerebral congestion, with loss of consciousness and snoring (with delirium, answering all questions properly, pupils dilated).

Headache, as from concussion of the brain. Pressive and numbing pain in the forehead, especially after a meal. Headache when walking as if brain was shattered and shaken. Sensation of fluctuation or of commotion in the brain, especially when walking. Pressive, stupefying headache, especially in forehead, occurring in alternation with needlelike stitches, particularly on left side. Forehead feels as if screwed inward. When coughing, sticking in head over right eye. Violent, throbbing headache, waking him at night, with throbbing carotids (sides of neck); headache in base of brain, brain feels as if loose; constrictive obstruction in the forehead.

Congestion of blood to the head. Red, sparkling eyes; face purple-red, worse in the evening. Heat and tingling in the head. Inflammation of the brain with unconsciousness, heat and tingling in the head. Violent pulsation in the head, like waves; the head shakes. Worse from becoming cold and after eating; better by bending the head forward (stooping) and from heat. Heat of the head, with general coldness of the body, without thirst. Liable to catch cold in the head, principally from dry, cold air. Headache alternately with pain in the nape of the neck. Waving or shaking of the head from one side to the other, with loss of consciousness and red, sparkling eyes.

Intermittent fever: It is indicated when the chill spreads from feet to the spine and thence to the neck and is worse at night. Weak or thready pulse, great prostration. The lowering of the temperature is accompanied by slow arterial action, drowsiness or by delirious and excited talk. Picks at the bed, at clothing. Fears being poisoned; hallucinations. Fibrillar twitchings and so on.

Paralysis: It is indicated in paralysis of one or more muscles following maniacal attacks.

Ignatia amara

Made from the St. Ignatius bean, this is the premier "grief remedy." Grief of any kind, as long as it is still on the surface and not buried, can be alleviated and shortened with use of this remedy. Anyone who hates cigarette smoke is a candidate for this remedy.

Mental and Emotional State

Hypersensitive to emotions, pains or odors; car fumes, tobacco; may sigh more than normal.
Hysteria brought on by any kind of situation.

Physical Symptoms

Fainting after an upset.
Headache: Head feels elongated, throbbing in center.
Hiccoughs caused by emotional upset, eating or smoking.
Insomnia.
Nerves: From sudden shock or trauma; "goes to pieces."

Modalities

Better: While eating, change of position.
Worse: In open air, after meals, drinking coffee, smoking and liquids.

Iodium purum

This is iodine, an element, used in form of a tincture.

Mental and Emotional State

Cross, irascible, peevish.
Delirium.
Excessive mental excitement with great susceptibility.
Fear, shuns persons; anxious apprehensions.
Fixedness, immovableness of thought.
Heart palpitates "like lightning" when thinking of real or imaginary wrongs.
Hesitation and irresolution.
Illusions of moral feeling.
Indolence of mind, with great repugnance to all intellectual labor.
Loquacity and immoderate gaiety.

Restless agitation (with inclination to move about), which will neither permit the patient to remain seated nor to sleep. Irresist-
ible impulse to run. Feels she will fall if she walks.

Sudden maniacal impulses to murder.

Tearful disposition and mental dejection; depression, sadness,
heartache and anxiety.

Physical Symptoms

Arms and hands: Pains in the bones of the arms, worse when lying down and disturbing the sleep. Weariness in the arms in
the morning in bed. Convulsive movements and trembling of
the arms, hands, fingers. Numbness of the fingers, tearing
pains in the fingers, jerking of the tendons of the fingers. Inflammation of finger or toe. Constant coldness of the hands,
which are covered with a cold sweat during labor. Picks at
bedclothes obsessively.

Breathing: Insupportable hoarseness and tingling in the throat,
especially in morning; voice becomes deeper. Membranous
croup, with wheezing and sawing respiration. Dry, barking
cough, especially in children with dark eyes and hair; child
grasps throat with hand. Croup, with much mucous expectoration, sometimes streaked with blood.

Inflammation of the throat, of the larynx and trachea, with
contractile pain of excoriation; pain in the larynx, with discharge of hardened mucus; contraction and heat in the larynx.
Increased secretion of mucus in the trachea, with frequent
hawking.

Chest: Dry cough, with pressure, shooting and sensation of burning in the chest. Cough in the morning; cough with expectoration of abundant and sometimes sanguineous mucus. Pains
in the chest and fever. Rattling of mucus in the chest, with
roughness under the sternum and oppression of the chest.
Cough resembling whooping cough, excited by an insupportable tickling in the chest, with anguish before the paroxysm
and excessive emaciation.

Difficulty of respiration; labored breathing; difficulty of ex-
panding the chest on taking an inspiration; suffocation. Shooting pain in the left side upon breathing. Loss of power to
breathe, especially upon going upstairs. Weakness of the chest;

congestion in the chest; burning, shooting tension in the skin covering of the chest.

Feet: Cramps in the feet, especially at night; jerking of the tendons of the feet; edematous swelling of the feet; acrid and corrosive sweat on the feet.

General: Liver, worse upper part of right lung.

Erratic pains in the joints; chronic rheumatism in the joints, with violent pains at night, without swelling. Sensation of torpor in the limbs; convulsive starting and twitching of the tendons. Distortion of the bones; pains in the bones at night. Trembling of the limbs, tottering walk.

Swelling and hardness of the glands. Hemorrhage from different organs. Powerful overexcitement of all the nervous system. Ebullition of blood and pulsation over the whole body, increased by the slightest exertion. Great weakness, even speaking excites perspiration. Atrophy and emaciation until reduced to the state of a skeleton (with good appetite); emaciation, ending in malnutrition, of glandular tissues (breasts, testicles, thyroid gland and so on). Edematous swelling, even of the whole body.

Legs: Cramplike pains in the legs when seated. Heaviness, swelling, trembling and paralysis of the legs; rheumatic tension in the thighs and knees. Inflammatory swelling of the knee, with tearing pains and suppuration; hot, bright red swelling of the knee with inflammation, pricking and burning; worse by touch and pressure; dropsical swelling of the knee; white swelling of the knee.

Modalities

Worse: In the night, before eating, fasting before breakfast. From wrapping up the head; can't even bear wearing a hat. Lying in bed, lying on the painful side. From food difficult of digestion. From outward pressure (as pressure of clothes and so on), in a warm room. When walking quickly. From warmth in general, in warm air, when getting warm in the open air.

Better: After breakfast, after eating (especially after eating bountifully); in a cold place, in the cold air; from uncovering the head; after rising from the bed.

Ipecacuanha

Made from the ipecac root, this remedy's sphere of action is nausea and vomiting. This is one of the minor whooping cough remedies and may help when there is bleeding.

Physical Symptoms

Asthma attack with constriction around the chest, shortness of breath, wheezing cough.

Bleeding: Bright red and hemorrhaging; bleeding from lungs with nausea; nosebleed.

Cough: Is constant, violent and with every breath. Coughing with blood coming from nose and mouth. Suffocative cough, and child or adult might become blue in the face.

Face: Eyes have blue rings beneath them.

Fever: Irregular, with heat and nausea.

Mouth: Much saliva is present.

Lungs: Chest seems full of mucus, but it won't come up with coughing. Bleeding in the lungs from coughing too much. Bubbling rales of coughing. Rattling sounds in lungs.

Nausea: Isn't relieved by vomiting; vomiting with constant nausea and face may be pale and twitch.

Pregnancy: For nausea and/or vomiting.

Sleeps with eyes half open.

Modalities

Worse: From eating veal; moist, warm wind; lying down.

Lachesis muta

Made from the venom of the Surukuku, or bushmaster, snake of South America, this is one of major Ebola virus epidemic remedies and can mean the difference between surviving or dying from it. (See "The History of Pandemics and the Ebola Virus," page 31; *Crolatus horridus*, page 226; phosphorus, page 257; and bothrops, page 214 for further information.) *Lachesis muta* is also one of the major remedies for invasive strep A, the flesh-eating bacteria. If you suspect this condition and if your symptoms match this remedy, take it on the way to the hospital—get immediate antibiotic treatment for this condition!

Mental and Emotional State

Highly talkative; unable to be coherent about time; can become very irritable and nasty, with a sharp tongue.

Sad in the morning, might be restless or uneasy and doesn't want to go anywhere; wants to be left alone.

Can't stand wearing tight clothes, especially around neck or waist.

Physical Symptoms

Alcohol: Craving for.

Fever: With hot flushes, but chilly in the back and feet are ice-cold.

Hemorrhage.

Hypotension: A sudden drop in blood pressure.

Lungs: Breathing almost stops upon falling asleep, sensation of suffocation or strangulation when lying down.

Menopausal hot flashes (See sepia, page 88).

Mouth: Gums are swollen, bleed easily and are spongy looking; tongue red, dry and swollen.

Nosebleeds with sensitive nostrils.

PMS symptoms: Mental, emotional and physical before onset of menses.

Septicemia conditions: *Seek immediate antibiotic treatment!*

Skin: Has a blue or purple appearance to it, hot and sweaty. Black and blue bruising and swellings. Bruises appear. Blackish colored skin, reddish colored skin.

Sleep: Patients sleep into aggravations of their symptoms. Sudden "starts" just as falling asleep. Sleepy and yet they can't fall asleep.

Stools: With blood in them, might look like charred straw with black particles in it.

Throat: Throat region has a sensation of a plug moving up and down; sore on the left side and worse swallowing liquids (but not food). Very dry, swollen; membranes may be reddish or blackish. Mucus sticks and can't be swallowed or coughed up. Tonsils and throat purple colored. Can't stand anything tight around the neck. Larynx is especially sensitive; can't stand anyone touching his throat or neck. Dry, suffocating types of cough with a tickling sensation in throat.

Venom poisoning by any insect or reptile.

Vomits black or red blood.

Modalities

Better: With discharges (mucus, coughing and so on), warmth (blanket/cloth/temperature).

Worse: Sleeps into aggravations, ailments appear during sleep. Left side; in the spring; warm bath. Pressure or constriction of any kind, especially clothing. Hot drinks. All symptoms worse at night and in the morning upon waking.

Laurocerasus

The common name for *Cerasus laurocerasus* is cherry laurel or common laurel. This remedy contains hydrocyanic acid; consequently, many of the symptoms are similar to those produced by that acid.

Mental and Emotional State

Aggravation in the evening.

Fear and anxiety about imaginary evils, despondency; insensibility and complete loss of sensation.

Loss of consciousness, with loss of speech and motion; dullness of senses.

Weakness of mind and loss of memory; inability to collect one's ideas.

Physical Symptoms

Breathing: Slow, feeble; moaning or rattling; almost imperceptible; panting; very difficult, labored breath, with sensation as if lungs would not be sufficiently expanded or as if pressed against spine. Spasmodic oppression of chest; gasping, suffocating spells, clutches at heart, palpitation.

Chest: Spasm of chest, veins of hands distended. Threatening paralysis of lungs; pleurisy if small bronchi are irritated. Suffocative cough; pain in pleura severe and localized. Pulse soft, but quick.

Coughs and spits a great amount of phlegm, sprinkled over and through with distinct clots of blood.

Pains in external parts of thorax on moving; burning in chest on taking an inspiration. Slow, weak, anxious respiration; rattling, snoringlike respiration; obstruction to respiration in region of stomach; asthmatic respiration as if lungs were incapable of being sufficiently dilated or as if they were paralyzed.

Pressure on chest; constriction of chest, with oppression; burning and stitches in chest. In lung affections where the patient coughs and spits a great amount of phlegm, which is sprinkled over and through with distinct dots of blood; the dots may be close together or considerably scattered.

Coldness of inner parts, heat of single parts; internal chilliness and external heat.

General: Want of reaction; vital powers are low; want of vital heat.

Internal inflammation.

Limbs: Painless paralysis of the limbs. Drawing and tearing pains in limbs. Pinching with sensation of tearing; stinging and tearing in the limbs.

Lungs: Acute suppuration of the lungs; suffocation, sickness, drowsiness.

Skin: Turns blue. Toe- and fingernails become knobby.

Spasmodic and continuous contraction of muscles; muscle spasms. Convulsions, with foam before the closed mouth; convulsive and spasmodic jerks, by fits.

Sphincters: Lack of power in regard to the action of the sphincters.

Throat: Scraping in larynx, with increased secretion of mucus, hoarseness. Spasmodic constriction of trachea; spasmodic infection of the larynx, heart affected. Hoarseness, roughness and scraping in throat and pharynx (back of throat); deep bass voice; spasmodic constriction of the trachea (windpipe).

Little, short cough, excited by a tickling and scraping in throat; abundant gelatinous expectoration with small specks of blood.

Trembling, especially of hands and feet, during exercise in open air.

Vital energy: Want of vital energy and of reaction; sense of fatigue in whole body; a slow, weak pulse. Weak, apathetic, lies in bed in morning; sudden weakness with excessive nervous dejection; fainting. Painlessness accompanies the symptoms; painlessness of the ailments.

Modalities

Better: At night and in the open air he feels better; in general better from sleep.

Worse: In the evening.

Ledum palustre

Made from the herb marsh tea, *Ledum palustre* works in the realm of puncture and nail wounds.

Physical Symptoms

Animal scratches or bites.

Black eye or any type of bruising.

Cold feeling of a persistent nature, lacks "animal heat," yet finds the warmth of a bed unwelcome.

Fractures: Can interchange with arnica (page 208) and ledum to reduce swelling and absorbed blood.

Insect bites.

Wounds always have a cold feeling to them.

Modalities

Better: From cold, putting feet in cold water.

Worse: From heat of bed; all symptoms worse in the evening.

Mercurius corrosivus

This remedy, *Mercurius corrosivus sublimates*, or corrosive sublimate, is used in form of a trituration or solution. Its chemical name is mercuric chloride, $HgCl_2$.

Mental and Emotional State

Anxiety, preventing sleep.

Depressed, low-spirited.

Ill-humored, during which nothing pleases, alternating with hilarity; greatly depressed, very ill-humored.

Stupor and delirium.

Weak intellect, he stares at persons who talk to him and does not understand them; mind sluggish, with torpid digestion.

Physical Symptoms

Arms: Arm much swollen up to shoulder, red and covered with vesicles (fluid-filled blisters). Rheumatic pains in left shoulder and shoulder blade. Deltoid muscle feels relaxed.

Coldness: Feeling of coldness, especially of head. Shivering, provoked by slightest exercise and also by open air (even when weather is warm); sometimes with cutting pains and rectal spasms and pain. Heat on stooping and feeling of relief on raising the body again.

Dysentery.

Fever: Pulse small, weak, intermittent, sometimes trembling. Chilliness from least movement and in open air, generally with colic; chilliness in evening, especially on head; chilliness at night in bed; heat when stooping and coldness when rising.

General: Painful drawings in the bones (like those that precede an intermittent fever) with heat in head. Pain in bones of upper and lower jaws. Inflammation of lymph glands.

Twitches, convulsive contractions; convulsive twitching of muscles of face, arms and legs; convulsions of limbs. Violent starts, with shaking of whole body, on going to sleep, trembling. Paralysis of upper and lower extremities. Lies on back with knees bent up.

General edema.

Glandular swellings.

Great debility.

Hands: Gray color of nails.

Legs and feet: Lower extremities drawn up in bed. Sticking pains in hip joints during rest, better in motion. Stitches in right hip joint. Sensation as if legs had gone to sleep. Muscles of thigh and calf feel relaxed; cramps in calves. Feet icy cold.

Skin: Burning and stinging heat in skin; great heat of skin at night with anxiety, preventing rest. External heat with yellowness of skin.

Surface cold and covered with profuse perspiration, especially on forehead; cold perspiration, often only on forehead. Clammy, cold perspiration, offensive, toward morning. Whole skin covered with cold perspiration, with anxiety; night sweat.

Burning and redness of skin, with formation of small vesicles. Severe and stubborn eczema of sweating parts of body; rash; ulcers.

Smallpox.

Swelling of glands (neck).

Naja tripudians

From the cobra (reptilia class, order squamata, suborder colubrina, family elapidae) comes this remedy, in form of a preparation where the snake's venom is utilized to make a tincture and triturations.

Mental and Emotional State

Affected easily by wine or other alcoholic drinks.

Comatose.

Forgetful: Very forgetful, absent-minded.

Insensible and speechless.

Loss of consciousness.

Mind: Wandering of the mind. Stupid and confused feeling; consciousness almost of being quite lost.

Sadness: Sad and serious, irresolute; melancholia, makes himself wretched brooding over imaginary wrongs and misfortunes. Better in the evening. Sadness with irresolution; with distress about sexual organs; with headache and inability for exertion as if everything were done wrong and could not be rectified; with increased perception of what one ought to do and uncontrollable inclination not to do it, causing restlessness.

Suicidal insanity.

Physical Symptoms

Breathing: Stertorous and difficult. Cough with tightness and fullness in larynx; irritation and tickling in larynx and trachea. Hoarseness; short, hoarse cough; short, puffing cough every minute, at 4 PM. Dry, hacking cough. Blood spitting; spitting of blood that had no tendency to coagulate. Expectoration of whitish, viscid mucus in morning on waking. Respiration very slow, shallow and scarcely perceptible; labored and difficult; gasping for breath.

Chest: Uneasiness and dull, heavy pain in chest. Lancinating pains, worse on deep inspiration.

Asthmatic constriction of chest, cannot expand lungs; followed by mucous expectoration.

Pain in left pectoral muscles in forenoon; occasional pain on top of both breasts. Most acute pain and oppression in chest as if a hot iron had been run in and a hundred-weight put on top of it; instantly better by hartshorn and water.

Heavy pain over lower half of right chest with stabbing on deep inspiration; cannot cough for the stabbing. Worse lying on left side, better lying on affected side. Dull pain to right of sternum; tenderness over sternum and in throat.

General: Ptosis and paralysis of the iris, with profuse diarrhea. Purple sores on the lips, gums and tongue. Pupils slightly dilated. Skin clammy and disagreeably cold.

Pulse: Languid, thready and rapid; pulse imperceptible at the wrist.

It is also to be administered when there is impending paralysis of the heart and the patient is blue. He awakes from sleep gasping. The pulse is intermittent and thready.

Throat: It is indicated when the larynx is invaded. The patient grasps at the throat with a sensation of choking. The fauces are dark red. There is fetid breath and short, hoarse cough, with a raw feeling in the larynx and upper part of the trachea.

Modalities

Worse: Lying on left side, after sleep, after menses; air cold, air drafts; pressure of clothes; alcohol.

Better: Being in open air; sneezing; smoking.

Nitricum acidum

This is nitric acid, or hydrogen nitrate (HNO_3). Preparations are in form of dilutions with distilled water. Being sensitive to touch runs through the entire symptomatology, including the symptoms of the mind.

Mental and Emotional State

Anxiety: Anxious all day and especially in the evening and during night, as if engaged in disputes. Anxious about his disease, thinks he is going to die.

Despair: Easily affected. Inclination to weep; hopeless despair. The mind is weak, there are no ideas.

Discontent: Discontented with himself and inclined to weep violently; despondent and sad.

Excitability: Nervous excitability, peevishness. Irritable, fits of rage and cursing; inveterate ill-will unmoved by apologies;

quarrelsome. Easily excited, much affected by peevishness; easily irritated at trifles.

Thoughts: Difficult to exert the mind or to collect the thoughts; memory weak. If she exerts her mind, thoughts vanish.

Physical Symptoms

Abdomen: Very sensitive.

Bladder: Very offensive urine; frequent urging at night with scanty micturition. Stinging in the orifice of the urethra, burning and smarting during and after micturition. Urine cold when passed. Urine deposits a red sediment. Urine has a strong odor, like a horse's urine. Urine albuminous, with pain in the region of the kidneys; urine bloody. Chronic inflammation and ulceration of the urethra with burning and stinging pains; inflammation of the bladder.

Bones: Inflammation and painful sensitiveness of the bones; ulceration of the bones.

General: Sensitive to touch.

Head: Feeling of rush of blood to the head with much heat in head. Pulsating headache as if the head was tightly bound; better by actually binding the head tightly. Sharp, shooting pains in the head become better when lying down. Sharp pains in the head with great sensitiveness to noises. Pains as if in the bones of the skull. Pressing and drawing pains in the left side of the head, extending to the ears and teeth.

    The hair falls out freely. Moist eruption on the scalp. The scalp is sensitive, even to the pressure of the hat. Head is sensitive to the slightest jar, to the rattle of wagons in the street or even to the step of one walking across the floor. Head is very sensitive, even to the pressure of a hat; sensitive to combing and to being lain on.

Respiratory: Voice hoarse, especially after long talking, with scratching and stinging in the trachea.

    Cough usually short and dry, caused by a feeling of constriction in the throat; worse at night, preventing sleep until toward morning. Feeling as if the chest were tightly bound, often with stitches in the small of the back; dry, barking cough in the evening after lying down; cough causes anxiety and vomiting of mucus and food.

Stitches in the sides of the chest; whistling rales on inspiration. A feeling of soreness in the chest when coughing and breathing; chest seems filled by a rush of blood, with heat and anxious palpitation.

Skin: General yellow complexion. Dark spots, like freckles. Redness and heat in the hands and feet as though they had been frozen or like chilblains. Stinging or burning pains in old ulcers or in warts; burning, itching, stinging, shooting, lancinating, splinterlike pains in ulcers, worse at night.

Discharges thin, acrid and offensive, of a brownish or dirty yellow color. Gangrene blisters on toe; scabby, moist, itching, offensive eruption, paining as from splinters when touched. Humid, stinging eruption on top of the head and temples, also in beard; bleeding easily when scratched and feeling very sore when lain on. Single burning, moist sores on scalp. Burning, itching or stabbing pains, worse at night, from change of weather or during perspiration.

Dryness of the skin; itching nettle rash, also on face and especially in open air. Blackness of pores; reddish-brown spots (scattered over body, especially in dark-haired people) and deep-colored freckles in skin; copper- or violet-colored spots.

In a moderately cold temperature, limbs become as if frozen, inflamed and itching. Skin cracks; wounds and ulcers, with lancinations as by splinters or with burning pains (especially when they are touched), which bleed easily. Ulcers with sanguineous and corrosive suppuration; pains in old scars in a change of weather; tightness of skin; swelling of lymph glands.

Stool: Profuse discharge of blood; constant pressing in the rectum without any evacuation. Long-lasting pains that are very exhausting. Diarrhea, frequently slimy, offensive, green, acrid. Stools bloody, with tenesmus, fever and headache; stools consist only of mucus, with cutting pains and straining, also with burning in rectum; constipation with evacuation of hard, scanty masses, with burning and cutting in the rectum and anus. Following the stools great irritability of mind and general exhaustion.

Throat: Inflammation and ulceration of the throat, with white patches and sharp pains as from splinters, on swallowing. Constant desire to hawk mucus from the throat, with sharp, stinging pains and with soreness as if raw and ulcerated.

Swallowing difficult on account of inflammation and sharp, stinging pain; violent, shooting pain on swallowing; extends to ears and causes a wry face.

Modalities

Worse: Night, touch, during perspiration, walking.
Better: Open air, when riding in a car.

Nux vomica

Made from the poison or marking nut, which contains strychnine. This is the "addiction remedy" that can help someone say no to an addictive substance, whether it is cigarettes, social drugs or any other kind of addictive substance. It is also a well-known posttraumatic stress disorder remedy (see also aconite, page 202; arsenicum, page 209; *Merc. viv.*, page 248; sulphur, page 266). *Nux Vomica* is also a great indigestion remedy. It is a "modern life" kind of remedy, especially for type A personalities. When a person parties a lot, overeats and drinks too much alcohol, this is the remedy to consider.

Mental and Emotional State

Insomnia occurring after mental strain or cannot sleep after 3 AM; mental strain.

Nerves: Constantly frustrated, critical, fussy and hypersensitive.

Premenstrual tension with flashes of anger/temper, irregular cycle plus pain during first couple of days.

Physical Symptoms

Colds from exposure to cold weather/wind.

Colic from overeating.

Constipation.

Cough: With gagging, retching; feverish and chilled.

Diarrhea from indiscriminate eating, alternating with constipation.

Eyes: Photophobia (sensitivity to light).

Fainting from sight of blood or from strong odors.

Hay fever: Long bouts of unrelieved sneezing, nose stuffed all night. Irritation of eyes, nose and face; if it doesn't work within an hour, consider arsenicum (page 209).

Headache: With vertigo or feeling as if head were split with a nail.

Hemorrhoids, itching.

Indigestion due to excessive eating or drinking with heartburn one to two hours after eating.

Travel sickness, nausea, along with splitting headache.

Vertigo, with loss of consciousness momentarily.

Modalities

Better: After taking a nap, in the evening; while at rest; in damp or wet weather; from strong pressure on affected part.

Worse: From mental exertion; after eating too much; from touch; spicy food, stimulants of any kind, narcotics or social drugs; dry weather, cold. All symptoms worse in the morning, starting about three or four o'clock.

Opium

Opium is the gummy exudation of the unripe capsule of the poppy, *Papaver somniferum*, N. O. *Papaveracea*. It is used in form of a tincture.

Note: Per FDA law, in the U.S., only MD/homeopaths are allowed to carry this particular remedy. Unfortunately, no other type of homeopaths are allowed to have *Opium* in their practice.

Mental and Emotional State

Contradictions: Carelessness or great anxiety and uneasiness; inconstancy and fickleness. Strong tendency to take alarm and timorous character; rash and inconsiderate boldness.

Tranquillity of mind, with agreeable reveries and forgetfulness of sufferings. Stupidity and imbecility; loss of consciousness.

Ideas: Great flow of ideas, with gaiety and a disposition to indulge in sublime and profound reflections.

Vivid imagination of the mind, increased courage, with stupefaction and dullness; very easy comprehension.

Mania: Illusions of the imagination; mania, with fantastic or fixed ideas. Patient believes, contrary to fact, that he is not at home. Delirium with frightful visions of mice, scorpions and so on and with desire to run away.

Rambling speech; talkative delirium, with open eyes and red face. Furious delirium; fright with fear, is followed by heat in the head and convulsions.

Physical Symptoms

Breathing: Troublesome hoarseness, as if caused by an accumulation of mucus in trachea, with great dryness in mouth and white tongue. Rattling breathing; respiration deep, unequal; deep, snoring breathing with open mouth. Weak and low voice.

Noisy, snoringlike breathing and rattling inspiration. (There may be occasional snoringlike breathing, for instance, coming on and lasting a little while after a convulsion—but wait and see whether that does not presently die away; if there is continued snoringlike breathing, give *Opium*.)

Dry cough, with tickling and scraping in larynx, better from drink of water; with gaping drowsiness, yet cannot sleep. Cough with profuse sweat on whole body. Violent, dry, hollow cough, worse after repose. Cough during deglutition or when taking an inspiration, with suspended respiration and blue color of the face. Cough with expectoration of blood or of thick, frothy mucus.

Difficult, slow and intermittent respiration as from paralysis of the lungs. Pneumonia. Obstructed respiration and stifling, with great anguish. Spasmodic asthma; fits of suffocation on making an effort to cough.

Chest: Aching in chest, with shootings in sides during inspiration. Tension and constriction in chest; heat and burning pain in chest, especially in region of heart. Suffocative attacks during sleep; tension and constriction of chest; heat in chest.

Bronchitis after catching cold or getting wet, with high fever, labored breathing, blood-streaked expectoration and pressure on chest. Constant cough at night, must sit up on account of shortness of breath and dread of suffocation.

Face: Face bloated, dark, red and hot; lower lip and jaw hang down.

General: Absence of all pain. Blood thick, frothy, mixed with mucus. Great oppression. Burning about heart, tremor. Feeble voice. Anxious sleep, with starts. Legs cold, chest hot.

At times feels as if he was not in his house, which he expresses by saying, "I wish I could be in the house with my family." Although in a desperate condition, he is not much alarmed and wants to sit up a great part of time because bed feels too hot; whole body, except lower extremities, perspires profusely and sweat is very hot. Gropes with his hands about bed as though hunting something.

Pneumonia: Double pneumonia; infantile pneumonia, where the pulmonary inflammation is disguised by symptoms of cerebral congestion and oppression. Cyanotic color of upper part of body, with slow, snoringlike breathing; difficult intermitting breathing as from paralysis of lungs. Suppuration of lungs occurring in those greatly addicted to using intoxicating liquors. Breathing labored, with rattling and snoring. Cough very difficult and attended with smothering spells; face becomes blue during cough. Congestion of blood to chest or pulmonary spasms, with deep, snoringlike, rattling breathing; spitting up of blood.

Modalities

Worse: During and after sleep, while perspiring, from warmth; from stimulants, from spirituous liquors; from fear, from furious fit of passion; at night.

Better: From cold, from constant walking, from open air.

Phosphorus

Made from phosphorus, this is a remedy that should be handled with great care and by an experienced homeopath. To take this remedy too often can invite disaster, as it can destroy red blood cells. A little of this remedy goes a long way. It is one of our great respiratory/lung remedies, and it is used for arresting hemorrhaging. Phosphorus is one of the major remedies for the filoviruses, such as the Ebola Zaire, Marburg and Sudan varieties. Besides *Crolatus horridus* (the major remedy to stop these filoviruses from killing a person, see page 226), bothrops (page 214) and lachesis (page 244), this is another remedy that should be kept on hand for the coming world epidemics. Phosphorus is the number two remedy, next to *Crolatus horridus*, that can make the difference between life and death if a person contracts a filovirus such as Ebola.

Mental and Emotional State

Irritated very easily; mind dwells on negative things; fear of things creeping out from under a bed or corner of a room, very sensitive to all impressions.

Mental "burnout"; writer's block.

Physical Symptoms

Chest: Heat sensation rising off of chest, bronchitis, pneumonia. Lungs congested with burning, heat; tightness across chest; oppression on chest, worse if lying on left side. Sharp, stitching pain in chest. Breathing is fastened and labored.

Colds: Both nostrils blocked or alternately one blocked.

Cough: With painful larynx, ticking sensation in throat, coughing up rust-colored mucus. Racking cough that shakes body and causes headache. Cough is racking, hard, tight and dry sounding and is worse in a cold room or when lying on left side.

Diarrhea with blood, with great weakness following the stool.

Eyes: Floaters, or black dots, before eyes; cataracts; eyes bleeding.

Face: Pale looking; blue rings under eyes. Red circles on cheeks and swelling of lower jaw.

Fever: With lack of thirst but ravenous appetite. Delirium with fever. Heavy perspiration, cold knees at night and chilly in the evening.

General: Use before surgery to cut down risk of abnormal bleeding. Heavy menstrual flow. Thirsty for cold water; loss of vital fluids, electrolyte balance. Sleep consists of short naps with waking up frequently. Vertigo with faintness. Nosebleeds. Scurvy.

Headache: Migraine quality, with nervelike pain, sensation of heat comes up the spine into the head. Congested feeling in head. Brain and mental faculties burned out and tired.

Hemorrhage: Bright red blood; rapid.

Hepatitis.

Limbs: Paralysis, with pains in joints, weakness and trembling with every movement; joints will suddenly give way.

Mouth: Gums bleed easily. Tongue red, dry and smooth. Mouth sore.

Nausea: Postoperative from reaction to anesthesia. Vomit black or bloodred. Postoperative vomiting: one dose of 30C in recovery.

Skin: Wounds bleed profusely even if they are tiny; they heal but break out again. Skin bruising, *purpura hemorrhagia* (bleeding under the skin, which turns red, then purple/blue, then brownish/yellow). Skin fungus. The skin of the forehead feels pulled too tight.

Uterine polyps.

Yellow jaundice.

Modalities

Better: In the dark; lying on right side; cold food; cold, open air; washing with cold water; sleep.

Worse: Touch; physical or mental exertion of any kind; warm food or drink; change of weather, from getting wet in hot weather, during a thunderstorm; lying on left side or painful side; climbing stairs.

Plumbum metallicum

Plumbum metallicum is the element lead (Pb), and the remedy is made by trituration.

Mental and Emotional State

Coma

Frantic delirium (bites, strikes), sometimes with demented aspect; fury. Mania; dread of assassination, poisoning; thinks every one about him or her a murderer. Weakness or loss of memory; dementia.

Silent melancholy and dejection; discouragement. Weariness and dislike to conversation and labor; weariness of life. Great anguish and uneasiness, with sighs; anxiety, with restlessness and yawning.

Slow of perception, increasing apathy; unable to find proper word while talking; imbecility.

Physical Symptoms

Arms and hands: Convulsive movements of arms and hands, with pains in joints; drawing and tearing in arms and hands. Wrist drop (paralysis of the extensor muscles of the hand). Weakness and painful paralysis of arms and hands. Dilation of veins on back of hands, arms and calves. Difficulty moving fingers. Red and swollen spots on fingers. Weakness and painful lameness of arms and hands; pain in atrophied limbs, alternating with colic; lightninglike pains, better by pressure. Arms shaky when attempting to use them.

Back: Tension in nape of neck, extending into ear on moving head. Tearings and shootings in loins, in back and between shoulder blades. Distortion of spine. Itching on coccyx above anus, going off when scratched.

Cold: Constant coldness. Shivering and clammy, offensive sweat.

Face: Sunken, cadaverous, pallid or yellowish complexion and features; dirty, sallow face. Greasy glossiness of the skin or puffed and bloated. Lips scaling off. Yellowish or livid hue of the skin. Ulcerations on the surface with unhealthy, livid appearance or brownish patches on the skin; occasional but rare and evanescent flushing.

Intense dry harshness of the hair; eyelashes fall out; head and facial hair falls out.

Sense of smell is either suspended or an offensive smell seems to be emitted by everything.

Jaws suddenly become rigid. Eyelids become spasmodically closed and the eyes distorted; eyelids hang down from palsy of the muscles and the pupils are contracted.

Limbs: Offensive sweat on the feet; feet swell. Fingers exhibit circumscribed swellings, with redness or purplish hue. Spine and toes are distorted.

Painful sensation of paralysis in joints of hands and feet. Paralysis of lower limbs; cramp in calves, worse at night; cramps in soles of feet; paralysis of thighs and feet; pain in great toe at night.

Drawing or tearing pains in the loins, between the shoulders and in the hips, knees and thighs or even in the arms and fingers, aggravated by lying down.

Deep drowsiness or absolute lethargy. Jerking of the limbs during sleep. Fingers are paralyzed and stiff. Feet feel as if they were dead when put to the ground; feet feel as if made of wood; numbness of legs and feet; thighs and feet as well as the joints of the feet, hands and hips are paralytically affected and give way; feet, and even the legs, are numbed and insensible. Violent pains in limbs, especially in muscular parts of thighs, worse evening and night.

Drawing in hip joints when lying down; sciatica with muscular atrophy, walking causes great exhaustion, with consecutive atrophy. Painful sensation of paralysis in hip joints, especially on going up stairs. Numbness of outer side of right thigh, from hip to knee.

Skin: In spots is very sensitive to contact and cold air; numbness, twitching; lightninglike pains indicate the neuritis.

Throat: There is want of muscular power in the gullet to effect the act of swallowing. There may be spasmodic tightness of the throat or a sensation of a lump rising in the throat.

Pulsatilla nigricans

Made from the windflower, this remedy is decidedly female or for people who are highly volatile, temperamental and change like the weather. It is also for any kind of runny, thin, clear discharges from any orifice of the body, including eyes and ears, and it is the mumps remedy.

Mental and Emotional State

Emotionally up and down, sensitive; cries easily or is easily moved. Nerves from bad news or emotional upset.

Physical Symptoms

Asthma.
Cold that is "ripe" or fully in evidence.
Eyes might have sties.
Headache of periodic type; from eating fatty food or ice cream.
Hiccough from drinking something cold.
Indigestion (bloated or gas) from eating fatty foods.
Lactation: Breast milk is scanty.
Premenstrual tension; period may be unpredictable, late or shortened.
Varicose veins.

Modalities

All symptoms are worse in the evening.

Pyrogenium

This is the leading hantavirus remedy. It is made from rotting meat that contained sepsis and is excellent for any kind of a septic or blood poisoning state, gangrene or any condition that poisons or eats away at the body. It might be considered a secondary remedy for invasive strep A (see *Crolatus horridus* on 226, lachesis on page 244, aconite on page 202) once it is under control through antibiotics, and it is a major strep A homeopathic remedy for cleaning up the blood and quickening the healing of the septicemia.

Mental and Emotional State

Anxiety is pronounced with insane notions.
Restless, cannot tell whether dreaming while awake or asleep.
Talkative in the extreme.

Physical Symptoms

Abdomen: Sore, swollen and with cutting pains; very offensive, painless and involuntary diarrhea; straining of the bladder and rectum.
   Vomiting looks like coffee grounds; vomits water back up when it becomes warm in the stomach.
Blood poisoning: Used for any septic state of this; *if suspected, seek immediate antibiotic treatment* along with this remedy if symptoms match.
Fever: Fever with chills. Septic fevers with cold and chilliness; startlingly high fevers that come on quickly. Sweating does not cause a fall in temperature; great heat with profuse, hot sweat.
Head: Bursting headache with restlessness.
Heart: Palpitation as if the heart were too full; can hear heart beating. Pulse is rapid and out of proportion to body temperature.
Limbs: Bones and limbs aching overall; bed feels too hard. Numbness of hands, arms and feet.
Mouth: Has terribly fetid, rotting, dead meat odor; breath smells horrible. Tongue is red and dry; has a smooth, varnished appearance.
Muscle soreness with great debility.
Sleep is light, almost a semisleep; dreams all night.

Modalities

Better: From motion, lying down, warm room.
Worse: Beginning motion, during the morning.

Rhus toxicodendron

Made from the herb poison ivy, this remedy works well in the area of sprains and strains that are better with movement. It is one of the leading hantavirus remedies and is considered a secondary remedy for invasive strep A (see *Crolatus horridus* on page 226, lachesis on page 244, aconite on page 202).

Mental and Emotional State

Delirium with fear of being poisoned; senses are numbed; great apprehension of night and will try to leave the confines of the bed.
Listless, sad; thoughts of suicide.
Restless in the extreme, with constant change of position.

Physical Symptoms

Airsickness.
Cough: Of a dry, teasing nature from midnight until morning, worsens during a chill.
Diarrhea with blood, slime or red mucus.
Ears: Bloody or with pus discharge.
Eyes: Red and swollen.
Face: Swollen with red rash; pains (nervelike) in face when chilled.
Fever: Comes and goes, with restlessness and trembling. Chill with dry cough and restlessness. Fever with great restlessness of body/mind. Thirst (for cold water), flu, fever, diarrhea, pains, stiffness.
Joints: Bones ache, stiffness or having to "warm up" before they feel loose and free. Joints are hot with painful swelling; limbs feel stiff, paralyzed; worse in cold, fresh air and better with heat applications.
Lungs: Coughing up blood; oppression on chest and can't get a breath without sticking pains.
Milk, desire for.
Nose: Bleeds on stooping; tip of nose red; swelling of nose.

Palpitations when sitting still; pulse quick, weak, irregular with trembling.

Paralysis, trembling after any kind of exertion.

Septicemia of any type, but *if suspected, seek immediate antibiotic treatment* along with using this remedy.

Skin: Red, swelling with intense itching; red rashes with burning sensation. Bruising to skin for no reason; skin tender/sore for no reason, burns or itches; or with pustules, swelling or blisters. Poison oak/poison ivy rashes.

Thirst is great but mouth and throat feel dry.

Throat: Sore with swollen glands, pain on swallowing; worse on left side.

Tongue: Has a red, triangular tip at the end of it.

Modalities

Better: Warm, dry weather; with movement, walking, change of position; rubbing the affected area; warm applications; from stretching and moving limbs.

Worse: During sleep; in cold/wet/rainy weather, after a rain; when lying on back, lying on right side; all symptoms worse in evening and upon waking the next morning.

Ruta graveolens

Made from rue and bitterwort, this remedy works chiefly on the ligaments, tendons and joints of the body. If the pain increases with movement and doesn't get better after moving around a bit, then consider this remedy.

Physical Symptoms

Bruised feeling in general, no matter what part of the body is affected; muscles feel bruised or sore.

Eyes: Feel as if bruised.

Joints: Stiff, worse with motion.

Ligaments: Bruised sensation.

Sciatica; worse lying down.

Sprains (use arnica, page 208, first and then *Ruta graveolens*).

Teeth: Dry socket after extraction.

Modalities

Worse: With movement.

Secale cornutum

Common names for *Secale cornutum* are spurred rye or ergot of rye. The fungus *Claviceps purpurea, tulasne*, is the cause of this disease in the rye (and in other grasses as well). Preparation for use is the tincture.

Mental and Emotional State

Confusion: Paralytic mental diseases. Treats his relations contemptuously and sarcastically. Wandering talk and hallucinations. Apathy and complete disappearance of the senses. Memory failed; forgets names of friends whom he or she meets daily. Confusion of mind, unpleasant foreboding; anticipates misfortunes as though about to lose something of great value. Mania with inclination to bite, with inclination to drown.

Sadness: Uncomfortableness and depression. Constant moaning and fear of death. Anxiety, sadness, melancholy; great anguish, wild with anxiety; great anxiety and difficult respiration. Apathy, indifference. Excessive sadness, gradually changes to cheerfulness, talks and acts foolishly; rage, followed by continuously deep sleep.

Physical Symptoms

Adapted to men or women of thin, scrawny, feeble appearance; irritable, nervous temperament; pale, sunken countenance. Shrivels up the skin, makes it dry and harsh; sallow complexion. Very old, decrepit, feeble persons. Women of very lax muscular fiber; everything seems loose and open; no action, vessels flabby; passive hemorrhages; copious flow of thin, black, watery blood; the corpuscles are destroyed. Many who escape immediate death are reduced to a state of malnutrition, wasting away, from which they never recover, are paralyzed, have limbs distorted and senses impaired.

In general, the sufferer retains a clear intellect and a good, even abnormally good, appetite to the last. The nervous symptoms of secale are convulsive. The body is at times rigid, and at times rigidity alternates with relaxation. This is especially seen in the hands, which are either clenched or have the fingers spread widely apart (a keynote symptom). The muscles of the face and abdomen twitch.

Bleeding: A predisposition to bleeding; the slightest wound causes bleeding for weeks.

Heat: With thirst and want to perspiration. Aversion to cover and to heat, yet is objectively cold. Anthrax becoming gangrenous. Burning in all parts of body, as if sparks were falling thereon. Great weariness.

Limbs: Tingling in the limbs and great debility, especially when the weakness is not caused by previous loss of fluids. Bruised feeling in limbs; drawing and tearing, with crawling in limbs. Numbness, convulsive twitching. Spasmodic distortion, only ameliorated by forcibly extending limbs. Tonic (tension) cramps and spasms; pains when in motion. Sanguineous vesicles, which turn to gangrene.

Skin: Sallow, lead-colored, flaccid and shriveled; rough and dry; loose and numb. Miliary (small nodules or lesions on the skin resembling millet seed) eruption, especially on chest and nape of neck; petechiae (small purple spots on the skin); purpura hemorrhage (bleeding beneath the skin that appears purple in color). Bruising; boils. Swelling and pain without inflammation; coldness, blue color, gangrene. Black, gangrenous pustules. Ulcers that turn black. Skin withered and gangrenous.

Blackness of outer parts, crawling on the skin as of insects; subcutaneous tingling (itching beneath the skin); skin shedding.

Sulphur

This, one of our greatest remedies, is made from the chemical sulphur. It is used in posttraumatic stress disorder (see also aconite on page 202, arsenicum on page 209, *Merc. viv.* on page 248, *Nux vomica* on page 254). Sulphur is sometimes used when well-chosen remedies don't address a person's symptoms, and it is very often used to finish off a constitutional case.

Physical Symptoms

Constipation.
Diarrhea in the morning.
Eyes might have sties.
Hands/feet have burning sensation in them.

Memory loss.
Skin dry and scaly; might be itchy or burning.

Modalities

Better: Dry, warm weather; lying on the right side; drawing up affected limb(s).
Worse: At rest, warmth of the bed; washing, bathing; from alcohol; all symptoms worse at 11 AM.

Veratrum album

Made from the herb white hellebore, this is a premier diarrhea remedy.

Physical Symptoms

Cramps in abdomen, legs or calves.
Crohn's disease.
Diarrhea with abdominal pains, cramps, sweating and exhaustion.
Irritable bowel syndrome (IBS).
Nausea with severe vomiting.
Surgery: Good for postoperative shock.

Modalities

Better: Walking, warmth.
Worse: Wet, cold weather; all symptoms are worse at night.

Zincum metallicum

This is *Zincum metallicum*, the element. The metal has an affinity with the central nervous system, the heart, the muscular system and mucous membranes. Depression of the higher centers produces an increase in reflex irritability. Other effects are general weakness; aguelike attacks with prolonged rigors; muscular pains and aches; nausea, vomiting, diarrhea; and widespread formication (sensation of bugs crawling on skin). Extreme prostration or collapse is a feature of acute poisoning with salts of the metal.

Mental and Emotional State

Irritation: Easily irritated by trifles, too tired to talk or listen to the conversation of other people, apt to jump at the least noise.

May appear preternaturally calm, especially in regard to death, of which s/he speaks with pleasure, though without any suicidal intent.

Memory: Is impaired and a fear may obtrude that he is going to be arrested because he has committed an imaginary crime. Loss of memory and restlessness at night, with frightful dreams.

Overactivity: The Zincum subject is likely to be brainy, hard-working; docile yet irritable; oversensitive, unable to throw things off and relax, either mentally or physically. Finally, this overactivity gives place to slowness and extreme exhaustion. The child is dictatorial, unsubdued by punishment. Incidentally, conditions calling for zincum may be induced by overwork and overstress or precipitated by a fright.

Physical Symptoms

Back: Spinal affections, burning whole length of spine, backache. Much worse from sitting and better by walking about. Spinal irritation, great prostration of strength.

Bladder: Can only void urine while sitting bent backward.

Feet: Sweaty and sore about toes; fetid, suppressed foot sweat. Sensation of coldness.

General: Child repeats everything said to her or him, cries out during sleep; whole body jerks during sleep; wakes frightened, starts, rolls the head from side to side; face alternately pale and red. Convulsions during dentition, with pale face. No heat, except perhaps in occiput, no increase in temperature. Rolls the eyes, gnashes the teeth. Weak, weary, wasted appearance with pallor, sunken eyes and a countenance devoid of expression. Sensation of coldness in abdomen. Vertigo. Zincum should be studied when the patient is restless and uneasy.

Extreme loss of strength may be manifest; the patient lies with eyes closed as if in coma and, when spoken to, hesitates, repeats the question to gain time and finally, speaking very slowly, gives a rational answer. Persons suffering from cerebral and nervous exhaustion; defective vitality; brain or nerve power wanting; too weak to develop skin eruptions or menstrual function, to expectorate, to urinate, to comprehend, to memorize.

Head: In the cerebral affections, in impending paralysis of brain; where the person's vital force is too weak to develop skin eruptions. Automatic motion of hands and head or of one hand and head. Aching in the forehead after reading, writing or studying. Rolls the head from side to side on the pillow.

Limbs: Twitching and jerking of simple muscles; weakness and trembling of extremities, of hands while writing. Weakness during menses. Automatic motion of hands and head or of one hand and head. Incessant and violent fidgety feeling in feet or lower extremities, even in sleep; must move them constantly. Cannot bear having back touched.

Muscles: Chorea (nervous muscular twitching) from suppressed eruption, from fright. Twitching of the muscles with paralytic weakness. Awkward gait, tendency to stagger in the dark or when walking with eyes closed.

Zincum should be remembered for those who suffer from nervous and cerebral exhaustion. There is chronic chorea embracing all the voluntary muscles of the face, trunk and limbs, so that the patient is unable to eat, walk or lie.

Skin: Chilliness is a feature, especially when out of doors, when touching some cold object. Sweats easily on slight pretext; at night perspiration may be profuse and continuous with a tendency to push back the bed clothes. Cannot tolerate any covering during sweat.

Sleep: Excessive nervous moving of feet in bed for hours after retiring, even when asleep. Sleep is broken and unrefreshing, punctuated by vivid, usually distressing or terrifying dreams. Liable to jerk awake in fear, or talk or walk in sleep. Complete inability to get to sleep may occur, with a tendency to hang the head down over the edge of the bed.

Stomach: Ravenous hunger, often complains of a weak sensation in the stomach at about eleven o'clock in the morning or noon. Great greediness when eating; cannot eat fast enough (incipient brain disease in children). Aversion to sugar, meat, fish and wine; the least quantity of the latter causes intense flushing. Thirst may be excessive, especially from noon to evening. There may be a voracious appetite or complete anorexia. Both eats and drinks with undue and unseemly haste.

Modalities

Worse: Aggravation is caused by any exertion, either physical or mental, from contact or jarring, by noise. Symptoms tend to

be worse from 11 AM to noon, after dinner in the evening and
during the menstrual period. Feels worse from drinking wine,
even a small quantity.

Better: Chest feels better after expectorating; bladder feels better
after urinating; back better after emissions; in general better
with menstrual flow.

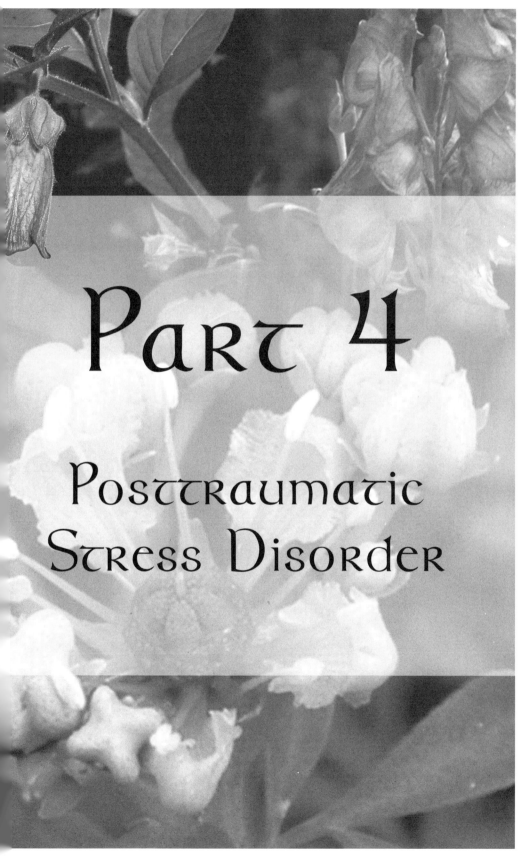

Part 4

Posttraumatic Stress Disorder

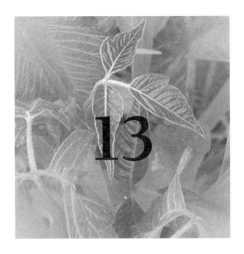

What Is Posttraumatic Stress Disorder?

Posttraumatic stress disorder, PTSD, is a lot more prevalent than one might think. Those who have heard this term usually connect it with Vietnam War vets. However, it's far more pervasive and widespread, although the theme of "war" is carried through—in many different ways. For instance, childhood abuse, incest/rape, spousal abuse, a raging parent, a teacher who strikes at a student, seeing or being a part of a horrific car accident, seeing or walking away from a plane crash or surviving a hurricane or earthquake can cause PTSD. These are all examples of "warlike" situations. Being a police officer, a paramedic, an emergency medical technician, a doctor or a nurse or a firefighter also sets a person up to be potentially exposed to PTSD.

Who is susceptible to PTSD? Everyone! With the World Trade Centers destroyed, the Pentagon attacked and more potential attacks by terrorists on U.S. soil, everyone in our country is at risk for *some* PTSD symptoms; to what degree is just a question of your vital force's ability to deal with sudden or prolonged trauma. Trauma is defined by *you*. Everyone is unique in how much or how long she or he can take trauma, and different trauma affects each of us differently. Our society nowadays is highly stressed.

Because of the nature of our everyday life, our vital force is in the "overwhelm position" more times than not. All that stresses our immune system and sets us up for all kinds of physical symptoms such as colds and flu. It also sets us up to be more susceptible to trauma, which is just another, more intense degree of stress. And that is when we become susceptible to PTSD symptoms. As you read this section of the book, you might find yourself in here.

My intention is not to go over previously covered ground or necessarily approach PTSD from the psychological point of view. Although the psychotherapeutical community is discovering new "tools" to help heal PTSD, I want to look at alternative methods of consideration to create cure. Because I have a Native American lifestyle, have been trained as a shaman and am a medical astrologer as well as a trained homeopathic practitioner, I want to explore PTSD within these unique frames of reference instead. This is not to say that these alternative medicine tools are the answer for everyone, but if a particular tool strikes a chord deep within your knowing, then you should explore it further at that point.

In the navy, I knew a lot of marines where I was stationed at USNAS Moffett Field, California. In 1965 half of my friends were shipped off to Vietnam. In January of 1966, my husband, a marine, was shipped off to that faraway place. When I got out, I waited in California for my husband's return. He was in the thick of it: Da Nang, Con Thien, Quang Tri—names of places that any Vietnam vet will instantly recognize. My husband then, in the last few months of his sixteen-month tour, become a sniper. And he was very good at what he did.

In the meantime, about half our marine friends who had gone over to Vietnam were severely wounded or had died and were not coming back. The few who did always stopped by to see me in San Diego, where I had an apartment and worked for a stock brokerage firm as a teletype operator. I gave them a bed to sleep in; real, home-cooked food; friendship; and a place to adjust to coming out of the bush back into the real world. It was then, as I was awakened in the middle of the night to their screams, their night terrors, their shrieks of absolute panic, that I began to see my father's previous PTSD behavior in them.

Over and over, I would spend nights, awakened, throwing on my robe and going to the other bedroom to try and help. Sometimes our friends just needed to talk after having been jolted awake by reliving their horrific experience. Sometimes they would collapse into my arms, holding me so tightly I thought I couldn't breathe as they sobbed and shook. Other times they pulled away, not wanting to be touched, not wanting to talk and asking me to leave them alone—they had nothing to say, they'd be all right.

These men all mirrored aspects of my father's personality, the way he lived his daily life. Most of our friends would stay at least a week with me; they'd tell me that they trusted me, that they could let their guard down, that they could be themselves. They were afraid to go home to the family or spouse; they weren't ready to face them just yet. I provided a safe place in their hellish storm of combat they'd managed to survive after 13 months in the Vietnam bush.

I learned so much sitting on the edge of the bed those dark, fathomless nights, about what war really does to a person; I learned throughout the months and the tears I sometimes cried with them and other times swallowed; and I saw my father's behavior more and more. I began to wonder if war did the same thing to all people, varied only by degree and intensity. I learned that war is horrible, that it is not the glorified John Wayne movie where right always wins. In war there are no winners, just survivors—mostly wounded survivors who are torn apart on spiritual, mental, emotional or physical levels.

By the time my husband came home, I was an expert on what war did to men. Unfortunately, my husband was the stoic type. He never talked about it; he never wanted to. He shoved all the horror he'd seen in the I Corps area of Vietnam, near the demilitarized zone, in the background and repressed it. Our marriage of five years quickly disintegrated because the war got between us and he refused to deal with it; in the end, it destroyed our relationship and our marriage.

I riled at the world. These men wouldn't go to "shrinks" or therapists for help. They distrusted them too; they distrusted anyone who hadn't been in the military. I kept in touch with a number of our marine friends after they'd left the service and went into civilian life. Many had the same problems my father had. They were unable to keep a job or cope within normalized society; they raged and were violent; they suffered from insomnia and restlessness; they were unable to keep a marriage together; they became loners outside of society's boundaries. I found myself wondering if there was anything that could help these men. I also realized that my father's war wounds had changed him irrevocably, and what saddened me the most was that I never knew what my "real" father had been like before his war experiences and being traumatized. I had to rely on his sisters and brother to tell me what he was like before—an entirely different man, one whom I would never know, one who had been destroyed by war. What a keen, eloquent loss! I can count on one hand those moments where he seemed to be free of the PTSD symptoms and I had the good luck to see the man beneath—and those times are special, even to this day.

Back in World War II, they called what my father suffered from "battle fatigue" or the "10,000-yard stare." After the Vietnam War, the psychiatric community finally came up with a group of symptoms that mirrored what war did to men and women and called it posttraumatic stress disorder, or PTSD.

In 1970, when I discovered homeopathy, I read *Boericke's Materia Medica and Repertory* and many articles on PTSD, and I recognized my friends and my ex-husband in those pages—their personalities, their "quirks" caused by the war horror they'd survived. I realized then that a homeopathic remedy could have helped them; could have healed their gaping, bleeding wounds in their psyche; could have helped them return to their original personality. I grieved when I realized that *Mercurius vivius* would have, in all probability, cured my ex-husband of his wounds.

However, I realized that it wasn't too late for other veterans—and that was the good news. Over time I also came to realize that I had an overlay of PTSD as did my other three siblings, because we grew up in that type of household. We showed many of the symptoms, and no wonder! My father had brought the war back with him. Our home was a war zone! Why shouldn't we all have suffered from PTSD? We did!

Let's look at PTSD; let's get familiar with it, because you know what? You don't have to go through a war or live in a warlike household in order to become a victim of PTSD. *Anyone* can get PTSD, whether you're part of the military or a civilian—it makes no difference. And as a matter of fact, many households around the world are combat and war zones—only, they are called dysfunctional family environments instead. Childhood abuse, whether verbal or physical, can create PTSD-like wounds in the child.

Spousal abuse is another kind of war where someone—usually the woman—receives endless verbal and/or physical abuse. This is no less a war zone; it is no less combat where a person cannot properly defend him- or herself, and the outcome is the same: trauma, sudden or prolonged, that eventually causes PTSD symptomology.

How Do You Get PTSD?

PTSD can be caused in different ways. Sudden stress, living in a war zone, exposure to inhumane treatment can cause PTSD, and whether or not a person experiences it and to what degree often depends on the individual's vital force.

Sudden, Unexpected Stress

Posttraumatic stress disorder can be caused by sudden, unexpected stress. For example, 9-11 caused massive PTSD, not only among the people at the towers of the World Trade Center who survived it, but among the entire population of the city of New York. Globally, anyone watching this horrific scene unfold on television could also be affected.

No one can tell ahead of time who is and who is not susceptible to PTSD. Trauma is defined by the individual psyche. In other words, what I may see as trauma may not affect another person at all or vice versa. There are hundreds of thousands of New Yorkers who now have some form of PTSD symptoms, and chances are they are the last ones to realize this. PTSD "stains" our lives, which is why I'm writing about it and hope that people will look at themselves, their subtle or not-so-subtle symptoms, and do something positive about it so they can have a PTSD-free life as an end result.

Examples of other situations where you might experience sudden, unexpected stress are seeing or surviving a bloody automobile accident, a train wreck or a plane crash; living through an earthquake, a flood or some other kind of natural disaster, such as a tornado or hurricane; experiencing an explosion; or being involved in a fire or seeing one wreak havoc. The attack on the Pentagon and World Trade Center is ripe for creating PTSD symptoms, but you don't need to have been there to "get" them; we are all vulnerable to such global trauma.

Being in a War Zone

All men or women who have gone to war—whether in armed combat; on the streets as a police person, firefighter, paramedic, ambulance attendant; or in a dysfunctional family—qualify. War veterans have earned their PTSD symptoms from encountering the gory, superstressful, bloody horror of war—up front and close. Their lives may or may not have been threatened.

Just living in a war zone is enough to trigger PTSD in some people. Terrorist attacks can create it. Living in a war-zone neighborhood or the inner city can trigger the symptoms. Living in places such as Yugoslavia, now carved up into fiefdoms, is another good example (all people in that area have suffered some form and exposure to PTSD). Israel is under constant threat of attack and I'm sure many of the people there suffer from PTSD symptoms.

Exposure to Inhumane Treatment

If a person is exposed to inhumane treatment—and this includes verbal or physical abuse (such as in form of spousal abuse), incest or rape or actually being a prisoner of war (POW)—PTSD symptoms will manifest. Torture comes in many forms. If one lives 18 years in a dysfunctional family, that is a special hell and torture in its own right. One doesn't need to be put in a cage somewhere in Vietnam to garner the same PTSD symptoms. Either environment will create them. If an individual views atrocity, that can trigger symptoms. Again, it doesn't have to be a war zone or combat—it can be a train wreck, an airplane disaster, a terrorist attack. As an example, the Oklahoma City bombing has, quite literally, created a city of PTSD survivors.

Many police and firefighters view human remains at accident sites all the time, and they do not always receive help in dealing with what they view. Some do get help, fortunately, but others do not. Human or animal atrocity affects all of us; the question is just to what degree. At some point, we all have an inner boundary where inhumane treatment, torture or atrocity will affect all of us.

Now the latest trauma, the terrorist attacks on our Pentagon and the destruction of the World Trade Center in New York City, has created a massive PTSD epidemic in the United States.

What Determines How Susceptible You Are to PTSD?

The psychological and constitutional elements of ourselves, which are collectively known to the homeopath as the "vital force," will create more or less susceptibility to PTSD symptoms. Ten people can view a plane crash. There will be 10 different, varying levels of reaction to it. Those whose vital forces are more susceptible to this type of trauma will be more profoundly affected and they will be the ones coming away with PTSD symptoms. Others may be less affected. Four children in an abusive household will have four different coping mechanisms and reactions to the war-zone environment, and each vital force will respond a little differently to it—but they will all walk away wounded with PTSD. It's just a question of how much damage has been done and where. Some people's psyche/vital forces are more resilient than others'. However, the more long-term the war zone that is encountered, the more certain it is that one will be affected. At that point, it'll just be a question of how much.

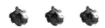

Any of the above described situations, combined with physical abuse or bodily injury, will cause PTSD. Injury, particularly to the head region, will guarantee it. In homes where children are slapped, beaten or thrown around, they will have a high degree of PTSD symptoms unless they have a very tough, strong vital force. And even then, these children will still be wounded, but perhaps not as deeply as some other individuals who are more susceptible to such a combative environment.

PTSD symptoms can worsen, especially if there is no social net or fabric where the affected person can seek help or protection from the warlike environment or warlike person. Without an abuse shelter being available, without the means to talk to someone who recognizes the bottom line of the problem, survivors, if left in the traumatic environment, simply become worse over time. A military vet who cannot seek help is left to suffer in his or her personal hell that only deepens and stains that person's entire life more year after year. PTSD symptoms, if not caught and reversed, become only worse with time. This ruins marriages, children and the PTSD survivor. In a sense, a PTSD survivor is still in the war zone, accident or POW cage—it just isn't visible anymore.

Symptoms of PTSD

Symptoms of PTSD vary, depending on the individual. Those who are affected by the ongoing terrorist activity involving the U.S. are going to be dealing with some, perhaps not all, of the symptoms. (You will experience all symptoms if you were in New York City at the time of the attack).

Flashbacks

These can occur at any time. Flashbacks are uncontrolled, intrusive and can happen during sleeping hours or during the day. Such recollections of the event(s) are stressful to the affected person.

PTSD survivors can experience disassociated states of consciousness in which they relive the traumatic event as if it was actually once again taking place in front of them, around them. Sometimes called flashbacks, these experiences are usually triggered by something. For example, a car backfiring on the street can cause a Vietnam vet diving for the sidewalk because he thinks it's a rifle or mortar going off nearby; he will relive the entire episode because of that car backfiring. Sometimes there is no noise and the flashback appears anyway.

An odor may set off a rape survivor, with a particular smell reminding her or him of the rapist. My sister once told me that the chicken she had baking in the oven was burning, and when she went into the kitchen, she had a flashback of seeing and smelling the Buddhist monk who had set himself on fire—and she had seen the whole gruesome event. The burning chicken brought it all back to her in that moment, along with the horrific emotions she had experienced while viewing the event.

A flashback takes total control over the individual, and the person is helpless to stop its occurrence. The inner torture someone experiences in that situation cannot be adequately put into words.

Chronic Anxiety

Along with the flashback, those suffering from PTSD can also experience chronic anxiety, hyperalertness, insomnia, the inability to concentrate. Some people experience memory impairment; huge chunks of their memory may be lost or they may have problems with short-term memory.

Nightmares or night terrors can predominate the hours during sleep. Sometimes those suffering from PTSD are afraid to go to sleep, or they fear the twilight or dark coming on at the end of each day. They are afraid to sleep and will eventually go into a sleep deprivation mode. With prolonged sleep deprivation, they will get a whole new list of symptoms added on to what they are already laboring under to carry.

Phobias

Some survivors of PTSD develop a phobia if they are forced to recall the traumatic event(s). Being forced into such exposure will only open their PTSD wounds even wider. At that point, they can become disassociated in order to survive the re-exposure or they can become phobic. For example, they can experience claustrophobia and do not want to be in a closed room but must escape and go outside, in the wide open spaces and fresh air.

Others might experience just the opposite, seeking the protection of an enclosed area, which is the only place where they feel safe. They may hide in a special room or space and not move from there for hours or days, until they feel safe enough to come out once again.

Emotional Roller Coaster

PTSD survivors may also experience emotional roller coasters, their emotional barometers swinging from euphoria one moment to rage or depression the next. They can become restless, constantly moving around, always walking from room to room, unable to sit still for any length of time. They will take off for the mountains—to hunt or fish is their excuse—but really, it is to be alone, to feel safe in the wilds.

Irritability may be high and obvious. Their hands may tremble or they may feel an inner trembling within their body, even if their hands remain stable and unaffected. Worst of all, there can be episodes of unexpected explosive anger or vitriolic rage. This may or may not escalate into violent, physical behavior against the unlucky person or child who is at the wrong place at the wrong time.

Hyperalertness

Some people turn to drugs or alcohol as a way to anesthetize themselves against this backdrop of nightmarish pain and memory. It is a way for them to put distance between themselves and the traumatic event(s). Some drink alcohol to sedate their extreme hyperarousal state. Their hyperalertness means being too sensitized to noise in particular, but an odor can set off a string of events just as easily as can a word, a shout, being touched by another person or some other kind of perceived threat. They can't handle someone walking up behind them, and often they'll cringe, whirl around and go into a defensive position.

If you want to easily spot someone with PTSD, check out a restaurant. Many of those suffering from PTSD cannot handle crowds at all, but those who can tolerate them for a short amount of time will be found sitting in the corners of the room, with their backs to the wall so no one can come up behind them. It also gives them the fullest view so they can watch everyone. They choose the safest position in a public place—against the wall, with their backs up against it, or in a corner seat. Because of this hyperalert state, which is really too much adrenaline and cortisol pouring constantly into the bloodstream, that keeps them on alert, they must seek quiet and be alone in order to come down or take the edge off this state.

I have found that adrenal exhaustion is often behind a number of PTSD symptoms, and many in the medical world haven't put this together yet. If one looks at adrenal exhaustion symptomology (chronically, it is known as Addison's disease, but there are milder forms of this that go unrecognized or undiagnosed), one can see it parallels that for PTSD: physical weakness, fatigue, low blood pressure, weight loss, dehydration, anorexia, nausea, vomiting, diarrhea, dizziness and a subnormal temperature. Mentally, those suffering from PTSD become insomniacs; they feel as if the body was in pieces, floating around them; they feel disconnected, quite literally, and spacy or as if the real world was not real at all but some waking dream they are having.

The other side of the coin to continued hyperalertness is the opposite medical state, known as Cushing's syndrome, where too much cortisol is being manufactured and pumped out by the adrenal glands because, on the inner psyche level, the person is still in a combat-preparedness state. And it doesn't matter if the individual was in the war overseas or experienced the war within the home—it can still pour too much cortisol into a person's bloodstream, creating this hyperalert state. The symptoms are: muscle-wasting weakness, skin is thin and wounds heal poorly, high blood pressure, purple streaks on the abdomen, kidney stones, osteoporosis, reduced resistance to infection, temporal balding, menstrual irregularities (amenorrhea) for women, impotence, excessive hair growth over the body, edema, *diabetes mellitus* and a plethoric appearance. Many will have adipose fat, especially "fat pads" and what is known as a "buffalo hump" on the back.

Detachment

There can be a numbing to the emotions, to the point where the affected person doesn't feel anymore. This is a symptom of shock, but the shock doesn't wear off as it's supposed to do after the trauma has occurred. Shock helps us protect ourselves from some overwhelming event in the moment it occurs to or around us. We unconsciously protect ourselves by distancing ourselves from the scene we just lived through, and this is known as disassociation—splitting off or away. As this occurs, many have said they see themselves floating above their body, watching the scene as it unfolds; they are quite literally out of their body, but it is their astral body that has left the physical form in this instance. Each time they are threatened, their astral form jerks out of their physical body and they may, or may not, remotely view themselves and the incident. Sometimes they just feel "floaty" or "spacy" or "like a balloon floating on the air," detached and away from the scene of the pain and torture.

I have found that I have this ability and inevitably, any time I'm truly threatened by something—nowadays it's usually a physical threat—I see myself above me. The latest occurrence of this happened in August of 1996, when my horse fell in a stream, slammed into the bank and then flipped over backward, carrying me with her. I viewed all of it. I didn't feel the impact as we landed on her left side against that steep, bush-covered bank. I didn't feel the pain of a thousand pounds of horse slamming my entire left side into the bank or her nearly rolling over on top of me. I felt no pain when she reared upward, trying to get back on her feet, lost her balance and fell over backward. I saw myself kick away from her, shoving with hands and feet and moving to the right or where she was going to fall. I could have died that day, but when I'm out of my body like this, I've always been protected from dying and injury. I walked away from this particular event with some bruises, which I took care of homeopathically, and that was all. So leaving one's body does have its pluses!

Shock symptoms for PTSD survivors do not wear off; they stay with them. PTSD survivors have been emotionally overwhelmed with what they saw, experienced and lived through. They live in a limbo state where there is no happiness, but no sadness either. It is a gray zone, an emptiness, an inner hollowness—an emotionless twilight zone. These individuals will tell you that they feel emotionally dead. Sometimes emotional detachment occurs along with this numbing state, and even if something traumatic, gory or horrific happens, they have no emotional reaction to it at all. As a result, they often feel estranged from others.

What PTSD Survivors Need

Ed Schmookler, PhD, from Albany, California, has a background rich in knowledge and experience as a therapist for posttraumatic stress disorder (PTSD) survivors. With his permission, I'm utilizing a paper on the topic he wrote and placed on the Internet, "Trauma Treatment Manual."

First and foremost, a PTSD survivor needs a sense of safety. For instance, if I look back on my life, I see I've chosen to live out in the country, usually on a farm, as far away from people as I can get because I felt safer there. Today I live in a desert canyon that few can find and where few people live.

In order to begin the healing process, every survivor of PTSD must find his or her safe place. It may seem strange to people who don't understand or feel what we feel, but what safety is, is a matter to be decided by the PTSD survivor. Safety can be going fishing or a hike in the woods. Usually, it is going off alone somewhere. Safety means providing ourselves with a place to think, to ruminate, to get clear or, if we've numbed out or used up the last of our emotional reserves, to try and get back in touch with the inner voice we know is there. It can also mean allowing nature to reenergize us, and we can do that only when we have peace and quiet.

If we say, "Leave us alone," do that. Respect our space. If we are feeling overwhelmed and walk out or away from you, the family, the group or situation, don't judge us. Just give us our space to retreat, to find that place of safety that is either within us or somewhere/something special—a certain room, a rocking chair, a closet, the woods, a walk along a road, a ride on a horse, doing gardening and so on—where we can wrestle with our inner PTSD demons.

Find Your Safe Place

Anyone with PTSD has learned not to trust any longer. In the case of a woman who was raped by a man, it might be a distrust of that particular gender. This woman might no longer trust any man—not even her brother, her father, her husband, her friend, even though none of them is the one who injured her. The loss of trust can also manifest in a general distrust of everyone, which can be seen in combat veterans. To them, even children are suspect, because in Vietnam, little children would carry live hand grenades to the unsuspecting marines or soldiers and kill or maim them. The combat vet learns to trust no one when incidents like this occur.

When I began to understand what had happened to me, I realized how it had stained my whole life as well as my second marriage. I was very lucky, because my second husband, David, is really a guardian angel in disguise. He gave me a safe place to be—with him, on our farm out in the middle of nowhere. He respected my need for privacy, for horseback rides for hours by myself and for spending vacations in remote, isolated areas instead of in cities or on tours with lots of other people. His kindness and acceptance and understanding of my needs eventually created a safe environment for me to start opening up my own PTSD Pandora's box and seek help. If Dave had not respected my needs and boundaries, I doubt I would be over the bulk of my PTSD symptoms today.

Define what is "safe" for you. That is the place to start; that is where the true healing begins. Where you feel safe is where you will finally be able to relax—even if you relax just a little bit. With that relaxation comes the slow process of PTSD symptoms being allowed to surface, little by little, into your consciousness. And when that happens, I suggest you have a good therapist to handle your PTSD ready and waiting, as well as a homeopath who can work in concert with you and your therapist, because you may need one or more remedies as your trauma layers expose themselves.

I would suggest this: If you are a survivor of childhood abuse/incest or rape, your therapist should have a background in these areas. If you are a PTSD survivor of combat (a military vet), choose a therapist who has a background in this—better yet, find one who has been there. Vets trust vets; it's as simple as that. Also, if you are a woman who was raped by a man, do not choose a male therapist, because your trust in men was broken by the male rapist; go to a woman therapist instead. Or if you suffered incest by a woman, then think about going to a male therapist, because your trust in women is broken. Sometimes this element can be overcome, but the worst is that even on an unconscious level, you will distrust someone who is of the same gender as the person who hurt you and you won't open up and be vulnerable with that therapist, or it will take you much longer to do so.

If you are affected by the Pentagon/WTC tragedy, you too are a survivor. The thing is, you didn't have to be at ground zero to "get" PTSD from this assault. Our psyches are highly impressionable and the more sensitive we are, the more we are likely to be affected by such a trauma. Even if we live 3,000 miles away from where it happened, it touches us.

I learned this lesson the hard way. Although my PTSD father had broken my trust in men, I went to a male psychiatrist, who positively put me on guard. I could hardly speak to him; he was so clinical, he kept me at arm's length, and he seemed so big and threatening to me. I left after three sessions and sought out a woman psychologist who had a background in childhood abuse/rape. Within three years, she had helped me turn my life around, and she also gave me the warmth and nurturing I needed to trust myself to open up.

It Is About Boundaries

PTSD survivors need to know you are going to respect whatever boundaries they need to put up in order to survive on an hour-to-hour or day-to-day basis. A trauma means that our normal life boundaries have been smashed and destroyed; our sense of innate protection, of "that can't happen to me," is suddenly shattered once and for all and we never feel safe again. Therefore, we begin to erect boundaries or walls from the place where we do feel safe to operate out of so we can live in society and try to get along or at least cope.

A good example of this is that I ask Dave to leave me alone when I'm working on a novel. I'm able to escape into my other world, where all things end positively and on a hopeful note. When we were first married, 28 years ago, he made the mistake of walking into my office one day while I was writing. I literally leaped three feet off my chair, whirled around midair and came down in a crouched, defensive position, my hands and arms raised above my head to protect myself. He was shocked and stood rooted to the spot over my unexpected behavior. I was shaking and breathing hard, my heart was pounding in full anxiety reaction as I remained in that frozen position of defense. Then he "got it." He realized instinctively that my request for this boundary hadn't been some inane, purposeless request on my part. That particular incident galvanized us both. He helped me open up over time and talk about my reactions, about my need for a closed door to my office and about him knocking on the wall long before he would come to my office to let me know he was coming so it wouldn't scare or shock me out of my creative state.

Never force your way of doing things on a PTSD survivor—that person will simply retreat from you and hide in a thousand different ways. Whatever her or his boundaries are, understand that these are very real needs in order for her or him to feel safe. Only when you respect these boundaries will there be a prayer of hope that the PTSD survivor will open up and struggle to become vulnerable—not only with her- or himself but also with you and the family over time. A lot of patience is needed on this point.

There were times, particularly when I was first married to Dave, that I didn't want to be held. I didn't want to snuggle. I didn't want to be touched—not sexually, not in any way. He didn't understand why (and I didn't either at the time), but when I pulled away, he wouldn't try and make me stay in his arms or he would withdraw his hand from my arm and respect my need not to be touched. It's very hard on the spouse and/or the children to understand this, but if you touch us without our consent, it creates trauma all over for us. It is telling us that, again, we have no control over ourselves, our body. We see you as the invader, the abuser, the rapist, the enemy in combat all over again. That is how you, the toucher, are perceived by us, the PTSD survivors.

Again, this is about boundaries, about who has control over us. The one thing we want back so badly is control over our environment, our body and ourselves. Each time a boundary is broken, we are retraumatized to a minor—or major—degree, depending upon the individual involved and her or his vital force. It is a violation of our being, particularly so in cases of abuse and rape. At its worst, we cannot handle intimacy at various levels or stages, and this is especially true for rape survivors.

Some veterans need to be held, for the arms of the person holding them become a boundary, a safe harbor for them. Intimacy may be a way of helping them to open up and start the healing process. Other veterans see intimacy as the enemy. They cannot tolerate being touched, much less held. They pull away if you put your hand out to touch them on their arm or shoulder in a friendly fashion. They can snarl at you, bark or become raging if you try and hold them or touch them. Don't do it. Back off. Give them what they need, because otherwise they see you as breaking down their boundary and, once again, this is perceived as trauma—not humanity, love or nurturing as you might see it. Your best, heart-felt intention won't work here. Just because you feel better when you are held, don't project that value on all PTSD survivors. It will not necessarily make them feel better; on the contrary, it may end up having a destructive, opposite effect on them.

On Judging and Listening

The more my PTSD symptoms became the focus point of my second marriage, the more I realized how different my actions/reactions to everyday things were from Dave's. I began to observe our differences quite closely after the office incident. I had thought my reactions were normal; he said they weren't. He said it was normal that I could walk up behind him any time I wanted and it wouldn't bother him—but it sure would send me up a wall if he did that to me! We had a lot of exploratory talks about this, and neither one of us realized what my problem was. We only knew that our reactions/actions were exact opposites. I thought I was normal and he was abnormal! (Of course, when you live in a

PTSD family, you would automatically think that. Dave had not; he'd come out of a more socially "normal" family life, certainly not a PTSD one!)

One of the most important things Dave did was that he never judged me. He accepted me just the way I was and didn't try to change me. Instead, he asked me what I needed so that we could live in harmony despite our differences. Whether he knew it then or not, by not standing in perpetual judgment of me or my actions/reactions, he provided another key to helping me unlock the PTSD-damaged part of myself and begin the healing process.

Don't be judgmental with the PTSD survivor. Don't say, "Well, you're wrong. Nobody else jumps at a car backfiring. Why should you?" Or, "Why can't you go out dancing with me? A guy is supposed to go dancing with his girl." Or, "Why do you always have to walk away from me when I'm angry? Why don't you stay and stick it out?"

The types of judgment and scenarios are many. Some PTSD survivors run at the first threat of an angry word, a warlike expression on your face, the tone of your voice or your (nonverbal) body stance. Survivors of violence usually do one of two things: They run away from the violence/fight/argument or they lose control, become raging, vitriolic and stand their ground against you. In the extreme, they may become physically abusive toward the person who is screaming, yelling or perhaps trying to talk in a reasonable tone of voice to them and trying to discuss something, and they perceive this event as a heated argument or worse—a verbal attack against them, which sets them off into a defense mode or posture in order to protect themselves from this perceived threat.

One of the greatest healers, at least for me, was Dave's undivided, focused attention on me when I wanted to open up and talk. He's a wonderful listener and I value that trait much more now than at the beginning of our marriage. However, not every PTSD survivor wants to open up and talk. At the other end of the spectrum is the loner who is closemouthed and can't say anything besides maybe one-syllable words like yes, no.

Being a good listener for PTSD survivors is one of the greatest gifts you can give us. In our being able to talk about it, you become our sounding board. That doesn't necessarily mean that we want you to fix "it"—a kind ear is often enough for us. I remember shortly after we were married, I'd wake up in the middle of the night, usually around three o'clock, with anxiety attacks. My heart was pounding, I was drenched in sweat, I was breathing so hard I thought my lungs would burst. Dave would struggle awake, sit up and ask what was going on. I'd sit there, arms clenched around my knees, repeating: "I don't know, I don't know. I'm just scared. Scared . . . " And he'd turn on a light and sit patiently, not touching me because sometimes I didn't want to be held after such an event (sometimes I did, but I always initiated it, not him—the respecting of the boundaries).

Over the first year of our marriage, each time I was awakened out of these nameless night terrors—which happened at least once or twice a week—Dave would calmly sit and listen. Eventually, I began to get more and more in touch with *what* was causing them in the first place. Before that time, I hadn't had a clue; all I knew was that they'd just happened ever since I'd left home. By being a good listener, Dave allowed me to delve into levels of myself that, over time, yielded a tremendous amount of direct, conscious information. And as this information became available, the night terrors subsided and after five years went away, never to return. That is the gift of listening and how it can help us.

Let It Happen in Its Own Time

A PTSD survivor can numb out, but at some point, her or his feelings will probably start coming back. It's important to realize that time will decide, along with the vital force, when the reappearance of one's feelings can happen.

The burying of feelings is an effort by our vital force to protect us, because it knows we couldn't handle the emotional avalanche, that it would destroy us, so it is actually a survival and coping mechanism. Usually, like for a new seedling poking its head above the ground for the first time, progress during the reemergence of our feelings is slow. It's important to not push those going through this into feeling more before they are able to handle it. Don't urge them to cry more, yell more or express themselves like you do—because they can't. Be patient with them and their reexploration of their wounded emotional superstructure.

The healing that takes place within each of us will unfold on its own schedule—not yours, not mine. Many times, being alone helps PTSD survivors think or feel things through. Try not to push us, cajole us into something or deride us. Don't try to help us if we don't ask for help. If we ask for your help, give it. Someone who doesn't have PTSD can easily see what we can't. Unless you're asked for advice, don't give it to us. Healing is a matter of self-exploration and self-awareness and self-discovery for us. It won't do any good for someone to come along and tell us what we need so we can "fix" ourselves. The "fix" is inside us.

If you want to know how to help, then ask us. Ask us if it's all right if you talk to us about what we're feeling or thinking. Getting permission helps PTSD survivors stay in control and it reassures us that you respect our boundaries. Being a know-it-all and giving us your two cents' worth on what's wrong with us or how we should go about repairing ourselves is considered an encroachment upon our boundaries. Hold your advice until and if we ask for it.

Random Acts of Kindness

Spouses or children of PTSD survivors often want to know what they can do to help. Looking back on my own experience, I find that Dave's unobtrusive, accepting presence was healing. The environment most of us need is not a therapeutic one (although in some cases, that may be necessary, at least temporarily), but rather, a continuum or fixed rut kind of flow that helps us minimize the number of surprises in our life. After all, it's unexpected "surprises" that got us into trouble in the first place! A place that has a set time for breakfast, lunch and dinner, for example, is the type of rut I'm speaking about. This may seem ridiculously simple, but it works. Fixity, a daily regime give us stability. Once we've got stability, we can focus on other wounded parts of ourselves.

Just being a good listener and giving us your full attention if we need to talk is a great healer in and of itself. And if we want to talk, listen with neutrality. What we might share with you could be emotionally revolting, powerful or traumatic, but don't allow your emotional reactions to overshadow our own. By mixing and matching, that stops our flow—and usually, we PTSD survivors don't talk too much about what happened to us.

Use the opportunity to be a sounding board; you don't have to fix things, just let us stumble through it. Your emotions may be triggered too, but try not to allow them to interfere in that moment, if you can help it at all. The kindness of being a good listener, being emotionally detached enough to keep your emotions from interfering with ours when we're ready to share and keeping your heart open during these precious few and far between times are what you can do to help a PTSD survivor heal. It's simple and straight from the heart.

What Good Has Come out of PTSD Trauma?

The watchfulness and the powers of observation a PTSD survivor has are remarkable. I've discovered that this is a useful asset for me as a homeopathic practitioner, because I perceive the little things, even the slightest of nuances—a change in the tone of voice, a very slight body language signal—that most people wouldn't see or wouldn't think are important. This ultra-awareness helps me usually figure out in a fairly short amount of time which homeopathic remedy a person needs.

Another added feature to PTSD is that our hyperalertness borders on more than just being in touch with a primal intuition ability. I call this our all-terrain radar ability. I can feel people's auras; at times I know what they're thinking before they speak. I can feel not only their energy but also their emotions. Fortunately, I can turn this "radar" off at will, but it comes in handy to me as a practitioner, because I can feel the root cause or core problem that has sent a person's vital force out of balance, for instance.

I'd been a walking PTSD survivor for 35 years before I realized how much my extrasensory abilities could be of use. I had joined the fire department in a rural Ohio community, where I served for three years. In any given year, I'd make 400 out of 600 runs. I drove fire trucks and tankers; entered burning structures; attended many grisly auto accidents, coal mine fires, wildfires, an airplane crash; looked for lost elderly people; and experienced many other traumatic situations.

I was the only woman in the department of 20 coal miners/truck drivers. Dave, my husband, was also in the department, but the only time I saw him was on night fires, when he was not at work. Most of my fire duty was during the daylight hours when I and one or, if we were lucky, two other men would show up at the fire house. That was the reason I had joined—to be a body available during the daylight hours, when half the fires occurred. Since this was a volunteer outfit, any man who was home during the day was usually sicker than a dog—otherwise, he'd be at work.

We always ran "lean" on day fire situations. I did the same work as any man, whether it was driving a fire truck or tanker or moving into a burning structure with a fire hose. I found that my phenomenally acute sensory ability not only saved my life many times, it saved other firefighters too. I could sense/hear/feel things on a more subtle level than they could, and it wasn't because they were men; it was because they weren't PTSD survivors like I was and they weren't used to operating off the subtle levels in order to survive.

I could hear, smell, taste on far deeper levels than most. I could hear the fire in a wall as it moved almost noiselessly through it. I could smell smoke where no one else could. I could feel fire before we encountered it. When we were in houses with our air packs on and oxygen masks strapped to our faces and we couldn't see anything, not even our gloved hands in front of our faces, my senses saved lives. At times I could feel a bad floor where fire had burned out the trusses beneath it, even though it looked safe to the firefighter next to me. I'd be aware of a slight shift in a room in the house where we fought the fire and would know that the ceiling was going to come crashing down on us if we didn't get the hell out of there! Feeling our way across a smoke-filled attic, I knew where the weakness was in the trusses before we crawled over them and fell through to the floor below. On an icy slate roof in the middle of winter, three stories up with a fire somewhere down below in the attic, I knew just where to put an axe through the roof to get to it.

Fire was a great teacher to me. It used everything I learned as a PTSD survivor to survive it and to help my partner and other firefighters survive. At the end of the first year at the department, many men wanted to back me up on a hose going into a burning structure, because they'd seen proof of my peripheral abilities to know fire. They knew they were safer with me and often called me a "bird dog," because I could sniff out a situation beforehand.

The other use of my PTSD-won abilities was at accident sites where screaming, shrieking, panic and hysteria were abounding, with blood and possible life-and-death situations on top of it all. I could detach emotionally from the grisly scene, think ahead to what needed to be done, as in a triage situation, and calmly go around doing what I had to do. My emotional reaction never got in the way, which was highly useful because many firefighters lost it and couldn't think coherently or ahead like they needed to in order to do their duty effectively. Afterward, after the adrenaline charge, I would come back into my emotional self. I worked through emotions at that point because I had homeopathic help to do it with, which I'll share with you in the next chapter of this book.

Another use of my extrasensory abilities was at wildfires. Anyone who read about the hot shots and smoke jumpers who got trapped in that ravine on Storm King Mountain in Colorado has a good idea of what a wildfire or forest fire can do. I respect fire greatly. I've seen it at its worst. I also know it's a living being, fully capable of moving, changing and transforming just as any of us are or can be. That may sound like a silly statement, but anyone who has dealt with fire knows what I'm speaking about.

We had wildfires in Ohio every spring and fall. I got to hate them. Imagine going up and down hills in 40 pounds of turnout gear and a helmet, and then carrying roughly 40 more pounds of water on your back in what is known as an Indian tank. Eighty pounds of gear, usually on a hot day, and then to be chasing a fire that is whim to wind, temperature and humidity over a hundred acres or more is a prescription for disaster in the making. I always carried homeopathic remedies on me for heat exhaustion and sunstroke, two things that struck many a firefighter. My PTSD radar was put to good use when I could sense a change in the fire direction.

Picture this: You are down in a 200-foot rocky, brush- and tree-lined ravine. The fire, which is in a grassy field, is moving toward you. You're getting hung up on brush, stumbling, chasing the fire. The wind changes—no one notices it except you; you feel/sense it. Looking up, you know that this "little grass fire" can suddenly turn and explode down into the ravine, and there are five of you down there, negotiating the territory and trying to scramble up the other side to reach the fire. Not a safe place to be!

This actually happened, and when I felt the wind shift, I yelled at everyone to get the hell out of there as fast as we could—and to move toward the approaching fire. My people, who knew of my abilities, listened. Personnel from another fire department working with us ignored my warning. The wind shifted, violently. It changed from a mild, little breeze to a sudden, 20-mile an hour blast. The "little grass fire" suddenly blew up on us. By the time we had scrambled on our hands and knees up to the top of that ravine, we were facing a 30-foot wall of flames. Unlike hot shots, we didn't have any silver tents to throw over ourselves to outlast the heat and flames. My senses told me to leap through the wall of fire. I had no idea how wide that wall of flames was—it could be just a few feet thick or much more.

Our turnout gear was flame retardant, but it was going to burn if put against too much flame and heat for too long. We all had our plastic visors down across our faces to protect our eyes. I yelled at our men to follow me—and leaped toward that wall of fire, my thickly gloved hands pressed against my lower face to protect it. I shut my eyes, held my breath and jumped! I felt the fire and heat envelop me, embrace me, whip around me. I left my body. I saw that the wall of flames was roughly six feet wide. I remember landing hard and stumbling forward, coming out the other side of the wall of flames rolling head over heels. The rest of my team came with me. The guys down in the ravine weren't so lucky; a number of them had to go to the hospital for burns because the whole ravine blew up from the fire as it leaped over it and trapped them. Our people did not even get singed, which was a miracle. I thanked my PTSD, because it had saved our lives and stopped us from getting burned.

Your PTSD symptoms can serve you in a positive way; the hyperalertness and vigilance can pay off. I've heard more than one police officer tell me wryly that "a little paranoia" is healthy—police officers distrust to a higher degree than those who don't have PTSD symptoms. Nowadays, especially for women, a little paranoia is good. We have to watch wherever we are when we're walking alone, hiking or even going to a car in a parking lot after dark! I inevitably am looking around, sizing up situations and people around me. That's another use of our heightened abilities.

After 9-11 and with the very real ongoing threat of continued terrorism in the U.S., everyone needs to be a little paranoid and stay alert. Be watchful. Don't put your head down and walk. Keep your head up and notice who is around and what is happening around you.

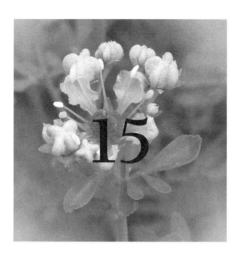

Homeopathy for PTSD

Homeopathy is a system of medicine that is beautifully designed to address powerful spiritual, mental and emotional shocks and trauma to ourselves. No less, natural essences, which come from nature in the form of mother tinctures, can also be powerful adjuncts. When someone has her or his case taken by a homeopath, one remedy is selected and given one time. This is known as classical homeopathy. Provided it's the correct remedy, or *simillimum*, a step-by-step cure process will take place known as Hering's Law of Cure, or what I term "retracing." For more information on this, go to "What Is Hering's Law of Cure and How Does It Affect Me?" on page 18.

The Dangers of Retracing with PTSD Survivors: What Should Be in Place

For PTSD survivors, this retracing can be a delicate balance that the homeopath has to monitor carefully or more often than s/he would when working on cases that do not involve trauma. This is especially true if there is mental or emotional trauma involved. Here, on the most delicate level, the spiritual-mental, is where psychotic damage can occur during the experience, and this is also retraced. So for those people who have had such experiences as "wigging out," "going insane" or "flipping out," these symptoms come back up to be gone through and experienced one more time. It won't be as intense or last as long, but the homeopath has to put in place certain safeguards for the survivor *ahead of time*, before the survivor takes the remedy.

We homeopaths can know ahead of time because we have taken your case. It is vital, especially for a PTSD survivor, to tell the homeopath everything. To not mention something out of shame, humiliation or fear that we will judge you can later on do harm to you and leave us, your homeopath, out in the dark, wondering what is going on with you and your remedy.

Finding the Right Homeopath for a PTSD Survivor

It's equally important to choose a homeopath with whom you can create a bridge of trust and faith. Go to page 360 in Appendix B for information on how to find a homeopath near you. If you don't get along, go find another, more compatible homeopath. PTSD survivors have been through the mill already, and to stick with a homeopath who isn't creating that trust/faith connection is only going to prove disappointing for the survivor in the long run. I would strongly suggest to any survivor to have a phone consult or an in-person consult with the potential homeopath, to make sure you are comfortable with the person, her or his personality and way of working with you. If the person doesn't feel right to you, don't set up an appointment and keep looking for the "right" homeopath. Perseverance pays off, so don't give up.

Ask the homeopath if s/he has had training or experience with PTSD or abuse. Ask how long s/he has been in practice. Knowing what I know about PTSD, I would want an individual with no less than 10 years of homeopathic experience and *some* background in this area (training, education or personal experience of PTSD). Dealing with PTSD is like dealing with a loaded gun with the safety off, a volatile Molotov cocktail or wired C-4. One just doesn't know what is going to happen with the survivor, especially when one gets into rocky areas emotionally or mentally during retracing. It takes a homeopath with a lot of experience, maturity and years in practice to not panic like the patient and to think clearly and without getting emotionally involved in the symptoms.

The Importance of Homeopathic Potency Given to a PTSD Survivor

I would also ask the homeopath beforehand if s/he is a high or low "doser." Unfortunately, in the U.S., many homeopaths are trained to start a case with a 200C, which is a high potency. Ordinarily, this wouldn't be a problem. But with a PTSD survivor, it can become an overwhelming problem and can do more damage to you and your vital force than most homeopaths will ever realize. And if they do realize it, it's too late because the damage has been done.

It takes nothing away from the case to start out with a low potency, such as a 6C, 12C or, at the highest, a 30C. If it's the right remedy, 48 hours after you've taken it, you will begin to have an alteration in how you're feeling. A good homeopath will invite you to call her or him at the end of that 48-hour period and check in, because things will be happening. This 48-hour check-in reassures you but also puts that homeopath on warning that the remedy is working. Depending on the case, PTSD survivors need closer attention than most other homeopathic patients. Sometimes they need daily contact with their homeopath for a period of time while dosage and potency of the remedy are adjusted for maximum help with minimum discomfort for them.

If your homeopath isn't willing to cultivate that kind of care and attention for your case, do not go to her or him but find one who will; if the homeopath insists that s/he will see you in six weeks and not before, this is not a healthy sign. Most PTSD cases I've worked on needed my close attention and ongoing conversations, especially the first couple of weeks after having taken a remedy, until we could see more clearly how the vital force was going to work with the remedy and you.

Communication Is Everything

It's absolutely essential that PTSD survivors can pick up the phone and call their homeopaths. Frequently, PTSD survivors don't want to talk to anyone, which creates an impasse that can stop the case and curing before it ever gets started. That is why a strong faith/trust connection between you and your homeopath is so important. When a PTSD survivor is retracing a certain symptom or a set of symptoms, the homeopath can, upon occasion, help make the symptoms less intense. The PTSD survivor has to communicate with the homeopath before s/he can respond appropriately. Homeopaths aren't mind readers—you have to talk to them; you have to tell them what's going on inside your head, your heart or body before they can potentially take the edge off the retracing you're experiencing.

So many times when the going gets tough, PTSD survivors just curl up, hide in a corner, take off for the woods or disappear in some way (being out of body or spacy, daydreaming, using drugs or alcohol) while they suffer through such retracings. It isn't necessary any longer to go that path alone. There is help for you, but you have to reach out, pick up the phone and ask your homeopath for the help.

In the past, when PTSD survivors couldn't get the help they needed, when that help never came, many just curled up into a fetal position at some point and toughened it out by themselves. Over time, this response became a part of their conditioning: You get in trouble, no one cares or there is no help, so don't bother reaching out and asking. Fortunately, that's no longer the reality.

When retracings occur, homeopaths may use what is called an undercurrent remedy to work with this new set of symptoms that has arisen. I prefer to use flower or germ essences whenever possible, because these mother tinctures come from an organic source and are less likely to mar the picture of your vital force and the homeopathic remedy you are using. Other homeopaths may resort to vitamins, minerals, herbs or possibly, if nothing else seems to touch your retracing symptoms, a combination homeopathic remedy at a very low dose, such as a 6X or 6C, for example, for a short period of time.

There are many ways to manage a case. Mine is to give the patient one remedy, one time, and then we wait. When retracings arrive, I try flower essences first. If there is none to address a particular set of symptoms, I look at a low-potency homeopathic remedy instead. Most importantly, you should know that there is no need to suffer endlessly with retracing symptoms—but you have to communicate. Pick up the phone and call your homeopath.

Acute and Chronic Trauma Homeopathic Remedies

Aconitum napellus

Aconitum napellus (aconite) is one of the greatest of the acute and chronic trauma remedies we have in our pharmacopoeia. This remedy is for anyone who has suffered trauma (PTSD or otherwise) of any kind. A car accident, falling down (especially for the elderly), breaking a bone, taking a spill from a horse, enduring combat, living through a natural disaster, getting bad news, seeing a horrific accident of any kind (airplane, car, train), being a victim of terrorism, being a survivor of rape/incest or spousal abuse are just a few of the areas where this remedy can help.

Mythologically, Cerberus (the dog who guarded Hades, hell/underworld) was being carried away by Hercules. As his foamy saliva fell to the Earth, the plant aconite was created in its wake. Considering that combat veterans have felt like they marched, quite literally, into the "jaws of hell," this remedy is one that should be carefully considered for those who have deep, seemingly impenetrable PTSD/trauma symptoms that cannot be budged by traditional medical routes. High potency, in the 10M range, should be considered, but it should be given only by a professional homeopath.

For aconite to be considered, the person must have felt as if s/he was going to *die* during or shortly after the trauma. The trauma is usually sudden, comes out of the blue, is completely unexpected and strikes like a lightning bolt, which sets this person's central and peripheral nervous system up for the shock that follows closely on its heels. The person's fear of death is heightened to an intense, conscious degree.

Aconite is a premier remedy for central nervous system shock. People thus affected are restless; they can't stay sitting down in any one spot for long. They need the company of others around them, but not have them smothering them. They just want to know there's a warm body in the nearby vicinity, such as the next room.

Mental and Emotional State

Persons for whom this remedy can work have experienced sudden shock or trauma of any kind. At the top of my list are combat veterans, rape survivors or anybody who suffered some tragic, *sudden* crisis.

They feel anguished, afraid they are going to die. At the same time, they become obsessive about every little thing, almost hypochondriac, in response. Every worry is not a molehill, but a mountain the size of Mount Everest. They worry for others too.

They are forgetful, cannot think coherently, and they can't answer your questions, no matter how clearly, slowly you repeat them. They feel as if they are in a bad dream or sleepwalking. They cannot keep their attention; their attention wanders.

They are restless, can't sit or stand still. They are emotionally intense; their restlessness is obvious. They have great fear, anxiousness and worry. Their foreboding over the future is paramount, as is their fear of death and/or of dying.

They have panic attacks or anxiety reactions; the hands may get hot, the feet will be icy cold. They may or may not know what starts these attacks. It can be an odor, a sound, a word, a gesture or something they see in the newspaper, on television or in real life. During the attack, some parts of the body may feel thicker than others.

Sleep consists of nightmares or night terrors (a step up from a nightmare). They may talk, mutter and mumble in their sleep state. They will have anxious dreams filled with symbols of death and dying or with a replay of whatever originally caused their trauma. They will be restless and endlessly toss about. They may start (jerk) during sleep. If they have dreams/nightmares, they may wake up and feel anxiety in their chest from them.

Physical Symptoms

They experience heart palpitations known as tachycardia, or racing of the heart. There may be pain in the left shoulder or a stitching pain in the chest. Along with the palpitations comes an avalanche of anxiety. They may feel faint. There may be tingling in the tips of their fingers. Their pulse will be hard, full and tense or bounding; it can be intermittent. When sitting down, they can feel the carotid arteries (located on both sides of the neck, near your trachea/windpipe or your temporal arteries located at the temples on either side of your head) beating.

One cheek on the face may be red, the other white; or the face may be flushed completely. Upon standing up, the face may turn absolutely white and they will feel dizziness for a few moments. Shortness of breath is not uncommon.

Urine retention: When under stress, perceived or real, they won't be able to urinate for a long time afterward. They have a great thirst for cold drinks, although it can be for drinks at room temperature too.

They may tremble badly; they may shake and have an inner trembling in the trunk of the body. They may shake/shiver/tremble all over, or only their hands may tremble.

Modalities

Better

In fresh air. They have to get near a window, open the window or go out of doors. Fresh air always helps to stabilize their anxious state of being.

With a warm sweat. Going out and jogging or lifting weights or doing some form of exercise that builds up a mild sweat always makes this person feel better. I've often seen PTSD survivors who are avid joggers or weight lifters; by turning to physical exercise, they are, in one way, unconsciously sweating out the hellish demons that reside within them.

From rest. Their nervous system is in hyperalert and they lose a lot of sleep, so when they are able to get some rest, they indeed feel much better.

Having company always makes them feel better and more stable; although they won't stand for suffocative or cloying attention, they do like to know there are other warm bodies nearby in case they start feeling a little shaky, anxious or out of sorts.

Worse

Warm rooms make them feel claustrophobic, trapped, as if the walls were coming in on them and they have to escape.

Violent emotions that may come from a fight with their spouse or an argument with a stranger will always knot them up inside and make them feel 10 times more tense.

Music makes them feel sad, and they simply can't tolerate the sound at all.

The evenings and nighttime are when all their anxieties and panic begin to emerge. It is the night hours that are hell. They become jumpier, more restless, agitated, unable to sit still; they are always going outside to cool off or have a window open in the room they occupy. They become worse if you touch them (they jump); they can't stand noise in any form but want the silence of the great outdoors surrounding them; they can't stand bright light and often go into a dark room or one with very subdued lighting.

Arnica montana

Arnica montana (arnica) is of special help in traumas where tissue damage was sustained—whether in combat, spousal abuse, rape or an auto accident, for example. Cells retain the memory of our trauma, just as our ligaments, tendons and bones do. An area that has been physically injured will hold the trauma long after it is healed over. Arnica is one of the best remedies to think of first when that area still gives you problems although it shouldn't, which simply means that the body is still holding the trauma.

Mental and Emotional State

"There's nothing wrong with me." The person who needs arnica will always say this, especially after an auto accident. This person can be going into deep shock but still insist she or he is "fine" and, "Why don't you go help so and so?" If you see a combat vet having a reaction and you inquire, s/he will say, "I'm fine," and want you to drop it at that. If you don't, this person will more than likely stalk off to be left alone. A classic keynote for using this remedy is when the individual refuses help from the EMT, paramedic, nurse or doctor. Combat vets who use the stoic demeanor and insist, "I'm fine," or "There's nothing the matter with me," are also classic candidates for arnica.

They fear the approach of strangers. Particularly in severe dysfunctional childhood survivors, rape/incest survivors and combat vets is this a normal response and arnica should be considered. This is the remedy for the one who doesn't like being approached from the front, side or rear—from any direction.

They constantly mutter to themselves. At first you may think they are talking to you, but when you ask them, they just wave a hand at you or shake the head. I've seen this reaction more in those who experienced severe auto accidents and in combat vets, especially vets who have gone on for a long time without some kind of intervening help—they drop into what I term the "muttering mode."

"I'm not in shock! I'm fine!" so says the person who needs arnica. Especially veterans, after they wake up from a horrific nightmare or night terror, will roll away from you (if you're sleeping with them) and mutter, "I'm fine, I'm fine . . . go back to sleep." And if you reach out to comfort them, they will pull away from you and leave not only the bed but the room as well. Think of arnica!

After the trauma or accident, they answer all your questions correctly. They seem cool, level-headed and emotionally completely detached from what just occurred to them. The less emotions in the voice or facial expression, the more you may think of arnica. Especially right after a trauma—a few hours or a few days later—most victims have problems remembering what happened, in what order it happened and many other details of what went on at the site of the trauma. Arnica folks can answer the questions correctly and without any apparent emotion.

Fear of open spaces. This is a red flag. For combat vets who spend a lot of time in some room of the house where they feel safe and who rarely wander outdoors or into a large area, arnica may be the remedy of choice. Rape/incest survivors may have this same reaction. They don't feel safe out in the open where "others" might be watching them. That is how a combat vet feels—if you are out in the open, exposed, the enemy can kill you.

They want to be left alone. They shrink away from your proffered hand, your loving embrace, a few words of compassion; they do not want consolation in *any* form. These are the combat vets who will never come to the one they love for what they need most—support, nurturance and consolation. There is something in them that drives them the opposite way, and only time and patience (and hopefully, constitutional treatment) will bring such anguished vets back to those who have loved and suffered with them all along.

Sleep—when they sleep at night, the head may be hot to the touch and the rest of the body may be cold; this is a keynote. If they don't get their normal amount of sleep, then they are restless and can't go to sleep for several hours after hitting the bed. Their dreams and nightmares include: death, mutilation of bodies, parts of bodies, atrocity-filled replays of the past, anxiousness. They also suffer from night terror. They may have an involuntary stool (usually diarrhea) during sleep or one of these horrific nightmares, which is another keynote for considering arnica. They might also suddenly rouse out of a deep sleep, filled with fear.

Their fears are many: fear of anyone approaching them; fear of being touched, injured; fear of becoming sick, of dying of a heart attack. They suffer from fear upon awakening. They fear the night, crowds and public places and won't go anywhere near a mall or shopping center. They want the woods, being out in the middle of nowhere in order to feel a little safer.

Nervousness is translated into the fact they can't stand anyone to touch them. It is the pressure of the touch that bothers them the most. The body is oversensitive to everything, and they cannot bear the least little bit of pain. In this state, there is an indifference or a lack of care about work or earning a living. They cannot remain at one job for very long before they quit or are fired. They just don't have the stamina and mental focus and concentration to do something for eight hours a day.

Most of the time, they will appear to be morose, indifferent, introvert—"dark" loners who can't stand being around people.

The Tortured Warrior—*Mercurius vivus*

Another remedy that should be considered for PTSD where the person has been leading a tortured life afterward is *Mercurius vivus* (*Merc. viv.*). There are many different types of mercurius, which is made from potentized quicksilver or mercury that is derived from cinnabar. Mercury, when broken down from this mineral, is highly poisonous. The one discussed here is known as *Merc. vivus* or also as *Mercurius solublis hahnemanni*. There are a number of other mercury remedies, so be careful not to confuse them.

Most of us know that mercury—that shining, globulelike, silver stuff—is used in a thermometer that rises and falls according to heat and cold conditions brought on by weather. You can take this same idea and apply it to a *Mercurius vivus* person: This individual is quite literally a "human thermometer," with ups and downs emotionally speaking. From a PTSD point of view, when the individual experiences the jumpiness, the paranoia, the suspicion, the obsessive/compulsive behavior or the absolute terror of night coming on, with symptoms worsening during the night, this remedy should be given a good look before moving on.

To me, *Mercurius vivus* personifies the wounded, tortured victim of war or any other event or atrocity of unbelievable, inhumane origins. I'd like to put this remedy, along with syphilinum, into the water of Yugoslavia. Bosnia and Serbia are, in my opinion, the very nature of *Mercurius vivus*—the torture, the inhumane deeds against other human beings, the twisted beliefs and distortion of religion that have fueled a hatred that knows no bounds, rules or ethics except utter annihilation of the other group. This is syphilis at its finest, unfortunately—an eating out of the human soul from the inside out until decency is destroyed. The twisted, sick, perverted hatred that eats and festers away from the inside of us eventually begins to destroy us.

So it is too with a combat vet or a survivor of some PTSD event that has broached our reality. *Mercurius vivus* can reach inside that which is, quite literally, eating us alive from the inside out and stop the inner destruction, the inner voices from the past, and set us back on a more harmonious path within ourselves. This is a powerful constitutional remedy and one that many combat vets could use. Let's look at it in detail.

Physical Symptoms

Generally speaking, *Mercurius vivus* types are light- or fair-haired. Their skin is considered unlined and smooth, with a translucent quality. Some can have a blotchy quality to their skin, but their flesh is always pale looking, sometimes of an almost sickly white quality or an earthy, yellow/sallow complexion with puffiness beneath the eyes. The skin may appear somewhat greasy looking or have a dirty yellow, rough and dry surface to it. Their cheeks may be red, swollen or hot. Lips are salty, dry and cracked in the right corner of the mouth.

There may be a touch of arrogance to their withdrawn, watchful nature, and they are always serious looking in their expression. Although there is a feeling of explosive tightness around a *Mercurius vivus* person, their faces belie this feeling; they look positively unruffled and free from the everyday stress or strain of life. In fact, you could say that they look completely detached or disconnected from the stresses of life. But that's not true. Inwardly, these people absorb the stress in their own, unique way. Just as a thermometer's mercury constantly goes up and down, so does a *Mercurius vivus* person.

Mental and Emotional State

On a mental level, *Mercurius vivus* types are restless and in constant movement, along with having a feeling of anxiety. They have a powerful desire for not only stability, but order. Many military and police types are *Mercurius vivus* people; here, a certain rigidity, inflexibility, order and discipline are standard operating procedures (SOPs), and this helps them feel more secure, even though their insecurity will always be present to some degree.

There is a natural suspiciousness directed toward others or situations that is inherent to *Mercurius vivus* types, and this can be advantageous if they are in the military or police force; it can potentially save them from getting killed. I've always said that a little suspicion and a tad of paranoia are healthy in today's environment, where we can barely trust strangers anymore, strangers of any age, and a *Mercurius vivus* person has this natural equipment already in place within. When a person who needs *Mercurius vivus* is put into a situation where her or his vital force is pushed out of balance, this paranoia becomes like the volume on a radio over time, getting louder and louder, until finally paranoia is all that exists in the individual's tightly focused and limited reality.

There's an incredible well of insecurity in them, and they can appear conservative and cautious when dealing with anyone. They may appear to be slow in thinking or speaking to you, but really, they are gauging you with their own internal radar to check you out to see if you are friend or foe. On the outside, *Mercurius vivus* types look like the "kids down the street," but inside there's a war going on that, if not helped early in life, can later on become a living hell and torment they carry around inside them—and this is when they can become abusive.

Usually, they are introverted, quiet (some would say, brooding), contemplative and conservative in bearing. When they listen to you, they are 100-percent focused mentally and emotionally, almost as if they are transfixed on every word you speak. This kind of attention can be flattering (who, after all, gives that much attention to anything anymore?), but some people can also react as if they feel a hunter is stalking them with this kind of undivided, powerfully focused attention.

Actually, if a *Mercurius vivus* person doesn't listen with all that focus and attention, she or he won't be able to speak! This is a keynote symptom for *Mercurius vivus* types. If they don't focus, their mind is scattered in 20 other directions and they'll never hear what you're trying to say; this is their way of compensating for the rash, helter-skelter activity of their thermometer-like mental activity.

The person's emotions are intense, like a Texas thunderstorm that blots out the sun on a hot summer day across the dry expanses of that state. Anyone who has watched one of these "frog stranglers" form across the baking surface of Texas' desert will immediately grasp and get a visual and emotional sense of what is going on inside a *Mercurius vivus* person every single day. In a powerful thunderstorm, there are huge updrafts and downdrafts—just like in a thermometer, just like a *Mercurius vivus* type's emotions. They feel intensely, volcanically and are helpless to do otherwise. And isn't it interesting that chief among their fear is . . . thunderstorms! They also fear being burglarized, and they fear for the health of their families; they have fear of becoming insane, of being poor, of dying.

Add PTSD events or a PTSD situation or a series of PTSD events on top of this, and all these symptoms become magnified to a high degree. Their fears turn up in volume, right along with their infamous paranoia and suspicion.

At a younger age, they may have been taught that violent expression of emotions is not good, so they put on this cool, calm, unruffled face that completely belies these horrific roller-coaster feelings. They may have problems and stammer as a result, be very shy or withdrawn. They will drool in their sleep and usually have many ear or throat infections while growing up. In being jammed down deep inside where they aren't given any expression, things begin to ferment for years. At some point, all this garbage of dark emotions, especially anger, has to vent somewhere and somehow, and this is where PTSD events can enter the picture and rip that placid mask off; the person is put into violent situations, which triggers their own, inner violence that up until that time was more than likely dormant.

Emotions that are either repressed or suppressed in *Mercurius vivus* types take on a bizarre twist: They become *impulses*. You would never know what they are thinking or feeling until suddenly, just like a lightning bolt out of that violent Texas thunderstorm, they will strike out at you. And when *Mercurius vivus* types strike out, they can easily kill—whether it was their original intention or not. I've always said about them that if they lash out, it isn't just to bruise a person; it's to maim the other or worse, to kill.

I've seen *Mercurius vivus* combat vets sleep with a gun under the pillow or carry a military-type knife on them at all times. The saddest of all, I saw my *Mercurius vivus* brother-in-law, who had been in the army special forces and went through two tours in Vietnam, take the pistol he always slept with under his pillow and use it against his wife. He was, typical of a *Mercurius vivus* person, having a night terror about one of his Vietnam firefights. His wife, who was awakened by his crying out and flailing around in the bed, reached out to touch and awaken him. He grabbed the pistol—which he kept locked and loaded—from beneath his pillow and shot her in the face. Later he told the authorities that he saw a Vietcong coming for him—he never saw his wife's face. To say the least, my brother-in-law was devastated by what he'd done because he'd loved his wife deeply and she'd seen him through a number of years of hell after his return from combat. And then he was sentenced to federal prison for seven years. It's one hell of a price to pay, one that shouldn't have had to be paid at all if I'd known about homeopathy at that time.

Mercurius vivus types usually know that their impulse to hurt or kill another is wrong, so they struggle valiantly to put on this societal face that makes everyone think they are the kids next door—so nice, so conservative and so proper. My compassion goes out to them, especially to the ones who grew up in abusive households to begin with. Their path is even more hellish and it is even harder for them to try and operate within the laws and social order of their community than it is for other *Mercurius vivus* types. I find that *Mercurius vivus* combat vets usually come out of such a household, and of course, like draws like: They get the horrific battles and see the worst of human beings, and so the inner destruction goes on. In them, the violence is just compounded in quantum leaps; they are a powder keg ready to ignite.

Mercurius vivus types are struggling with all these ugly, violent emotions deep within, which may manifest outwardly as compulsive disorders, anxiety attacks, agoraphobia, panic attacks, paranoia or other mental states of imbalance. There can also be depression and suicidal thoughts. In their later stages of imbalance, they have always reminded me of a wounded or trapped wild animal who is in a cage, pacing, constantly pacing, watching you warily with hackles up and teeth bared, growling and completely distrusting. And they won't growl or snap—they'll bite with the intent of killing their foe or perceived enemy.

That is why, when Dr. Gail Derin did her study on (and treated homeopathically) 30 Vietnam veterans for her thesis, "The

Remedies of War," *Mercurius vivus* was found to be one of the main remedies to cure vets from that war, besides sulphur, *Nux vomica* and *Calcarea carbonica*.

Mercurius vivus types, when raised in a war zone such as a dysfunctional family situation, have all the hallmark symptoms of PTSD. And they parrot the suspicion, distrust, apprehension, emotional volatility (an explosion just waiting to be triggered by some small, seemingly insignificant event) as well as paranoia. When they have reached the last stage of expression, the symptoms are abusive in their implementation. They can no longer contain or control their inner turmoil, rage, suspicions, paranoia or compulsiveness. They become violently destructive, with the intent to badly injure or kill the other person. There is fury coupled with an impending sense of doom; there are homicidal or suicidal impulses; there is the ability to fly off the handle at the least provocation, internal agitation and a desire to escape it by traveling or running away to another state or country. Their speech is hurried, perhaps even nervous or stammering. And there is an incredible restlessness—they can never stay in one place very long.

You will see an instability to their mental processes along with irresolution, and it shows up as constantly changing their minds (just as a thermometer changes from moment to moment). Their anger comes out in tirades. When night comes, their anxieties and apprehensions rise, to taunt and torture them with further mental anguish. They may perspire heavily during that time. The war they wage at night is one against inner demons that are so hellish they can never put a name to them—but they are eating them up, from the inside out. Only *Mercurius vivus* can stop this awful inner destruction.

PTSD and Anger

One of the outgrowths of PTSD can be anger, particularly when the person is a *Mercurius vivus* constitutional. There are times when this anger or rage wells up in them, in retracings or following Hering's Law of Cure, and the homeopath has to be ready to deal with it immediately. In these situations, an acute homeopathic remedy like anacardium, staphysagria, stramonium or belladonna may be needed to take the edge off the rage so it's controllable this time around.

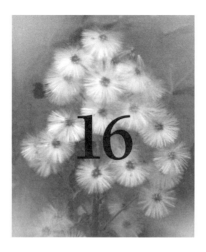

Shock and PTSD:
What Do They Have in Common?

What Is Shock?

One of the greatest underlying problems with PTSD—and trauma in general—is *shock*. Few people truly understand the power of shock on a body and how it can reverberate through every level of our being, from our cell structure on up through our vital force/auric field. Shock leaves no stone unturned; shock takes no prisoners. And because of this, shock needs to be addressed fully and understood to its highest ramifications.

A little child who runs down a sidewalk and falls experiences a mild form of shock. An elderly woman who falls down the steps of her porch does too, and so does the accident victim and the combat veteran. Good news can shock a person and so can bad news. Shock, depending upon the person and the individual's vital force orientation, brings suffering with it, to varying degrees and intensity levels. There isn't a person alive who isn't susceptible to shock—although there are people, especially those who have a supersensitized central and peripheral nervous system/brain, who become pallbearers for this mysterious occurrence. First, though, let's define shock.

Shock, seen from a strict medical understanding, is the circulatory system's inability to continue to circulate blood or adequately perfuse the organs and tissue. What does this translate to so that we can understand more? The cardiovascular system, composed of the heart, arteries and veins, moves the blood and its components all around our body. Blood moving back to the heart carries carbon monoxide and waste in the red blood cells and goes through the lungs. As we exhale, these waste products are then released through our mouth and nose, and those same red blood cells can then pick up fresh oxygen from our inhalation and carry it to the organs and tissue of our body. They too, need "fresh air" in order to survive. The red blood cells also carry nutrients—"food"—to our organs and cells. These exchanges occur in the capillaries of our body, where the old air and waste are taken out and the good air and food are then utilized. This is known as perfusion. Without this very necessary metabolic "dance," our body would quickly become acidic.

Another function of the cardiovascular system is that it allows a thin sheath of muscles to constrict and relax our arteries—controlled by our autonomic nervous system. And we've all experienced the consequences of what happens when these arteries don't contract. How many of you have stooped over to pick up something, and when you straightened up, you got very dizzy? In fact, you might even have felt like fainting. Maybe you did! The arteries never fully contract, nor do they ever fully relax during shock. The dilation (opening/relaxing) and constriction (closing) of the arteries is an ongoing process, occurring every moment we live.

If we suffer a shock, the arteries may dilate and the volume of blood (six liters in an adult) settles downward in our body. The perfusion, which is so intrinsic to life, isn't able to go on as it did before. The heart, for example, requires *constant* perfusion. The brain, spinal cord and central nervous system can't go without perfusion for more than four to six minutes without permanent damage to these systems; the kidneys will be damaged after forty-five minutes without adequate perfusion; and our muscles become permanently damaged after two hours. In other words, no part of our body can go without perfusion—and shock causes the loss of this vital function.

By understanding this underlying concept, you begin to grasp the power of shock and how it can either permanently injure an organ or system in our body, or kill us within a very short period of time. I strongly believe that just as we learn cardiopulmonary resuscitation (CPR) and have to take a two-day course and get "carded" for it, there should also be a one-day course on shock, the different types of shock and what to do about it. Armed with just a minimum amount of first aid, we could save many more lives, especially at auto accidents or with the elderly.

Later, when the physical body is stabilized, the shock that is still stuck in our cells, bones, muscles, memory or vital force can be addressed with homeopathic intervention, the use of a particular flower essence or therapy.

Signs and Symptoms of Shock

Following is a list of symptoms to watch out for if you suspect a person is experiencing shock:

1. The person appears restless, anxious or may sense some kind of impending doom.
2. The person has a weak, rapid pulse (known as a "thready" pulse), or the pulse may be very difficult to feel.
3. The person has cold and wet skin. (Usually, we refer to this as "cold, clammy and pale.")
4. Profuse sweating (diaphoretic) is common.
5. Paleness of the skin and later cyanosis (the skin turns blue, especially around the mouth and eyes) reflect the lack of oxygen getting to the tissues of the body.
6. Breathing may be shallow, labored, gasping, rapid or possibly irregular. (This is especially so when the person has suffered a chest injury.)
7. The person's eyes are not only dull looking (that "nobody's home" look), but the pupils are also dilated (wide open/black or dark appearing) and the eyes appear flat or lusterless. The "sparkle" is extinguished.
8. The person may become exceedingly thirsty, especially for cold drinks. (Do *NOT* allow someone in shock to drink water! See page 317.)
9. Nausea or vomiting may occur due to injuries but can also occur as the shock deepens, so this is a red flag that the shock is turning worse.
10. The person's blood pressure begins to fall. This is one of the last and most serious signs of shock setting in.

11. There may be an altering or loss of consciousness in some cases of rapidly developing or severe shock. The person may faint or become unconscious.

What Can I Do to Prevent a Person from Going into Shock?

First, if possible, call 911. Or if there are two of you, have the other person call 911 and stay with the victim who is in shock. Everyone should carry a blanket or two in the trunk of the car, along with a little box that has latex gloves, gauze dressing and roller bandages. (Since I am a homeopath, I carry a "black bag" in my car at all times. In it are latex gloves, a stethoscope, blood pressure cuff besides other items.) If you at least carry a blanket, that will help enormously.

1. Make sure that the person's airway is open, and that means that the person is able to breathe. If you have your CPR card, you know what to do and how to do it, so I'm not going into it here. If you don't know, you should contact your Red Cross representative or your fire station and find out when the next CPR class is going to be held—and go! You won't be sorry. The information and techniques you learn in that class can literally save a life, especially when people are in shock.

2. Control any obvious external bleeding with a sterile compress and direct pressure on the wound. (This is why you wear gloves; with today's transmissible viruses such as HIV and AIDS, you need these gloves. Medical houses sell the total-protection type that EMTs and paramedics in the field use, and these are the ones I suggest you buy.) If you have someone with you, have him or her get the blanket out of the car and put it over the person.

3. Elevate the person's arms and legs (providing they are not broken). You would *NOT* do this if the person has a head injury; in that case, keep the victim lying flat. However, if there is no head trauma, you can elevate the legs slightly. This helps the blood to run back into the center of the body, especially back into the chest and brain so that the very necessary perfusion can be maintained. You can use rolled-up towels

to put beneath the person's ankles and wrists, or be creative with whatever happens to be handy. It's very important to get the blood back into the trunk of the body. You only have to elevate six to twelve inches to perform this life-saving technique.

4. Be sure to avoid rough handling of victims. Stay with them, talk to them and monitor how their eyes look, their skin color, their breathing and levels of consciousness. Do *NOT* give them any food or water, no matter how much they plead with you, even though they usually get violently thirsty. Unfortunately, if you cave in to their request for water, they can lose consciousness immediately afterward or vomit it back up. Either way, you have caused the shock to deepen, and the vomit can possibly go into their lungs and cause even worse problems than before. So be strong and say *no* to liquids or food.

If you can do this much for a victim, you've done plenty until EMTs or paramedics arrive on the scene to take over for you. And you can pat yourself on the back knowing that you didn't allow shock to continue its damage in that person.

Shock and PTSD Survivors

Dealing with the physicality of shock is one thing. Dealing with the residue it leaves behind like an invisible imprint upon our emotions, mind and, potentially, our spirit is quite a different story. Here, homeopathy, flower essences and other tools can play a part in dissolving it, removing it from our cellular and vital force/auric field memory.

A shock can stay lodged for decades in our cellular tissue, our muscles, even our bones and especially our brain cells, which is our memory. If you don't think so, look at any Vietnam vet; in many, you still see signs of shock, with anxiety and restlessness being the most obvious.

The less obvious signs are digestive problems—nausea, vomiting, diarrhea—or shallow, irregular or gasping breathing. Just think of the night terrors they awaken from! They hear a sound or inhale an odor, and the adrenaline starts pumping. They can break out into a cold sweat, breathe erratically, become pale and their level of consciousness can change—and all these are classic symptoms of shock.

Homeopathic Remedies

Veratrum album

One of the most underused remedies for shock and trauma is *Veratrum album*, or white hellebore; most have been taught to look toward aconite or arnica for shock/trauma. It's interesting that even back in the time of the Greeks, Hippocrates used white hellebore for evacuations and proclaimed that it was necessary in order to create cure. It's little wonder, since this herb promotes expulsion of any kind from our body and is well known as the remedy of choice in chronic diarrhea. The entire herb is highly poisonous and grows in the mountainous regions of Europe.

This remedy reminds me of those combat veterans who have been completely destroyed by their experiences in war. Their faces are pale; their brows are beaded with cold sweat; they have dark rings around their eyes, which are dark and clouded looking. Their features can be pinched or distorted; they can be frowning or have a terrified look to them. Their cheeks are sunken, and their skin can display blue or gray color around their lips or eyes. They are prisoners of their shock and PTSD; their central nervous systems are "shot" by their trauma.

One word I like to use for this remedy is "collapse." Just think of what shock does to people—they literally collapse in front of you on every level; there is a taking down or dismantling that occurs because of shock. Following the homeopathic law of "like cures like," if we want to stop a person from collapsing, we use a remedy that creates collapse in a healthy person. *Veratrum album* has no peer in this arena.

It is also well known as the remedy to use for those who undergo surgery and come out "shocky" afterward: They are cool to the touch but perspire heavily (cold sweat); there is blueness around the mouth and eyes or even to their general skin cast; and they are weak. Postoperative shock can be halted with *Veratrum album*, which gives you an idea of its power and fortifying ability to the vital force when under fire from shock symptoms.

Persons who need *Veratrum album* have a highly sensitized nervous system and mind, and if they experience a powerful shock or a series of shocks, their vital force takes the blows in these two major areas. Symptoms such as general weakness, collapse, exhaustion along with profuse cold sweating (especially on the brow) with a burning sensation inside (and yet they are freezing cold) are a few keynotes to look for. These individuals are always worse in humid weather, colder or cool temperatures, when moving around and at night. They are highly restless and, one might say, hyperactive. They just can't remain still, and their moving around can sometimes be seen as mania.

The mind of a person who needs *Veratrum album* is a torture chamber to be imprisoned within. Often these individuals are melancholy and they'll sit there, head hanging down, brooding in silence. They may not notice anything or anyone around them. People might say they are sullen or appear indifferent to their surroundings. They may sit there doing some kind of repetitive action, such as tearing a page from a magazine into little pieces or picking away at a fiber on their clothing.

At other times, when these individuals come out of their shell of silence, they can be hard, tough and seemingly incapable of feelings for others. One moment they are talking and philosophizing; the next, they may break into hysterical laughter. They may appear manic, hyperbusy, talkative, restless and rude. At their worst, they can be haughty, critical of others and careen between anger and violence. The picture of *Veratrum album* is, for me, a grenade with the pin pulled, and the only question I ask is, "When will it explode?" That is the feeling around someone who needs this remedy and who has suffered horribly from PTSD and shock. These individuals can appear jealous and then suddenly become quite loving and amorous. They may kiss and hug you inappropriately or be hypersexual at these times. And so they swing from manic behavior to sullen, withdrawn, intense silence.

The *Veratrum album* PTSD survivors swing between two extremes of behavior. They are "in their head" and they over-mentalize everything. They can construct castles in the air with their mind and create another universe, if they wish, which will be a place of safety for them compared to the world they are forced to live in with us. In this stage, they may also not be able to tell you the truth. They manipulate others with their lies or with their altered reality—which seems real enough to them. It is the only place where they can feel safe with their central nervous system wrecked by the shock factors of PTSD and trauma.

I once had a Vietnam veteran patient who desperately wanted to try constitutional treatment to cure himself of his mania. He'd suffered badly during the war from shock, and when he came home, he hid at home. Little by little, over the years, he carefully constructed this world of mental rules where if he followed them religiously, he wouldn't flip out or go psycho. He'd been in therapy almost 15 years and was getting nowhere. He also had irritable bowel syndrome (IBS). He took *Veratrum album* 30C. In one dose, it cleared up the IBS he'd had for over a decade, and he was amazed and grateful for homeopathy's miraculous cure of this condition.

I wasn't surprised, because he was a veratrum constitutionally. When it came time to take a more powerful dose of the remedy, he managed to sabotage himself time and again by refusing to follow instructions, until I refused to work with him. He really didn't want to get well—he preferred this complicated intellectual world he'd built inside his head instead. And why not? He was able to function and he chose to remain at that level of function. A homeopath can't *force* anyone to heal if she or he doesn't want to.

Veratrum album's keynotes are many and quite obvious. This remedy is well known for its excesses, and you can read that into all levels, not just the physical one. Veratrum people have excessive perspiration, diarrhea and vomiting (projectile vomiting). They can get diarrhea from drinking cold water on a hot day. They have intense thirst, which is no wonder, since they are always sweating out so much liquid! They may end up with green-colored urine, green vomit, green diarrhea—which is also a keynote.

They are cold. Their breath feels cold. They have cold sweat and a cold face. They may say they feel their blood "running cold" through the body, or they may experience a cold chill that wracks them from head to toe. Their skin may turn blue or cyanotic or even purple in color. If they touch you, you realize that their hands are icy cold, and so are their feet. One of the keys to shock is being cold, which is why you cover the victim with a blanket. And for *Veratrum album*, one place where all this coldness is lessened, is being in a warm room or near a fire. *Veratrum album* persons are always better with heat.

In the last stages, people who are classic candidates for *Veratrum album* as the remedy turn to religion so they can be saved, because they've been unable to save themselves with the constructs and powers of their mind. However, in this out-of-balanced state, they turn to religion with a fever pitch. It is their salvation, even though they despair of ever being saved. They may move into constant prayer or praying and at some point feel that they are anointed to "save the world." Their religious fervor and manic tendencies combined create a person who goes around with Bible in hand, proclaiming that she or he is the only one who can save us and is the second coming of Christ or one of the disciples who has returned to save us all.

These individuals also scold us for our ways, pointing out our faults to us, and they are self-righteous when doing so. Sometimes they will say they see the world burning up and on fire—a literal hell. This haughtiness, that they are better than the rest of us, combined with zealot religious fervor make these persons seem like the fire-breathing, pulpit-pounding preacher from the 1800s. Their delusion is so deep at this point that somewhere within them, they know that Spirit/God is the only one who can save them and so they move in that direction—but in an out-of-balance expression of it.

Another area of problems for *Veratrum album* candidates is cramping. While they are having a bowel movement, their lower legs may cramp. Women's menstrual cramping can make them faint—and fainting is a keynote for *Veratrum album*. Sciatica may act up on them and send shooting pains, like electric flashes, down their legs. Their feet and knees may feel heavy, as if they were stones.

The sleep of *Veratrum album* candidates is equally disturbed. They awaken at night, trembling, or they start at any noise or sound—even in the soundest of sleep. Dreams or nightmares awaken them feeling frightened and scared. These are anxious dreams, of robbers or of being hunted and being unable to escape. When they do get to sleep, it is a long, uninterrupted and very deep slumber.

They have unique cravings that help us decide whether or not this is the remedy that can help. They love sour things, such sour fruit (lemons/limes), sour drinks, salt, ice, fruit in general and sardines. They don't want warm food and instead prefer cold food. And although they love fruit, it ends up disagreeing with them and they get stomach distension as a result. Potatoes and green vegetables aren't on their short list of favorites either. Interestingly, they crave ice water, but it too can give them problems after they've slugged down great quantities of it—they can vomit it right back up.

Veratrum album's symptoms are better with heat of any type, such as from a blanket, sunlight or fire; being held (if they want physical contact); consuming hot drinks; lying down; consuming meat and milk. They are worse with exertion; cold drinks; fright from pain; wet, cold weather or humid, chilly weather; at night; before and after menses; from touch or pressure; if pride is injured by another (they hate being criticized); change of weather.

Veratrum album could, in my opinion, be of great help to a number of combat veterans or people who have suffered severe traumatization of some sort and where the shock has not worn off with time but rather has become entrenched and goes deeper and deeper with time. This is one of the key remedies to halt the total destruction of shock that occurs if left untended.

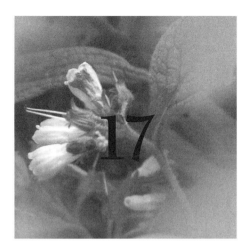

Flower Essences for PTSD

We've seen the pervasive devastation that PTSD can wreak on a person's life. Literally, no corner or facet of a life remains untouched by it; rather, it's simply a matter of *how much* it is staining the fabric of a person's life and to what depth. Because everyone's vital force is different, different healing tools must be considered. What I will share with you here is not the whole answer. Indeed, for some it won't mean anything at all, whereas for others a certain homeopathic remedy or flower essence will resonate when they read about it.

Psychotherapy, homeopathy as well as soul recovery and extraction (SR/E; see page 340 in chapter 18) are perhaps the three greatest tools toward real cure of PTSD symptoms. Everything else, including flower essences, becomes an adjunct tool that can lend support to the larger, more powerful ways of healing mentioned above. Any healing method undertaken must have the trust and faith of the person who is employing it. For instance, if a person doesn't believe SR/E will help, it won't. The same is true for homeopathic treatment. We all must resonate to what we inwardly know will help us heal. There are different answers for each of us and, luckily, there are many tools out there too!

Flower essences are an adjunct to homeopathic treatment and frequently, one of my shamanic facilitators will suggest them when a particularly traumatic piece is brought back via SR/E for a client.

Flower essences take the edge off. The best news is that they don't suppress or interfere with a homeopathic remedy, which is why I've continued to develop them for use. If you resonate to any of the flower essences presented in this chapter, it will more than likely help you.

Some essences are more powerful than others. A star (✷) indicates the powerful ones, with an accompanying warning—*do not take those without professional help being available.* You may want to take a flower essence (or more than one, depending upon how you resonate with them and how your symptoms match the accompanying symptom picture) before an SR/E or during therapy. If you are under the care of a therapist or homeopath, please consult with her or him first before taking any essences; get permission and guidance.

What You Love Can Help Heal You

As said before, in homeopathy we have the law of similars: "Like cures like." Since 1993 I have been conducting provings on many flower and gem essences, and over the years, I have discovered a remarkable thing, the "language" of the flower. In other words, I can look at a person's personality and characteristics and say that a specific flower (bush, tree or plant) can help support that person toward good health. Here's another way to put this: *What you love will help you.*

Let me give you an example: Let's say that your most favorite flower in the world is the red rose. You can purchase the red rose flower report and find out all about yourself physically, mentally, emotionally and spiritually. If you agree with the report and what it offers you, then you should take the red rose flower essence that we make. By taking it, the energy and vibration of what you love most (this red rose flower) will begin to help bring your vital force back into harmony. Sometimes it creates near miracles; other times the benefits are more subtle. However, the benefits are there and will help you toward inner balance and harmony within yourself. And that is a good thing.

So what you love can help you. It's that simple. Life isn't really as complicated as we like to think, and sometimes the plants of nature are powerful advocates and supporters of us. And if someone has PTSD symptoms, that person's favorite flower can do nothing but help her or him back to good health in the long run.

The flower reports will become available to the public in November 2004. Just go to page 386 to find out how to order them at that time.

Flower Essences for PTSD Symptoms

Bear Grass

Bear grass (*Xerophylum tenax*) is a flower essence that comes from the Rocky Mountains; it is an incredible healer in many senses. Bears are known to be powerful medicine among the Native American, and no less powerful is this plant that has their name, this bulb plant that blooms only once every five to seven years high in the Rocky Mountains.

From the provings that have been performed on it thus far, it can be seen that bear grass is going to have far-reaching implications. First of all, it has white or yellow white flowers and can therefore deal with any and all chakras of a person or animal. The yellowish cast to bear grass strongly suggests that it can help in the realm of mental disorders and dysfunctions, especially in cases of brainwashing—abusive family situations where powerful conditional patterns make it hard to break from past, learned experience. Bear grass has the ability to move rapidly through blocks and to immediately dissolve them. Many of the provers report feeling this energy work, usually as a warmth in the region where the block was located. There is no question that this flower essence can clear the way for relearning and breaking old, established habit patterns.

For PTSD survivors, this can translate into the essence working directly and quickly in areas where there still is tension, denial, suppression or repression of either memories or emotions. It is not traumatic as crested prickle poppy (see page 330) can be in the dream state; anyone can utilize this remedy.

✿ Bromeliad, Red and Yellow

This is for those individuals who are supersensitive to light, sounds and odors. If they get into a crowd-type situation or get too closely crowded, they may lose their temper, become highly agitated or angry. This essence helps to tone down the supersensitiveness as well as the edgy quality of someone's irritability, which always moves into an angry outburst toward another or a situation. Frequently, this type of individual is quiet and shy and you wouldn't think them capable of an explosive, angry outburst — but that's because they are literally sitting on a time bomb within themselves.

They may also swing to the other extreme and be extremely egotistical, braggarts, bossy, militaristic and pushy toward others. It's all a bluff, of course, but they can look like the raging lion upon occasion and subdue others with their powerful presentation. They are paper tigers, scared inside. However, if pushed, they won't always back off, and that's when they may allow some of this ugly fear to vent itself. This person can become highly aggressive and even physically threatening. Red and yellow bromeliad is known to take the edge off such behavior. However, to retrain such a person and vent her or his behavior in more positive ways, other, more primary tools that are acceptable to this individual need to be employed.

Children who after experiencing or witnessing a terribly traumatizing situation begin acting out their aggression, do well on this essence. It's not unusual for a child to be out of control, striking out, hitting, biting or kicking days or weeks after she or he experienced a PTSD episode. Red and yellow bromeliad backed up with SR/E, homeopathic treatment at a constitutional level or psychotherapy can help remove this trauma so that such children don't end up carrying it around with them the rest of their lives.

Broom Snakeweed

Broom snakeweed is Escoba de la Vibora, *Gutierrezia spp. compositae,* and its nickname is "confrontation of fears essence." This plant's plane of expression is emotional and mental, and it primarily works on the solar plexus chakra (yellow).

This powerful flower essence may be of use as an adjunct to homeopathic treatment of a person who has a lot of fears and whose fears have turned inward. Many women who have been abused in a marriage can use this flower essence. Children who have suffered abuse, trauma or PTSD where it has turned them into cowering "cowards" who run away at the first sign of confrontation or trouble also do well with it.

Fear is our greatest inhibitor when it comes to looking at our own internal demons, and it stops us from evolving and growing as a consequence. This flower essence has the power to work directly with our fears—no matter what they are—and to help us stand our ground. That can also mean standing our ground within ourselves and not only when confronted with some external event that is scaring us to death or immobilizing us with fear until we're paralyzed. Broom snakeweed can dissolve the paralyzing effect of the fear, helping us to meet it squarely—eyeball to eyeball—and stand our ground.

The most amazing thing happens when we are able to stand our ground and face our fears: Eventually, the fears dissolve. They may lessen to a high degree or disappear totally with time. Broom snakeweed helps this to occur much more swiftly, thereby alleviating our fear of confrontation.

Negative Qualities

If there ever was a remedy for someone who has been abused or traumatized by shock or PTSD, this is it. This is for anyone who is afraid of confrontation of any kind. The inability to confront may turn the person into a passive-aggressive (PA) individual, and broom snakeweed is excellent for PA personality types who manipulate others to do their bidding.

Positive Qualities

Broom snakeweed allows a person to stand up and confront her or his abuser or fear. It helps people who get fearful before a confrontation (internally or externally) to deal with it without that gut-wrenching fear stopping them. It is excellent for people who are worried, first and foremost, of what others may think of them: They're able to stand up and speak clearly for themselves, consequences be damned. It turns a mouse into a lion, without aggression. This essence imbues individuals with their own, inner truth and allows them to speak it without fear of recrimination or judgment.

Note: This remedy is excellent once the woman has left the abuser and she is at a safe house or shelter. Do *not* give it to her if she's in the abusive home where her abuser could, if provoked by her fearless stance, turn on her and injure her badly or possibly kill her or her children.

Broom snakeweed can help lessen the degree of fear response, and if the homeopath knows that the patient is retracing old fear/anger, the flower essence should be utilized during this time period.

Commentary

Sometimes in field work, the essence I'm retrieving "speaks" to me in many synchronistic ways, and broom snakeweed is certainly one of them. Suffice it to say, I had to confront my fears face to face. The most interesting facet of this confrontation was that as it was "going down," nine buzzards were circling above me. Since I have buzzard medicine, I knew it was the cosmos telling me symbolically that everything would turn out fine—and it did. It was a miraculous afternoon getting this essence!

The Native Americans gather this plant, an old herbal remedy from the Southwest, and use it as a "bath tea" to reduce the pain and swelling of their arthritis, in lieu of having to take aspirin. They will take a cup of the plant, boil it for half an hour, strain it and pour the liquid into bath water. By soaking in it, pain goes away. They will also drink a cup of the tea while taking the bath.

I've used this essence from time to time when I had to face my peer group to give a talk and experienced internal fears (butterflies). A couple of drops made the fear go away and made it very easy for me to talk to those people—without fear, without anger, just straight across the board in a mature, adult fashion and with calm deliberateness and an inner feeling of solidity.

What I like most about this remedy is that it doesn't bring up anger to use it as a bludgeon against someone else. Rather, broom snakeweed harnesses the anger, melds it, molds it into a *strength* that you can use in the most positive of ways. This is an excellent remedy for children who are being bullied by other kids at school or for those who work with a condescending boss who doesn't respect them, for example.

There are times in all of our lives when we must "pay the piper," regardless of personal cost to us, and speak our truth. This essence will help you do it with your own morals, values and principles well in place—in a balanced way. And truth is far mightier than any sword of abuse. Looking at this bush, which is scattered all across the Southwest, one would think it was a weed. To me, it is a silent testament and a reminder that none of us ever need to be afraid of speaking our truth that comes from our heart and soul, and that none of us ever need to allow our internal demons and fears to stop us from living our truth. In the spring, our deserts, valleys and canyons are fragrant with this wonderful, light-smelling flower that bathes slopes in a blanket of bright yellow. Let each one of us wear our blanket of truth, no longer afraid of reaction, abuse or our fears in any form.

Century Plant

Century plant (*Agave parryi*) is designed to gently move a person who is blocked by a PTSD trauma into wanting to make the necessary changes so that it no longer holds her or him in a tight, unrelenting grip. This is a powerful flower essence, yet it is one of the quietest and most gentle of all the PTSD remedies. Century plant is about transformation, slowly but surely. It helps in the worst cases and frequently, I combine it with crested prickle poppy (but this combination is only used when a homeopathic practitioner, shamanic facilitator or therapist is in place first).

Known as the "breakthrough essence," it helps shore up an individual's desire to heal from the PTSD. Another essence I frequently consider along with century plant is bear grass (see page 325). I've never seen blocks dissolved as rapidly and thoroughly as with this essence. Bear grass lives up to its name as being a master healer in the essence world, and when teamed with the bulldog quality of the century plant, it is a particularly powerful, yet gentle combination.

Corn Plant

Corn plant (*Dracaena fragrans*) is a recent proving. To put it succinctly, this essence has the ability to bring out and discharge our own darkness (anxiety, fears, paranoia and so forth) and replace it with a sense of profound peacefulness, calmness and centeredness. It stabilizes a person very quickly.

This recent proving was done just before the terrorists hit the Pentagon and the World Trade Center, so it appears to be the most powerful of all the essences I've mentioned above and is the one I suggest for everyone to try.

❊ *Crested Prickle Poppy*

Crested prickle poppy (*Argemone pleiacantha*) is one of the most powerful PTSD tools I know of. It, more than any other, can work rapidly toward bringing up those memories we've repressed or suppressed. This essence should not be used if the individual is mentally or emotionally unstable, as it can send a person into a psychotic break. This essence works swiftly with us by bringing up our "shadow" contents from deep within our subconscious, where the worst of the PTSD symptoms continue to lurk and poison us. It does this by bringing up, in our nightly dream state, shadow dreams where we think (or know) that whoever is chasing us will kill us.

The dream nature of crested prickle poppy is not one of clothing things in mysterious, unidentifiable dream symbols. No, when we're dreaming with this essence, it's straightforward and needs no interpretation; the dreamer will know what the dream means right away. For those who think they have never dreamed (you do but don't recall it) or who forget their dreams as soon as they wake up, this flower essence will help remember and recall after waking.

This is an essence for those who really want to work aggressively through their PTSD and get it done and over with. It is not an essence for the faint of heart or for those who are sitting on the fence, not sure if they really want to plumb the poisonous depths of their unconscious. It takes a lot of courage to face our own closet of skeletons and manmade monsters from our past. This flower essence will do it.

A note of caution here: Take crested prickle poppy 20 minutes before going to bed, putting four drops beneath your tongue. Never take this flower essence at any other time of the day, because it can make you spacy so that you won't pay proper attention to your driving, for example. Keep a pen and paper nearby so that you can begin a dream log. Take this essence for 30 days, go back over your dream log and you'll see a very obvious message forming—repeatedly. If the dreams become too much, then stop taking the essence for 5 days and start again. It is within your power to begin to allow the poisons to vent under controlled conditions.

I've written a book on the provings we've done on this incredible resource entitled *Crested Prickle Poppy Proving* (see Appendix D). It is a definitive guide to all the symptoms it can deal with, which are considerable.

Yarrow

Yarrow (*Achillea millefolium*) is a must for those who have PTSD symptoms that are specific to not feeling safe in certain places or situations. There are specific colors to address different safety issues or these raw feelings of vulnerability: White yarrow is for a general, overall sense of no safety, a vague sense of danger that is felt almost everywhere. Yellow yarrow is about the mind or mental faculties that combine with our solar plexus, the seat of our fears and anxieties. Pink yarrow is about not feeling safe around those who love us—we just can't reach out and trust them as much as we'd like to.

Often I suggest a yarrow combination of all colors to strengthen the person's will and help create healthy, more positive boundaries for the individual. This essence is particularly good for loners who stalk off into the forest or hills to be alone. The reason for wanting to be alone is that their personal boundaries have been destroyed years earlier, and they are so raw and open on other levels that they cannot protect themselves appropriately in places such as a shopping mall, a grocery store or other places where there are crowds of people.

Noise, odors, psychic bleeding or hemorrhaging (you feel weak, your mental faculties sputter to a halt and you may be forgetful) or any other negative energy is combated by the power of yarrow. Not only does it help to slowly but surely rebuild a person's own boundaries, it also allows people to speak up for themselves and to use the word "no" and mean it. Many codependent women who aren't necessarily burdened with PTSD symptoms need this remedy.

Flower Essence Comparison

Petrified sequoia tree imbues us with a zenlike acceptance of ourselves, mind- and bodywise. Colville (yellow) columbine connects heart and mind and integrates the two so completely that standing in our truth is no longer plagued by fear. Shasta daisy helps us to trust our own intuitive, higher knowing despite the chaos, shouting or commotion going on around us. Corn plant, which helps eradicate the darkness (our fears, anxieties, paranoia and so forth) and puts it in place, helps create calm, peacefulness and feeling centered and stable.

These are but a few flower essences that might be considered for dealing with PTSD. There are many more, but they must be fitted with an individual's specific symptoms. Those reviewed here have powerful abilities directly tied to addressing trauma and PTSD symptoms in particular.

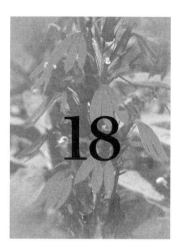

Shamanism and PTSD

As we have seen in the previous chapters, anyone can become a survivor of various symptom pictures for posttraumatic stress disorder (PTSD) as a result of having experienced trauma. There are many ways to approach the healing course of PTSD symptoms. The psychological community, for example, works via therapy, and of late some new tools have been developed within this community, among them eye movement desensitization and reprocessing (EMDR), traumatic incident reduction (TIR) and visual kinesthetic dissociation (VKD). All of these methods have brought some success with some individuals, and if you are interested in any of these types of treatment, contact your therapist for details.

Trauma in any form is not going to be cured by just one tool, however; human beings are far too diverse and unique as individual beings for that. To help PTSD survivors heal, we need many tools, from many areas. Sometimes this tool is psychotherapy; other times it is prayer, hands-on healing, sweat lodges, Rolfing, polarity therapy, Gestalt therapy, vision quests, herbs, vitamins and minerals, traditional drugs, homeopathic treatment, Bach flower treatment or another tool.

One tool that has rarely been written about but that deserves a lot of attention and exploration as a possible road to becoming healed from PTSD symptoms is shamanic intervention. I don't claim to be an authority on worldwide shamanism. I can approach this subject only through my own experience and observation and will share how shamanism helped me with my PTSD symptoms.

What Is Shamanism?

Before I go into that, I need to point out that I'm going to use the word shaman to denote both male and female. Sometimes "shaman" denotes male and "shamaness" denotes a female, but for simplicity's sake, I'll use "shaman" for either gender.

Shamanism is a gift, a skill, a talent that's as old as humankind on Mother Earth. Being a shaman does not mean you have to be of Native American blood; it has nothing to do with your skin color or nationality. Over the years, I have learned that all countries have shamans and that they can be male or female.

In the "olden" days, shamans were a working part of their communities: By day, they were out in the fields working, they were parents, they did all the things everyone else did to help keep the community alive and well. By night, they donned the shaman's cap and journeyed in behalf of the people of their village.

Shamans still have one foot solidly rooted in Mother Earth and our third-dimensional reality and the other in those less visible dimensions that intersect the third dimension and flow in and around us all the time. Shamans are, symbolically speaking, a fulcrum point between the seen and unseen worlds. They are messengers, journeying for others and bringing back messages for them. For example, they may bring a message from a loved one who is deceased.

Shamans journey in an altered state of consciousness, at will, in a fully controlled manner. It's important to note that shamans can shut off this psychic ability in them when they want to close it down. Some shamans, especially those from Third World cultures, use hallucinogenic drugs as a device to make the leap from third-dimensional reality into the other dimensions. (When Timothy Leary and his group started experimenting with LSD decades ago, they had found a substance in that drug that "trip-levered" open that particular psychic valve/door in our brain that allows entrance into these other dimensional realities.) Other shamans use sound to journey. For example, the constant, unbroken beat of a drum will place me and my facilitators into this altered state so that I may journey. It is not astral traveling or astral projection, which is an entirely different metaphysical process. What I was taught is soul recovery and extraction with drumming as a source to move into what shamans call nonordinary reality.

Shamans are trained for decades, usually in the format of the "wounded healer archetype" and the "shaman archetype." To become a shaman, certain earmark events must first occur in one's life, and one doesn't usually become one until around age 40 (although there are exceptions to this). From the time they are born, shamans are on a shamanic path, even though they usually don't realize or know this until much later. They typically go through one or more life-and-death experiences or have a near-death experience (NDE), so they know what the other dimensions look like and what the death experience is all about. They may have been very sick as babies or children, or they may have taken on a chronic disease and then cured themselves of it later on in life.

Shamans go through a period of "insanity," because to work in the other dimensions, they must know what these dimensions look like, what they are composed of and who inhabits those places. This can happen in the form of a nervous/emotional breakdown, a psychotic break from reality, schizophrenia or multiple-personality dysfunction, to mention a few examples. Shamans go through one of these forms of "insanity" as journeyman apprentice shamans and come out the other side whole and healed, in order to move forward in their shamanic development.

Shamans cannot have a fear of death or dying, so they go through this process repeatedly until it's no big deal any more. They must work through all their major fears, whatever they may be, before they can be successful at what they do. Many people are in training as shamans and don't know it, but to see such events unfold in their lives is an indicator to me that they are on that path.

How Do We Lose and Recover "Pieces" of Ourselves?

From a shamanic viewpoint, when we encounter something that scares, shocks or traumatizes us or when we experience grief or loss of a beloved person or animal, place or thing, a part of ourselves can—but does not always—split off as a result. In essence, it is *trauma* that creates this splitting-off process. PTSD certainly ranks high as a major reason for soul loss of one or more of our pieces. This splitting off of a piece means it is energy, in some form. I don't try to define it; to me, it's just an expression of energy. Whether it comes from one's soul, one's spirit, one's aura or a layer in one's aura, I really don't know, and I'll let you try and decide that for yourself.

This piece becomes "stuck" in one of many dimensions at that time frame or reference point/age when the trauma occurs. If we lose enough pieces of ourselves, it sets us up for disease on a physical, mental, emotional or spiritual level or a combination thereof. It can, in homeopathic vernacular, put us out of harmony, or balance, within our vital force.

How Can Shamans Help?

By recovering the piece or pieces and bringing them back to you, the shaman teaches you how to reintegrate them back into yourself. To keep our craft humble, I like to refer to what we do as being cosmic bird dogs—we hunt and sniff around in other dimensions, find and locate the missing pieces and, like a good retriever, we gather them up and bring them back to you! Sort of like playing fetch or hide-and-seek. Another duty we perform is helping you integrate these parts of you back into yourself, your vital force, your aura, and therefore, we stay in close touch with our clients shortly after a journey.

In what shape or form shamans bring back a piece to you varies, depending on the shaman. Sometimes the piece is in the form of a symbol and sometimes it is a color. Some shamans, like myself, literally see the trauma you endured on a movie screen. They see the entire event—what you were wearing, what people said, what everyone involved felt and so on. These shamans bring all this information, including the missing piece(s), back to you.

"Are there other ways to recover my lost pieces?" you may ask. Absolutely! You can also recover pieces of yourself. You can get your pieces back through many different models of intense therapy or prayer work, through a certain event occurring or reoccurring, through your own soul growth, with age/time or by using any of the other tools that we can use to heal ourselves. I have seen pieces return with homeopathic constitutional treatment.

Taking a shamanic intervention route, to me, is faster and quicker—it shaves off years of therapy and saves a lot of money in the process! If you aren't comfortable with shamanic intervention, you should not employ it as a tool to help you heal. On the other hand, if you are comfortable with the process and concept and have faith and trust in it, shamanism may be a tool to explore as a possibility.

Hot and Cold Journeys

Shamans can journey "hot" or "cold." (I like journeying cold.) "Hot" means you have told us: "I want this piece of myself brought back," and you identify the trauma and the age you were when it occurred to you. "Hot" means you're asking us to go after a specific incident where you were traumatized by a person, place or thing and to recover the piece or pieces for you.

"Cold" means we don't want to know anything about you or your potentially lost pieces or trauma. Cold journeying has a greater, more profound effect on you, because first of all, you know we don't know anything about you, your loss or situation beforehand; and secondly, when we bring back the piece or pieces and identify them, your age and other details, you know it's true and that we did our job. When a cold journey brings back pieces only you could know about, the healing is immense and profound on every level. Let me give you some examples.

Three Shamanic Case Examples

Many years ago, a very famous painter contacted me for help. He said that in the previous five years, he hadn't been able to paint like he had before. He'd read my book and told me he had many symptoms of missing pieces (which I'll go into later). I stopped him and said that I didn't need to hear any further information about him or his problem than what he'd just shared with me. Rather dumbfounded, he asked if I was sure I didn't need more information. I said yes, I was sure, because if I was allowed to "cold" journey for him (to do this, we have to get approval from the person we journey for as well as an approval from our spirit guide), I'd know all I needed to know. We made an appointment that he'd call me on a given day, at a given hour. In the meantime,

I'd journey on his behalf. (By the way, we do most of our journeys long-distance, meaning you don't have to see us in person. You might live halfway around the world, but when we're in our journey state, time and distance don't exist. This enables us to help people around the world without them spending a lot of money traveling to see us in person or vice versa. However, not all shamans have this unique capability.)

When I went into the journey for this painter—after having received permission—I was shown a double-hung window, half open to let the breeze in. White, delicate curtains framed the window. A man stuck his head out the window to call someone outside the house. I saw the window come smashing down on the back of his neck, injuring him. I then saw this wildly spinning yellow triangle outside the window, seconds after the physical trauma had occurred. My guide told me to recover the triangle and bring it back to the painter and then instructed me to do extraction work on his neck where the injury had occurred. (Extraction means to take out or replace something in the person's vital force/aura.)

When the painter called, I told him what I had seen and described his trauma. He was thunderstruck. Yes, he had injured his neck exactly as I'd seen it, and for the five years since then, he had not been able to paint his beautiful, other-worldly scenes anymore. Not only that, but he'd been to pain clinics around the world and used both traditional and alternative methods to get rid of the chronic pain that had ensued from that accident, and nothing had worked to relieve his daily misery.

He nearly cried when I told him about recovering the golden yellow triangle. He told me that this triangle was what he used to envision a new picture, in his mind, with his eyes closed, before he'd begin painting. As he'd lapse into this light form of meditation, the golden triangle would grow larger and he'd see himself going through this "door," and on the other side, he would see these incredible, wildly beautiful landscapes from other dimensions—which is what he painted. He would, in a shamanic way, transport himself into another dimension via the golden triangle, memorize what he'd see, bring the image back through the triangle into his physical body, and then he would get up and paint it.

The happy ending to this story is that since recovering this lost piece, he has been painting as before the accident, and the pain in his neck is gone.

My brother, Gary Gent, is a Vietnam War veteran. He was in the army and stationed in Saigon. Luckily for him, our sister Nancy was also living in Saigon at the time, so Gary was more fortunate than most: He had family there, which helped him immensely. However, two weeks after having come stateside, he was in a motorcycle accident that nearly killed him (the shamanic path—near-death experience). He was driving, his girlfriend was on the back (neither was wearing a helmet), and a pickup truck turned the corner at 35 miles per hour and struck them. Gary's girlfriend escaped with cuts and bruises, but Gary ended up in a coma, the rear of his skull badly injured. He lay in a coma for nearly two weeks, and the doctors thought for sure the tissue surrounding the brain stem injury would swell up and shut off the blood supply to his brain, thereby rendering him brain-dead.

I remember those awful days. My mother and father drove down to Modesto, California, where the accident had happened. I knew some homeopathy then, but my mother couldn't find the remedy (*Arnica montana*) that I wanted her to give to Gary. So she laid hands on him instead as she had done with all of us kids when we were sick. I'm sure it made the difference. A week later, Gary came out of the coma, and the doctors considered it a miracle he'd survived, much less wasn't mentally retarded. The only loss he suffered was his loss of smell.

Many years later, I journeyed for Gary and retrieved the piece of him he'd lost at the spot where the accident had taken place. I saw the motorcycle, its color, the color of the pickup and everything that had happened. I brought this piece back to him. When I described the scene, he told me I was accurate in all details. Because of that retrieval, about 50 percent of his ability to smell has returned.

Tyo Llorente, the Basque shaman, ran a journey for me. She did cold journeying like I do. She came back with a piece of me from my rape. She described my attacker in detail, and she confirmed that I'd lost the piece due to the violation. The most profound change that I experienced after that was that I no longer jumped when someone came up behind me. It was the most amazing thing!

Homeopathic Treatment and Soul Recovery and Extraction (SR/E) Applications

I had lived part of my life in this PTSD mode and neither homeopathy nor therapy had cured it, but the journey had. What I have discovered over the years is this: Homeopathy was able to help those pieces of me that were already with me as well as my vital force/aura, but it could not cure those missing parts that were somewhere out there and that I had yet to integrate. Therapy performed in a similar fashion. It was the shamanic intervention that brought those pieces back so they could be dealt with homeopathically, through therapy and with flower essences that completed the bulk of my healing.

When I work with new clients and if they are open to shamanic intervention, I will mention the possibility. If they want it, then I like SR/E to be performed first before I take their constitutional case, since inevitably, the symptom picture changes and sometimes dramatically so. I like to wait three months after the SR/E, because it usually takes that long to integrate any returning pieces. By that time, the vital force and aura have settled down, and the symptoms have changed and stabilized. At that point, I take the client's case.

There are instances where a homeopath knows darn well she has the right remedy, but the person's vital force is not responding. This is the time to think about getting a journey done for the client, because there is a missing piece. Once that piece is returned and integrated, the well-chosen remedy is given, and this time it will work! There are also instances where the homeopath has tried several remedies and the vital force is not budging or responding. In such cases, a journey will oftentimes unstick the whole affair, get the vital force working and integrating so that the picture shifts or changes. At that point, the homeopath can retake the case, prescribe a remedy—and it will work.

Indicators of Soul Loss

Over the years, I have noticed certain tell-tale signs that signal, at least for me as a shaman, that an individual might have experienced soul loss. I'd like to share these signs with you and at the same time emphasize that the following is not a complete list. Rather, it is only a compilation of my observations, so there could well be more. I'd also like to share the words we use daily in our speech that indicate soul loss, but you wouldn't realize it. These phrases are red flags for you to evaluate if you truly have suffered soul loss or not.

Signs That Signal Soul Loss

1. Schizophrenia

This is a condition that manifests when many pieces are taken. Usually, it is due to severe, repeated childhood traumas, and the spirit is shattered into many, many fragments or pieces. Because the pieces are missing and not within the vital force/aura, the "leaks" in the aura are so many that the person can no longer filter out the other dimensions that surround her or him. It is like being a radio and receiving 50 radio stations simultaneously—there is music, noise, talk—with no way to shut them off or turn them down.

2. Multiple Personality Disorder (MPD)

This is also known as the "three faces of Eve." Individuals with MPD have suffered through great emotional/mental trauma, usually in utero or during their baby or childhood years, and have developed compartmentalized personalities to deal with the ongoing traumas. Wether the trauma exists now, in their current life, or not does not matter. As each piece is flipped off due to trauma, a new personality emerges from the person's psyche in its place to fill the hole, or vacuum, left by the piece being lost due to trauma. As each piece is recovered, the personalities begin to disappear.

3. Depression

Any type of depression that is diagnosed as ongoing or chronic applies here. When we lose enough pieces or lose one main piece, we become depressed—grieving and potentially angry over the loss of those pieces or that piece. This also includes manic depression.

4. Inability to Ground Oneself

Here is someone who is constantly daydreaming, shows a lack of interest in daily life and wants to escape by watching TV, drinking alcohol, consuming drugs, checking out otherwise; this is someone who is considered to have a "space cadet" mentality. This person usually runs around frantically, is completely disorganized and has little self-discipline. Ungrounded people have literally, in the astral sense, pulled up and out of their physical body, usually from the knees upward. It is simply too painful for them to be 100 percent grounded and connected to the third-dimensional reality. They also "lift off" because there are pieces missing and they feel terribly vulnerable; they try to escape that feeling of vulnerability and loss by leaving their body.

5. Detachment

Here is a feeling as if the person is standing outside her- or himself and seeing the world pass by without being connected to it in any way. This may be accompanied by sociopathic behavior, where the individuals exhibit no morals, values or principles. In fact, there is no sense of anyone else existing except they themselves and what they want out of life. Emotions are numb, and sometimes there is physical numbness somewhere in the body as well. There may also be a sense of helplessness, giving up or feeling immune to human or animal suffering in general.

6. Blocks of Memory Loss

Any time you cannot remember a certain age or stage of your life, soul loss has occurred. That piece—or those pieces—that retains that memory is no longer there for you to recall what happened. Usually, loss of large blocks of memory (say, from ages six to twelve) show that trauma has occurred, soul loss followed and memory loss is the result. This pertains particularly to combat vets, "trauma junkies" (emergency medical technicians, paramedics, police officers and firefighters; especially those involved in the Pentagon and World Trade Centers disasters) and to those who have experienced a severe auto accident, hard labor during pregnancy, a weather event such as a tornado or hurricane or an earthquake, to mention but a few examples.

7. Chronic Illness

If enough pieces are lost, acute or chronic illness can occur. This can start at the time you were born or at a specific age in your life. Soul loss can occur to the baby in utero, during labor/birth or shortly after birth (caesareans are particularly traumatic for the baby). If this happens and there is soul loss, the baby has a long, chronic history of always catching every cold, flu and childhood disease—over and over again. For example, I was chronically sick from the time I was born, and at two years old, in 1948, I almost died. I had my tonsils removed at that early age. I then continued to contract every cold and flu and ear infection around until I was five years old. After that I contracted scarlet fever, which led to rheumatic fever and heart damage at the age of six. At age eleven I had mononucleosis, and at age twelve, hepatitis. This is the path of the shaman—learning about life and death through acute or chronic diseases and barely surviving them. The missing pieces can be returned and health can be achieved.

8. Addiction

This includes any type of addiction, including drugs, alcohol, codependence, food (anorexia as well as bulimia), sex, love, gambling and so forth. It also includes repetition of the same mistake over and over again, which is another form of addictive behavior. Choosing to continue marrying abusive men or creating difficult work situations over and over again are examples of such behavior.

9. Inability to Release

Following a divorce, a death of a loved one or pet, your life revolves around the past and it becomes an obsession that you cannot seem to release, stop thinking about or stop feeling about.

10. "Why Am I Here?"

Asking, "Why am I here?" It includes a sense of emptiness, of not connecting or being connected as you know instinctively you should be. It is a sense of knowing that you are not whole but being unable to express it that way. And it is a sense of not belonging, wanting to go home and knowing home is not Earth.

11. Continual Cycles of Colds or Flu

If this cycle begins at any age, no matter how many antibiotics are taken, there is soul loss involved. Contracting immune system diseases, such as arthritis, cancer or AIDS also indicates soul loss. If you are easily stressed, there could be soul loss; when stress reaches the immune system, it buckles quickly, due to soul loss. When the piece is not there to support and underwrite the immune system, cycles of illness ensue.

12. A Vague Feeling of Impending Doom

This feeling often appears after the loss of a piece. The individual begins to feel terribly vulnerable and may unconsciously sense that something is wrong or missing but not know what it is.

13. Obesity and Unexplained/Explained Weight Gain

This is a pattern I've seen repeatedly with those who were molested or raped as a baby or child, and they may or may not have memory of it. I have also seen the pattern in women or men who have been raped when they were older and they do remember it. Yet another scenario is a highly dysfunctional childhood where abuse was experienced. The result is the same: The person unconsciously either eats more food or the body, even without the use of more food, builds a protective barrier or padding to help deal with the vulnerability that this individual feels so sharply. Fat becomes a physical symbol of armor or protection against the unconscious knowing that a piece of them is missing (usually a number of important pieces) and they must do something to protect that hole or loss within.

The fat ("protection") can also be put on to make the rape or incest survivor look unattractive to avoid being attacked again. Any time violation occurs—whether in the form of incest, rape, mugging or combat—our body will in some instances (from a homeopathic view, especially the carbon and calcarea families), use fat as an armor of protection against this loss of pieces.

14. Abuse or Violence

It doesn't matter whether you are a baby, child or adult—if you experience abuse or violence, you can and usually will lose a piece or pieces. The worse the abuse or violence, the more pieces you will lose. And even if the abuser is now dead, she or he can still retain those missing parts of you. Abusers "steal" pieces of others because they've had so much of themselves stolen from another individual, and the only way for them to survive (so they think, usually on an unconscious level) is to take from others—and so the abuse cycle moves from one generation to another. PTSD also falls under this heading, and it can be an actual war that a person lives through or a "war" in the family while growing up.

15. Loss of Self-Esteem

The feeling of shame or humiliation and the lack of confidence are all signals of major soul loss. Women often suffer from this, since they usually live in a society that suppresses the female gender.

Expressions That Signal Soul Loss

Over the years, I've gathered a lot of sayings from those who have experienced soul loss. See if you find yourself among these expressions:

- I just don't feel whole.
- I know s/he has a piece of me.
- I feel as if there's a gaping hole here, in me (pointing to the area/region).
- I just feel lost, as if I have no direction, no goals.
- I can't sleep well at night.
- S/he stole a part of me.
- S/he still has a stranglehold on me.
- I feel as if s/he's still got a part of me even though s/he's dead or out of my life.
- I'm tired all the time; I just don't have any pep or energy.
- I feel as if I'm an extremist; I can't do anything middle-of-the-road but have to go to extremes.
- S/he hates me.
- I have dreams about this person; it's as if s/he's haunting me.
- I feel like I'm a slave to that person.
- I feel out of kilter, out of balance, but don't know why!
- I feel like a cripple, but I shouldn't!
- My senses feel dead; I don't feel any joy or sadness.
- I can't cry—I haven't for years.
- I feel as if s/he's controlling me and I don't have the strength to say no to her/him.
- I feel as if I'm being torn apart by all of them.
- I feel like a puppet just waiting for my family to jerk my strings.

Appendix A:
Homeopathic Antidote List

While you are on a homeopathic remedy, certain things you smell, eat or drink may neutralize, or "antidote," the homeopathic remedy you are taking. And of course, the same items may not antidote a remedy for another person! Antidoting of a remedy is very individual to the person who has taken a remedy. As a result, the list below can provide general information only. Please consult with your homeopath about her or his list (if your homeopath has one) and do not simply follow the one presented here.

For example, smelling perfume as they pass a department store counter will antidote some people's homeopathic remedy but will have no effect on others'. One woman who uses peroxide/bleach to change the color of her hair may antidote her remedy, but another woman will not. We don't know why this is so, but we see it happening all the time. Keep in mind that one person's antidote is not necessarily another's.

If you do antidote your remedy, try to figure out what might have done it and share your suspicions with your homeopath immediately. If you have antidoted, you will have a resulting relapse that may be short-lived (up to two weeks) and involve only a few symptoms; in a worst-case scenario, the relapse caused by the antidoting material may be complete, that is, all your symptoms will come back. If this occurs, you must schedule an appointment to have your case reevaluated and possibly retaken at that time.

Coffee

There is an oil (not the caffeine) in the coffee itself that will antidote the remedy. This oil is in the "real" coffee as well as in the decaf variety.

Go to your health food store and look for a coffee substitute; drink that instead. You may continue to drink any other caffeine-type products, such as cola, tea (make sure it does *not* contain peppermint, spearmint, camphor or eucalyptus; if it does, do *not* drink it as these items will antidote a remedy as well), vegetable and fruit juices and water.

Herb Tea

Herb teas that contain any of the mint family (spearmint, peppermint), eucalyptus or camphor will antidote a remedy. "Strong" herbs may also partially antidote a remedy. I suggest you stick with mild forms (many of Celestial Seasonings' teas use "mild" herbs, but make sure you don't choose a tea with camphor/eucalyptus or a mint in it!). Items such as orange peel, hibiscus or lemon herb are okay. However, when you get into strong herbs such as ginseng, cascara sagrada or golden seal, then you may run the risk of a partial antidote.

Camphor, Eucalyptus and Mint

This includes inhaling the odor of mothballs too. Skin or mucous membrane (placing it externally on your skin) application of camphor, menthol or strong herbal oils (such as eucalyptus, rosemary, lavender) can antidote a remedy.

Camphor is used in Vick's VapoRub, Tiger Balm, Blistex medicated lip ointment, Chapstick, Ben-Gay, Campho-Phenique, Deep-Down Pain Relief Rub, Vick's Vaposteam, Afrin menthol nasal spray, Vick's inhaler, Rhulispray, skin creams like Noxema and Caladryl. It is also found in other ointments used for topical treatment (applied to your external skin) of muscleaches and pains, in most lip balms, some lip sticks, cough lozenges, many mouth washes and shaving creams. Brief smelling of camphor can antidote a remedy. Also avoid concentrated Pine Sol cleaner, Listerine, tea tree oil and wintergreen. Read labels *carefully*! If you aren't sure, do not apply the substance to your skin or smell it; call your homeopath first.

Odors

Some people walk into a hair-dresser's establishment and the smell of the strong chemicals used there will antidote their remedy. Others walk by a perfume counter in a department store, and their remedy is antidoted. Any strong smell may antidote a person's remedy. Do the best you can to avoid *any* strong odors, knowing that it's impossible to avoid all of them, particularly if you live in a polluted city landscape.

Hair Coloring

If you get your hair bleached and chemicals applied to it, it will antidote your remedy. Even using a rinse can, for some people, partially antidote a remedy.

Strong Flavors

Vinegar is probably the biggest problem, since some homeopathic remedies are highly susceptible to antidoting with vinegar. And sometimes the person taking the remedy is susceptible to vinegar as an antidote to her or his vital force. Don't forget that vinegar is found in most grocery store salad dressings!

Dental Work

The high speed of a dental drill can and sometimes does approximate the frequency of a remedy and antidotes it. If you cannot avoid dental work during this time, inform your homeopath when the dental work is finished and s/he will send you the same remedy/potency to take again.

We do not yet know what laser or air-powered drills do to a remedy. My guess is that they will not antidote the remedy, but the jury is still out on these, as they are too new a technique for us to know for sure. Above all, if you need to go to the dentist, go right away and do not wait.

Vitamins, Minerals and Herbs

All of these items will "hide" or "cover" your symptoms. Your homeopath needs to see if the remedy is making inroads into your ailment/symptoms. To do this, any changes in the pattern of your symptoms must be carefully monitored. Any of these substances alters, hides or covers your symptoms and will interfere directly with the homeopath's ability to accurately follow your case.

Your homeopath will ask you to stop taking all of these several weeks or a month before your case is taken so that s/he can "see" your symptoms clearly. Your homeopath may have a list of supplements for you to avoid, so be sure to talk to her or him about this.

Traditional Medical Drugs and Over-the-Counter Drugs

Drugs are designed to remove specific or local symptoms. A resulting suppression of symptoms weakens your vital force as a whole and often clouds (hides) the homeopathic picture of your real symptoms. Drugs can dampen the work of the homeopathic remedy, which means you will take the homeopathic remedy at a lower potency and more often if your medical doctor requires you to stay on your drug(s). Remember, though, that it is most important to *stay on your medication(s)*. *Do not go off* them without your doctor's prior approval.

If it is not possible for you to be off your drug(s)—and as I said above, this must first be discussed with your physician who will make this decision for you; you do not make it for yourself—be patient and understand that the homeopathic remedy you are taking has to work through the drugs you are taking at the same time it is working against the ailment. Diabetes and asthma are two examples of diseases where medication must be taken and homeopathy works as a secondary support.

Consult your physician and homeopath *before* you decide to go off *any* drug! Do not make this decision yourself! Many drugs are the type you cannot just stop but rather must be carefully monitored and weaned off to not create damage to your body. The good news is that as the homeopathic remedy begins to cure your symptoms, you will be able to slowly go off whatever drug(s) you are currently taking—but again, not without the prior approval of your physician.

Other Treatments

The balance of symptoms on all levels is a delicate one that can be easily upset. Some treatments are likely to suppress symptoms, thus weakening the vital force; they might antidote the remedy or confuse the symptom picture and therefore make it more difficult for the homeopath to accurately follow your case.

Consult a homeopath before planning acupuncture, polarity therapy, psychic healing or any other treatment aimed at the energy plane of you and your vital force. Getting treatments such as a chiropractic adjustment, an osteopathic treatment, massage, acupressure, foot reflexology or cranial work is fine as long as no electrical stimulation is involved (and it can, especially in chiropractic or osteopathic work). The masseuse should be informed not to use any oil containing mint, camphor or eucalyptus on you but rather mild or ordorless oils to avoid antidoting your remedy.

Others

Avoid foods, chemicals or substances that you know cause a severe reaction in your system. Avoid the consistent use of electric blankets and electric waterbed heaters; use a timer to heat the bed during the day, before use. Avoid recreational drugs; they clearly antidote a remedy. Alcohol, in moderation, is usually not a problem. Lastly—I always tell my patients, "If you aren't sure, don't eat it, apply it to your skin or inhale it. Call me first and ask. That way, you will avoid most potential situations of antidoting your remedy."

And no matter how hard you try, you may well end up antidoting your remedy because something that you are susceptible to that is not on this list will do it, and we will only know after the fact, when your symptoms suddenly start to come back—and they shouldn't return, but the opposite should be happening: Your symptoms should steadily clear and go away over time.

Appendix B: Homeopathic Resource Information

Research

The following information comes from the National Center for Homeopathy (NCH) at http://www.homeopathic.org. You can also call the NCH in Alexandria, VA, at (703) 548-7790.

Controlled Clinical Studies Published in Peer-Reviewed Journals

C. N. Shealy, MD, R. P. Thomlinson, and V. Borgmeyer, "Osteoarthritic Pain: A Comparison of Homeopathy and Acetaminophen," *American Journal of Pain Management*, 1998; 8:89-91.

A double-blind study to document the relative efficacy of homeopathic remedies in comparison to acetaminophen for the treatment of pain associated with osteoarthritis (OA) among 65 patients; an Institutional Review Board (IRB)-approved protocol. Results of the study documented better pain relief in the homeopathic group (55 percent achieved measured relief from homeopathy as compared to 38 percent from acetaminophen); however, the superiority of this treatment, in comparison with the acetaminophen group, did not reach statistical significance.

The investigators concluded that homeopathic treatments for pain in OA patients appear to be safe and at least as effective as acetaminophen and are without its potential adverse effects, including compromise to both liver and kidney function. Many of the patients asked to continue with the homeopathic treatment.

M. Weiser, W. Strosser, and P. Klein, "Homeopathic vs. Conventional Treatment of Vertigo: A Randomized Double-Blind Controlled Clinical Study, *Archives of Otolaryngology—Head and Neck Surgery*, August 1998, 124:879-885.

This was a study with 119 subjects with various types of vertigo, half of whom were given a homeopathic medicine (a combination of four homeopathic medicines) and half were given a leading conventional drug in Europe for vertigo, betahistine hydrochloride. The homeopathic medicines were found to be similarly effective and significantly safer than the conventional control.

D. Reilly, M. Taylor, N. Beattie et al, "Is Evidence for Homoeopathy Reproducible? *Lancet*, December 10, 1994, 344:1601-6.

This study successfully reproduced evidence from two previous double-blind trials all of which used the same model of homeopathic immunotherapy in inhalant allergy. In this third study, 9 of 11 patients on homeopathic treatment improved compared to only 5 of 13 patients on placebo. The researchers concluded that either homeopathic medicines work or controlled studies don't. Their work has been recently replicated and is submitted for publication. (See "Is Homeopathy a Placebo Response?" *Lancet,* 1986, below.)

J. Jacobs, L. Jimenez, and S. Gloyd, "Treatment of Acute Childhood Diarrhea with Homeopathic Medicine: A Randomized Clinical Trial in Nicaragua," *Pediatrics*, May 1994, 93,5:719-25.

This study was the first on homeopathy to be published in an American medical journal. The study compared individualized high-potency homeopathic preparations against a placebo in 81 children between the ages of 6 months and 5 years suffering from acute diarrhea. The treatment group benefited from a statistically significant 15-percent decrease in duration. The authors noted that the clinical significance would extend to decreasing dehydration and postdiarrheal malnutrition and a significant reduction in morbidity.

E. Ernst, T. Saradeth, and K. L. Resch, "Complementary Treatment of Varicose Veins: A Randomized Placebo-Controlled, Double-Blind Trial," *Phlebology*, 1990, 5:157-163.

This study of 61 patients showed a 44-percent improvement in venous filling time in the homeopathically treated group when compared with placebo.

P. Fisher, A. Greenwood, E. C. Huskisson et al, "Effect of Homoeopathic Treatment on Fibrositis," *British Medical Journal*, August 5, 1989, 299:365-66.

This trial was double-blind with a crossover design, comparing *R. toxicodendron* to a placebo in 30 patients suffering from an identical syndrome identified as the admission criteria. It showed a significant reduction in tender spots, by 25 percent, when patients were given the homeopathic medicine as compared to when they were given the placebo.

D. Reilly, M. Taylor, C. McSherry, "Is Homeopathy a Placebo Response? Controlled Trial of Homeopathic Potency with Pollen in Hayfever as Model," *Lancet*, October 18, 1986, 881-86.

The double-blind study compared a high-dilution homeopathic preparation of grass pollens against a placebo in 144 patients with active hay fever. The study method considered pollen counts, aggravation in symptoms as well as use of antihistamines and concluded that patients using homeopathy showed greater improvement in symptoms than those on placebo and that this difference was reflected in a significantly reduced need for antihistamines among the homeopathically treated group. The results confirmed those of the pilot study and demonstrated that homeopathic potencies show effects distinct from those of the placebo.

A. , "Nuclear Magnetic Resonance Spectroscopy of Homeopathic Remedies," *Journal of Holistic Medicine*, 5, Fall–Winter 1983, 172-175.

This study and the one below show that different homeopathic remedies tested at different potencies had distinctive readings of subatomic activity, whereas the placebos did not.

G. W. and R. B. Smith, "Changes Caused by Succession on NMR Patterns and Bioassay of Bradykinin Triacetate (BKTA) Successions and Dilutions," *Journal of the American Institute of Homeopathy*, 61, November–December 1968:197-212.

This study and the one above show that different homeopathic remedies tested at different potencies had distinctive readings of subatomic activity, whereas the placebos did not.

H. et al, "Homeopathic Treatment of Neuralgia Using Arnica and Hypericum: A Summary of 60 Observations," *Journal of the American Institute of Homeopathy*, 78, September 1985:126-128.

This double-blind study was conducted on patients with dental neurologic pain following tooth extraction. An impressive 76 percent of those given the homeopathic medicines arnica and hypericum experienced relief of pain.

Other Clinical Studies of Interest

A. K. Vallance, "Can Biological Activity Be Maintained at Ultra-High Dilution? An Overview of Homeopathy, Evidence and Bayesian Philosophy," *Alternative and Complementary Medicine*, 1998, 4:1;49-76.

"The objective of this article is to critically review the major pieces of evidence on ultra-high dilution (UHD) effects and suggest how the scientific community should respond to its challenge. Such evidence has been conducted on a diverse range of assays—immunologic, physiological, behavioral, biochemical and clinical in the form of trials of homeopathic remedies. Evidence of UHD effects has attracted the attention of physicists who have speculated on their physical mechanisms. . . . It is argued that if the phenomenon was uncontroversial, the evidence suffices to show that UHD effects exist. However, given that the observations contradict well-established theory, normal science has to be abandoned and scientists need to decide for themselves what the likelihood of UHD effects are. . . . The difficulty in publishing high-quality UHD research in conventional journals prevents a fair assessment of UHD effects. Given that the existence of UHD effects would revolutionize science and medicine and given the considerable empirical evidence of them, the philosophies of science tell us that possible UHD effects warrant serious investigation and serious attention by scientific journals."

T. E. Whitmarsh, "When Conventional Treatment Is Not Enough: A Case of Migraine Without Aura Responding to Homeopathy," *Alternative and Complementary Medicine*, 1997, 1:2;159-162.

Following three years of unsuccessful conventional treatment, a 55-year-old male suffering from common migraine, which would commence with nausea followed by vomiting every hour for 12 hours and throbbing pain well localized to the left fronto-parietal area, was referred to Glasgow Homeopathic Hospital. Consultation with a homeopathic physician, who also has extensive experience in diagnosis and treatment of headache disorders, led to the prescription of a single homeopathic remedy (bronia), which was absolutely effective for the condition. On follow-up two months later, the patient has been headache-free and had lost no time from work. He had taken the bronia only for three weeks (that is, 12 doses). He remains attack-free three years after treatment. This case is offered as an open, admittedly retrospective study, comparing the best of conventional migraine therapy with appropriate homeopathic therapy in the same patient.

J. Lamont, "Homeopathic Treatment of Attention Deficit Hyperactivity Disorder: A Controlled Study," *British Homoeopathic Journal,* October 1997, 86:196-200.

Forty-three children were randomly assigned to either placebo or homeopathic treatment groups, and then those initially given a placebo were given an individualized homeopathic medicine. All subjects underwent a homeopathic interview to determine which individualized remedy was appropriate. Results show significant improvement once the patient began taking the homeopathic medicine.

K. H. Friese, S. Kruse, and H. Moeller, "Acute Otitis Media in Children: A Comparison of Conventional and Homeopathic Treatment," *Biomedical Therapy* 60,4,1997:113-116 (Originally published in German in *Hals-Nasen-Ohren* (Head, Nose and Otolyngarology, August 1996:462-66).

This study of 131 children allowed parents to choose homeopathic or conventional medical care from their ear, nose and throat doctor. In this group, 103 children underwent homeopathic treatment, and 28 underwent conventional care. They found that total recurrences in the homeopathically treated group were .41 per patient, whereas recurrences in the antibiotic treatment group were .70 per patient. Of the "homeopathic" children who did have another earache, 29.3 percent had a maximum of three recurrences, whereas 43.5 percent of the "antibiotic" children had a maximum of six recurrences.

Vittorio Elia and Marcella Niccoli, "Thermodynamics of Extremely Diluted Aqueous Solutions," *Annals of the New York Academy of Sciences,* June 1999.

An extensive thermodynamic study has been carried out on aqueous solutions obtained through successive dilutions and succussions of 1 percent in weight of some solutes up to extremely diluted solutions (less than 1×10^{-5} mol kg-1) obtained via several 1/100 successive dilution processes. The interaction of acids or bases with the extremely diluted solutions has been studied calorimetrically at 25C. Measurements have been performed of the heats of mixing acid or basic solutions having different concentrations with bidistilled water or with the extremely diluted solutions. Despite the extreme dilution of the solutions, an exothermic heat of mixing in excess has been found in about 92 percent of the cases, with respect to the corresponding heat of mixing with the untreated solvent. It is shown that successive dilutions and succussions may alter permanently the physical-chemical properties of the solvent water. The nature of the phenomena here described still remains unexplained, but significant experimental results are obtained.

J. Dittmann and G. Harisch, "Characterization of Differing Effects Caused by Homeopathically Prepared and Conventional Dilutions Using Cytochrome P450 2E1 and Other Enzymes as Detection Systems," *Alternative and Complementary Medicine*, 1996 2:2,279–290.

The target of the investigation was to ascertain differences in the effects of homeopathic potencies (D) and equally concentrated conventional dilutions (V) on p-nitrocatechol formation catalyzed by CYP 2E1. *Arsenicum album* and *Potassium cyanatum* (D) were compared to equivalent dilutions of As 203 and KCN (V). Significant differences in enzyme activity were found. The difference of influence exists and this may be attributable to the manufacturing process of homeopathic drugs, namely, the stepwise dilution with intermediate agitation.

P. C. Endler, W. Pongratz, G. Kastberg et al, "The Effect of Highly Diluted Agitated Thyroxine on the Climbing Activity of Frogs," *Veterinary and Human Toxicology,* 1994, 36:56.

This study and the one below show that a homeopathic medicine can influence the growth and development of tadpoles in water.

P. C. Endler, W. Pongratz, R. van Wijk et al, "Transmission of Hormone Information by Non-Molecular Means," *FASEB Journal,* 1994, 8, Abs. 2313.

This study and the one above show that a homeopathic medicine can influence the growth and development of tadpoles in water.

J. Benveniste, P. C. Endler, and J. Schulte, eds., "Further Biological Effects Induced by Ultra-High Dilutions: Inhibition by a

Magnetic Field," *Ultra High Dilution*, Dordrecht: Kluwer Academic, 1994, 35.

This study and the one below show that certain magnetic fields can neutralize the effects of a homeopathic medicine.

J. Benveniste, B. Arnoux, and L. Hadji, "Highly Diluted Antigen Increases Coronary Flow of Isolated Heart from Immunized Guinea Pigs," *FASEB Journal,* 1992, 6:Abs. 1610.

This study and the one above show that certain magnetic fields can neutralize the effects of a homeopathic medicine.

E. Davenas, B. Poitevin, and J. Benveniste, "Effect on Mouse Peritoneal Macrophages of Orally Administered Very High Dilutions of Silica," *European Journal of Pharmacology,* April 1987, 135:313-319.

This study shows that Silica 6C and Silica 10C induce a statistically significant increase in immune function as measured in macrophages in the blood of mice.

Meta-analyses of Clinical Studies in Homeopathy

K. Linde, N. Clausius, G. Ramirez et al, "Are the Clinical Effects of Homeopathy Placebo Effects? A Meta-analysis of Placebo-Controlled Trials," *Lancet*, September 20, 1997, 350:834-843.

This state-of-the-art meta-analysis reviewed 186 studies, 89 of which fit predefined criteria. Rather than count and compare the number of trials that show efficacy of treatment, the researchers pooled the data from the various studies to assess data. The results show that patients taking homeopathic medicines were 2.45 times more likely to experience a positive therapeutic effect than when taking a placebo.

J. Kleijnen, P. Knipschild, and G. TerRiet, "Clinical Trials of Homeopathy," *British Medical Journal,* February 9, 1991, 302:316-323.

This is the most widely cited meta-analysis of clinical research prior to 1991. It reviewed 107 studies of homeopathic medicines, 81 (or 77 percent) of which showed a positive effect. Of the best 22 studies, 15 showed efficacy. The researchers concluded: "The evidence presented in this review would probably be sufficient for establishing homeopathy as a regular treatment for certain indications." Further, "The amount of positive evidence even among the best studies came as a surprise to us."

K. Linde, W. B. Jonas, D. Melchart et al, "Critical Review and Meta-Analysis of Serial Agitated Dilutions in Experimental Toxicology," *Human and Experimental Toxicology*, 1994, 13:481-92.

This meta-analysis of 105 studies in toxicology shows that homeopathic medicines may be useful in treating toxic exposures. It was conducted by a similar group of researchers who recently published a meta-analysis on clinical studies in the *Lancet*.

Professional Societies and Associations

The following information comes from the National Center for Homeopathy (NCH) at http://www.homeopathic.org. You can also call the NCH in Alexandria, Virginia, at (703) 548-7790.

Academy of Veterinary Homeopathy (AVH)
PO Box 9280
Wilmington, DE 19809
(866) 652-1590 phone
(866) 652-1590 fax
office@theavh.org
www.theavh.org

The Academy of Veterinary Homeopathy has been established for the purposes of establishing standards for the practice of veterinary homeopathy and to advance veterinary homeopathy through education and research. Membership is open to licensed veterinarians and veterinary students in AVMA-accredited veterinary schools.

American Association of Homeopathic Pharmacists (AAHP)
33 Fairfax St.
Berkeley Springs, WV 25422
(800) 478-0421 phone/fax
info@homeopathyresource.org
www.homeopathyresource.org

This is an alliance of homeopathic manufacturers, pharmacists and other qualified parties. It serves the homeopathic community by promoting excellence in the practice of homeopathic pharmacy, manufacturing and distribution and provides outreach via education, public relations and research support.

American Board of Homeotherapeutics (ABHt)
1913 Gladstone Dr.
Wheaton, IL 60187
(630) 668-5595 phone
(240) 465-8077 fax
skyhawk1@bigplanet.com
www.homeopathyusa.org/ABHt
Established in 1960, this board is open to MDs and DOs; it awards Dht, Diplomate in Homeotherapeutics.

American Institute of Homeopathy (AIH)
801 N. Fairfax St. Ste. 306
Alexandria, VA 22314-1757
(888) 445-9988 phone
(888) 445-9988 fax
info@homeopathyusa.org
www.homeopathyusa.org
Established in 1844, the American Institute of Homeopathy (AIH) is the oldest national U.S. medical organization. Its members are licensed medical and osteopathic physicians, dentists, advanced practice nurses and physician's assistants who practice homeopathy. The AIH strives to promote the public acceptance of homeopathy while safeguarding the interests of the profession.

California Homeopathic Medical Society (CHMS)
169 E. El Roblar Dr.
Ojai, CA 93023
(805) 646-1495 phone
(805) 646-8159 fax
rhiltner@sbcglobal.net
www.homeopathywest.org
The California Homeopathic Medical Society is a nonprofit corporation dedicated to the encouragement of homeopathic practice, fellowship and personal growth. The CHMS was founded in 1877 as a professional association for homeopathic physicians and has extended membership to include other homeopathic practitioners and lay persons in the western United States.

Council for Homeopathic Certification (CHC)
PMB 187
17051 SE 272nd St. Ste. 43
Covington, WA 98042

(866) 242-3399 (toll free in US and Canada, PT) phone
(415) 869-2867 fax
chcinfo@homeopathicdirectory.com
www.homeopathicdirectory.com

The CHC has established the largest professional certification standard in North America and is open to all professional homeopaths, including both licensed and nonlicensed practitioners. The CHC serves to unite the homeopathic profession under a commonly agreed level of homeopathic competence. It provides the public with a clear choice in finding qualified professional homeopaths.

Council on Homeopathic Education (CHE)
13 Dutchess Terr.
Beacon, NY 12508
(703) 229-4343 phone
(703) 229-4343 fax
info@chedu.org
www.chedu.org

The mission of the Council on Homeopathic Education is to establish, maintain, ensure and improve the quality of education within the discipline of classical homeopathy. The council accredits schools and the sponsors of continuing education programs; it sponsors the North American Network of Homeopathic Educators and serves as a resource for educators and students.

Florida Homeopathic Medical Society
668 Lake Villas Dr.
Altamonte Springs, FL 32701
(407) 628-9708 phone
prswan@aol.com

Dedicated to classical homeopathic medicine, FHMS consists of licensed medical professionals and associate members (lay people who have taken 150 hours of NCH-approved coursework). FHMS encourages the recognition and acceptance of homeopathic medicine, offers fellowships for practitioners and plans to act as a representational voice for homeopathy in Florida.

Homeopathic Medical Society of the State of New York (HMSSNY)
6250 Route 9
Rhinebeck, NY 12572
(845) 876-6323 phone
(845) 876-2627 fax
homeopathicmd@earthlink.net

The Homeopathic Medical Society of the State of New York was established in 1862 as a professional organization open to MDs and DOs; it was formed for the advancement of homeopathic therapeutics. The society meets twice annually and distributes a newsletter to its members.

Homeopathic Nurses Association (HNA)
8403 Tahona Dr.
Silver Spring, MD 20903
(301) 445-0611 phone
margeaster@aol.com
www.homeopathicnurses.org

This is a support organization for nurses studying and integrating homeopathy into practice.

Homeopathic Pharmacopoeia Convention of the United States (HPCUS)
PO Box 2221
Southeastern, PA 19399-2221
(610) 783-0987 phone
(610) 783-5180 fax
hpus@aol.com
www.HPCUS.com

The Homeopathic Pharmacopoeia Convention of the United States (HPCUS) publishes the *Homeopathic Pharmacopoeia of the United States* (HPUS). It investigates substances for inclusion and sets standards for identification, testing and preparation of homeopathic remedies. The HPUS is recognized in the Food and Drug Act as the source of regulation of homeopathic drugs in the U.S.; it is a 501(c)(3) organization.

Illinois Homeopathic Medical Association
400 E. 22nd St. Ste. F
Lombard, IL 60148
(630) 792-9311 phone
(630) 792-9316 fax

This is a state professional homeopathic organization that promotes homeopathic research and education. Professional educational seminars are held once yearly in the Chicago area, featuring world-renown homeopathic educators, often with CME accreditation. There are yearly membership meetings in the fall. A trifold brochure describing homeopathy and listing practicing members is available.

National Board of Homeopathic Examiners (NBHE)
6536 Stadium Dr. Ste. L
Zephyrhills, FL 33542
(813) 782-2690 phone
(813) 782-3275 fax
info@nbhe.org
www.nbhe.org
Awards DNBHE, Diplomate of the NBHE.

North American Society of Homeopaths (NASH)
1122 E. Pike St. Ste. 1122
Seattle, WA 98122
(206) 720-7000 phone
(208) 248-1942 fax
nashinfo@aol.com
www.homeopathy.org

NASH is the professional homeopathic practitioners' association dedicated to support, promote and represent certified homeopathic practitioners and help enhance the role of the homeopathic profession as an integral part of our nation's health care. As the leading professional organization representing all certified homeopaths in North America, NASH aims at elevating its members to becoming the future leaders in the homeopathic profession. NASH offers *The American Homeopath Journal*, an annual NASH conference, NASH newsletters and conference/seminar discounts.

Ohio State Homeopathic Medical Society (OSHMS)
5779 Wooster Pike
Medina, OH 44256
(330) 784-4493 phone

This is a society of medical professionals supporting the advancement of homeopathic education and practice.

Texas Society of Homeopathy
4200 Westheimer Ste 100
Houston, TX 77027
(713) 621-3184 phone
(713) 877-8035 fax

info@txsoho.com
www.txsoho.com
The Texas Society of Homeopathy is a 501(c)(3) professional and lay homeopathic organization formed to promote homeopathic education in Texas and the surrounding areas. The annual conference features a special speaker and provides the availability of earning continuing educational and CCH credits.

Homeopathic Products and Services

The following information comes from the National Center for Homeopathy (NCH) at http://www.homeopathic.org. You can also call the NCH in Alexandria, Virginia, at (703) 548-7790.

An asterisk (*) in the following listing indicates that completion of the program alone does not grant a license or certification to practice homeopathy.

Arizona

Educational Organizations and Programs

Desert Institute School of Classical Homeopathy
2001 W. Camelback Rd #150
Phoenix, AZ 85015
(602) 347-7950 phone
(602) 864-1747 phone
(602) 864-2949 fax
disch@igc.org
www.chiaz.com/disch
A licensed nonprofit school in Arizona offering a 750-hour program in classical homeopathy (1/3 clinical). Clinical training with live clinics and personal case supervision; postgraduate training program; proving research and clinical research; large, diverse faculty with mentorship program. Distance learning courses available; 40 hours of CMEs available.*

Southwest College of Naturopathic Medicine
8010 E. McDowell RD #111
Scottsdale, AZ 85257
(480) 970-0000 phone
(480) 970-0003 fax
www.scnm.edu
Four-year naturopathic medical school including clinical training in classical homeopathy.*

California

Products and Services

Homeopathic Educational Services
2124 Kittredge Street #N
Berkeley, CA 94704
(800) 359-9051 (orders only)
(510) 649-0294 phone
(510) 649-1955 fax
mail@homeopathic.com
www.homeopathic.com

Provides a comprehensive assortment of homeopathic books, tapes, medicines, software and distance learning courses*, including a new eBook and eCourse on homeopathic family medicine, which includes up-to-date information on homeopathic research.

HomeopathyWest
1442A Walnut St #138
Berkeley, CA 94709
(877) 850-5078 phone
(877) 850-5078 fax
seminars@homeopathywest.com
www.HomeopathyWest.com

HomeopathyWest brings outstanding homeopathic educators from around the world to the West Coast. Its purpose is to promote high standards of practice, maintain a flow of creative ideas and encourage development of worldwide connections within the homeopathic community.

Jackie Wilson, MD, DHt, DABFP
Consultant in Homeopathy
536 Brotherton Road
Escondido, CA 92025
(760) 747-2144 phone
(760) 747-1709 fax
drwilson@cox.net
www.homeopathicdoctor.com

Consults on new drug monographs, drug testing and affordable clinical trials, helping companies efficiently develop homeopathic medicines compliant with FDA/HPUS regulations. Is a board-certified family physician and member of the Homeopathic Pharmacopoeia Convention of the United States.

Standard Homeopathic Company
210 W. 131st Street
PO Box 61067
Los Angeles, CA 90061
(800) 624-9659 toll free
(310) 768-0700 phone
(310) 516-8579 fax
shcinfo@hylands.com
www.hylands.com
Manufacturer of single remedies, combinations, topicals.
Hahnemann Laboratories Inc
1940 4th St.
San Rafael, CA 94901
(888) 427-6422 phone
(415) 451-6981 fax
info@hahnemannlabs.com
www.hahnemannlabs.com
Offers high-quality, high-potency remedies; home and professional kits.

Kent Homeopathic Associates Inc.
710 Mission Ave.
San Rafael, CA 94901
(877) YES-KENT (937-5368) U.S. and Canada only
(415) 457-0678 phone
(415) 457-0688 fax
kha@igc.org
www.kenthomeopathic.com
Creator of MacRepertory & ReferenceWorks for both Windows and Macintosh.

Santa Monica Homeopathic Pharmacy
629 Broadway
Santa Monica, CA 90401
(310) 395-1131 phone
(310) 395-7861 fax
info@smhomeopathic.com
www.smhomeopathic.com
Offers a complete homeopathic pharmacy, herbal remedies, vitamins, minerals, books.

Educational Organizations and Programs

Teleosis Foundation
PO Box 7046
Berkeley, CA 94707
(510) 558-7285 phone
(510) 528-1998 fax
teleosis@igc.org
www.teleosis.com

Teleosis Foundation is a nonprofit corporation that provides access to alternative medicine for the underserved and promotes ecologically sustainable medicine. It owns and operates the Teleosis School of Homeopathy, offering weekend seminars, professional programs in classical homeopathy, teaching clinics and clinical internships in New York, Boston and throughout California.*

Homeopathic Academy of Southern California
2136 Oxford Ave
Cardiff by the Sea, CA 92007
(877) 800-4197 toll free
(858) 794-0787 phone
homeopathicwellness@cox.net
homeopathic-academy.com

Homeopathic Academy of Southern California is a three-year, 500-hour certification program in San Diego. This most comprehensive program meets one weekend per month from September to June. The program includes a student clinic and a homeopathic mentorship program.*

Hahnemann College of Homeopathy
80 Nicholl Ave.
Point Richmond, CA 94801
(510) 232-2079 phone
(510) 412-9044 fax
hahnemann@igc.org
www.hahnemanncollege.com

Four-year comprehensive training program for medical professionals (home study).*

Institute of Classical Homoeopathy - San Francisco
2325 Third St. Ste. 426
San Francisco, CA 94107
(415) 551-1020 phone
(415) 551-1021 fax

ich@classicalhomoeopathy.org
www.classicalhomoeopathy.org
Classical Hahnemannian training offered in seminars and four-year program.*

Pacific Academy of Homeopathic Medicine
1199 Sanchez St.
San Francisco, CA 94114
(415) 695-2710 phone
(415) 695-8220 fax
health@homeopathy-academy.org
www.homeopathy-academy.org
Professional training over three years for students of all backgrounds.*

Caduceus Institute of Classical Homeopathy
549 Fredrick St.
Santa Cruz, CA 95062
(800) 396-9778 toll free
(831) 466-0516 phone
(831) 466-3516 fax
willa@homeopathyhome.net
www.homeopathytraining.org
Professional-level distance learning program for health practitioners and serious lay students. Carefully developed modules make homeopathy easier to learn. The foundation of the course is video tapes of actual classroom sessions. Onsite clinical training also available.*

Colorado

Products and Services
Mediral International, Inc.
10550 E. 54th Ave. Unit E
Denver, CO 80239-2131
(877) 633-4725 toll free
(303) 331-6161 phone
(303) 355-4155 fax
homeopathy@mediral.com
www.mediral.com
Classical single and combination remedies, private label manufacturing, custom formulation, nosodes, sarcodes, xenobiotics,

allersodes, professional and OTC products, test kits. All remedies are hand succussed. Exclusive manufacture of Dr. Recommends, Medrial and Nature Knows homeopathic remedies. "Tru-potency" manufacturing ensures consistently reliable natural pharmaceuticals for clinical practices.

Educational Organizations and Programs

Colorado Institute for Classical Homeopathy
2955 Valmont Rd. Ste. 100
Boulder, CO 80301
(303) 440-3717 phone
(303) 442-6525 fax
info@homeopathyschool.org
www.homeopathyschool.org

CICH offers a two-year certification program approved by the State of Colorado. Graduates receive the initials CHom, which signify a professional level of achievement. Students obtain clinical training and prepare for the Council for Homeopathic Certification exam. CIHC hosts nationally and internationally renowned instructors and uses interactive techniques for adult learners.

Connecticut

Educational Organizations and Programs

The School of Homeopathy, Devon
(Correspondence Course)
Director Misha Norland FSHom
82 E. Pearl St.
New Haven, CT 06513
(203) 624-8783 phone/fax
betsy@homeopathyschool.com
www.homeopathyschool.com

Comprehensive training in homeopathic philosophy and practice at the highest standards through North American Flexible Learning Program. Tutored correspondence study is supported by seminars, clinical workshops and in-practice supervision. Anatomy & physiology and pathology & disease courses are also offered and required for completion.*

Florida

Products and Services
Weise Pharmacy, Homeopathic and Natural Medicines
4343 Colonial Avenue
Jacksonville, FL 32210
(800) 554-6670 toll free
(904) 384-4642 phone
(904) 384-0569 fax
weiseg@bellsouth.net
www.weiserx.com
Homeopathics, herbs, supplements, hormones, aromatherapy, injectables, veterinary, books; custom compounding.

Budget Pharmacy
3001 NW 7th St.
Miami, FL 33125
(800) 221-9772 (orders)
(305) 649-3300 (information)
(305) 642-4486 fax
budgetrx@aol.com
Complete homeopathic pharmacy, compounding pharmacy, vitamins, minerals, books, mail order.

Alternative Medicine Family Care Center
2050 40th Ave. Ste. 2
Vero Beach, FL 32960
(772) 778-8877 phone
(772) 778-9509 fax
moxaman@attglobal.net
www.drdannyq.com
In the Hahnemannian spirit, all treatments are individualized. As appropriate to individual needs, any of the following will be utilized: classical homeopathy, acupuncture, Chinese herbs, N.E.T. (neuro-emotional technique), natural allergy elimination technique, enzyme replacement therapy. Trained with Dr. S. K. Banerjea (Calcutta, India), Dr. A. U. Ramakrishnan and Dr. Ed Floyd. Provides alternative medicine since 1986.

Illinois

Products and Services

Merz Apothecary
4716 N. Lincoln Ave.
Chicago, IL 60625
(800) 252-0275 toll free
(773) 989-0900 phone
(773) 989-8108 fax
service@smallflower.com
www.smallflower.com
Established in 1875, Merz Apothecary is one of the nation's leading suppliers of homeopathic remedies and products. Pharmacists are on staff at all times to answer questions. Merz Apothecary distributes Boiron and other lines and offers more than 15,000 natural health and personal care products.

Walsh Homeopathics Ltd
2116 ½ Central St.
Evanston, IL 60201
(847) 864-1600 phone
(800) 9WALSHS (992-5747) phone
Homeopathics, flower essences, herbs and vitamins for people and animals.

Maryland

Products and Services

The Apothecary
5415 W. Cedar Ln.
Bethesda, MD 20814
(800) 869-9159 toll free
(301) 530-0800 phone
(301) 493-4671 fax
apoth123@aol.com
www.The-Apothecary.com
Retail pharmacy, homeopathics, nutritional supplements; 20-percent discount mail-orders.

Washington Homeopathic Products Inc.
4914 Del Ray Ave.
Bethesda, MD 20814

(877) 483-8789 toll free
(301) 656-1695 local
(877) 656-1592 fax
www.homeopathyworks.com

Established in 1873 in Washington, DC; offers over 1,700 single remedies, consecutive potencies 1–30, high potencies and LMs; tablets, pills, dilutions, ointments, topicals, 70 combination remedies (since 1915); 65 of the most popular books; Bach, Badger Balms, HomeoPet, Pflueger products and more. Individual, professional, wholesale and distributor accounts; NCH discounts.

Massachusetts

Products and Services

Johnson Drugs
577 Main St.
Waltham, MA 02452
(888) 335-5577 toll free
(781) 893-3870 phone
(781) 899-1172 fax
info@johnsondrugs.com
www.johnsondrugs.com

Offers an extensive selection of homeopathic medicines, nutritional supplements and herbal medicines. Is Boiron USA's referral pharmacy and stocks potencies from MT Æ CM including LM potencies. A full-service pharmacy that also offers complete compounding services and fee-based consultations.

Educational Organizations and Programs

New England School of Homeopathy
356 Middle St.
Amherst, MA 01002
(413) 256-5949 phone
(413) 256-6223 fax
nesh@nesh.com
www.nesh.com

Offers beginner to advanced information via courses, seminars, books, tapes.*

Teleosis School of Homeopathy
5A Lancaster St.
Cambridge, MA 02140
(617) 547-8500 phone
info@teleosis.org
www.teleosis.com
Offers weekend seminars, professional programs in classical homeopathy, teaching clinics and clinical internships in Boston. The school is operated by Teleosis Foundation, a nonprofit corporation that provides access to alternative medicine for the underserved and promotes ecologically sustainable medicine.*

Michigan

Products and Services
Lexington Veterinary Clinic
5346 Main
Lexington, MI 48450
(810) 359-8828 phone
(810) 359-5046 fax
tgif@greatlakes.net
www.greatlakes.net/~tgif
Holistic veterinary clinic.

Educational Organizations and Programs
The Institute of Natural Health Sciences CHE Professional Accreditation
20270 Middlebelt Rd. Ste. 4
Livonia, MI 48152
(248) 473-8522 phone
(248) 473-8141 fax
instituteofmich@aol.com
250-hour homeotherapeutics course licensed by state board of education.*

Minnesota

Products and Services
Pavilion Classical Homeopathy @ Aveler Chiropractic Center
600 E. Main St.
Anoka, MN 55304

(763) 421-3722 phone
(763) 413-7042 fax
homeopathjt@aol.com

Educational Organizations and Programs

Northwestern Academy of Homeopathy
10700 Old County Rd. #15 Ste. 300
Plymouth, MN 55441
(612) 794-6445 phone
(877) 644-4401 toll free
(763) 525-9518 fax
info@homeopathicschool.org
www.homeopathicschool.org
Four-year comprehensive professional program including 665
hours supervised clinical instruction.*

Nevada

Products and Services

Dolisos America
3014 Rigel Ave.
Las Vegas, NV 89102
(800) DOLISOS (365-4767) toll free
(702) 871-7153 phone
(702) 871-9670 fax
dolisos@skylink.net
www.dolisosamerica.com
The U.S. subsidiary of one of the world's largest homeopathic manufacturers. Provides an extensive range of single
homeopathic remedies; offers nosodes, mother tinctures and
gemmotherapy, oligotherapy and organotherapy. Specialty
items include regionally customized allergy mixes, unique
children's combination products and a homeopathic flu prevention product.

New Jersey

Educational Organizations and Programs

British Institute of Homeopathy
At The Herb Garden
580 Zion Rd.
Egg Harbor Township, NJ 08234-9606

(800) 498-6323 toll free
(609) 927-5660 phone
(609) 653-1289 fax
britishinstitutehome@yahoo.com
www.britinsthom.com

Offers courses to learn the basic principles of Hahnemannian homeopathy at home, with a professional homeopath as a tutor.*

New Mexico

Products and Services

Natural Health Supply
NHS Labs
6410 Avenida Christina
Santa Fe, NM 87505
(888) 689-1608 toll free
(505) 474-9175 phone
(505) 473-0336 fax
nhs@a2zhomeopathy.com
www.a2zhomeopathy.com

Distributes a full line of remedies, kits, books and supplies for professionals, students and consumers in the homeopathic community. Laboratory division manufactures professional-quality remedies; makes many kits available for both professional and consumer use and also distributes glassware, educational materials and computer programs.

New York

Products and Services

Weleda Inc.
175 N. Route 9W
Congers, NY 10920
(800) 289-1969 ext 212 phone
(800) 280-4899 fax
rx@weleda.com
www.weleda.com

Prescription and nonprescription, homeopathic and anthroposophical medicines; natural personal-care products.

Apthorp Pharmacy
2201 Broadway at 78th St.
New York, NY 10024

(212) 877-3480 phone
(212) 769-9095 fax
Homeopathic single and combination remedies, mail order.

Educational Organizations and Programs

Homeopathic Resources & Services/Library
Homoeopathia (Historical Research)
PO Box 131
Old Chatham, NY 12136
(518) 794-8653 phone
kirtsos@aol.com
Preservationists of the history of homeopathy through its litera-
ture and artifacts; provides historical homeopathic research, collection development and appraisal services. Sells rare homeopathic books
and journals and purchases homeopathic books and memorabilia.

New York Luminos School of Homeopathy
158 Franklin St.
New York, NY 10013
(212) 925-4623 phone/fax
faculty@nyhomeopathy.com
www.nyhomeopathy.com
The NY School of Homeopathy, which has been educating
homeopaths since 1990, recently merged with Louis Klein to become the NY Luminos School of Homeopathy. Four-year diploma
program offers rigorous and thorough professional training, high
standards of excellence, monthly weekend classes with personal
attention and supplemental online instruction.*

The School of Homeopathy, New York
964 Third Ave. 8th Floor
New York, NY 10015-0003
(212) 570-2576 phone
(212) 737-2489 fax
kathy@homeopathyschool.com
www.homeopathyschool.com
Comprehensive Hahnemannian schooling, including clinical
training and supervision; licensed, unlicensed.*

North Carolina

Products and Services

King Bio Pharmaceuticals Inc.
3 Westside Dr.
Asheville, NC 28806
(800) 543-3245 toll free
(828) 255-0201 phone
(828) 255-0940 fax
tara@kingbio.com
www.kingbio.com

A physician-based company dedicated to the production of safe, all-natural medicines without side effects.

Pennsylvania

Products and Services

Thomas Happ - Consulting Chemist
107 Knapp Rd.
Lansdale, PA 19446-1716
(215) 368-8482 phone
(215) 362-4596 fax
happ@snip.net

Chemical analysis and documentation of United States Pharmacopeia (USP) and other homeopathic ingredients.

BOIRON
6 Campus Blvd.
Newtown Square, PA 19073
(800) BLU-TUBE (258-8823) orders
(800) BOIRON-1 (264-7661) consumer info
(610) 325-7480 fax
info@boiron.com
www.boiron.com

Boiron was founded in 1932 in Lyon, France, and today employs more than 2,600 people internationally; strives to give every physician and health care professional the opportunity to integrate homeopathic medicines in daily practice.

Arrowroot Standard Direct (ASD)
83 E. Lancaster Ave.
Paoli, PA 19301
(800) 234-8879 toll free
(610) 296-4212 phone
(800)296-8998 fax
customerservice@arrowroot.com
www.arrowroot.com
Offers mail order that is qualified to service health care professionals and consumers with a fully licensed FDA state-of-the-art laboratory and a PA-inspected natural pharmacy.

Texas
Educational Organizations and Programs
The Texas Institute for Homeopathy
1406 Brookstone
San Antonio, TX 78248-1425
(210) 492-3162 phone
(210) 492-9152 fax
texashomeopathy@aol.com
www.texashomeopathy.com
Intensive, professional, three-year-diploma course in classical and therapeutic homeopathy.*

Vermont
Products and Services
1-800-HOMEOPATHY
PO Box 8080
Richford, VT 05476
(800)-HOMEOPATHY (466-3672) phone
(877) 999-0090 fax
info@1800homeopathy.com
www.1800homeopathy.com
America's oldest mail-order resource, offers remedies, books, free catalogues.

Virginia
Products and Services
Annandale Apothecary and Health Center
3299 Woodburn Rd. Ste. 120
Annandale, VA 22003

(703) 698-7411 phone
(703) 698-7415 fax
pfhughes1@msn.com
Complete line of homeopathic remedies, kits, books and nutritional supplements.

Washington

Products and Services
Minimum Price Homeopathic Books
250 "H" St
PMB 2187
Blaine, WA 98230
(800) 663-8272 orders only
(604) 597-4757 phone
(604) 597-8304 fax
orders@minimum.com
www.minimum.com
Huge stock of books, tapes and software; knowledgeable staff.

Homeopathy for Health
422 N. Earl Rd.
Moses Lake, WA 98837
(800) 390-9970 orders/questions
(509) 766-0182 phone
(206) 350-1556 fax
health@elixirs.com
www.elixirs.com
Offers 2,500 remedies, complete lines of Natra-Bio, Standard, Boiron, BHI, Dolisos, Natural Care, Hylands, new and classic books. Complete online symptom/remedy search and *materia medica*. Phone consultations with Kathryn Jones, registered Health Counselor DiHom, 15 years experience. Free monthly newsletter, ships worldwide.

West Virginia

Products and Services
Homeopathy Works
33 Fairfax St.
Berkeley Springs, WV 25411
(800) 336-1695 (orders only)

(304) 258-2541 phone
(877) 286-0601 fax
info@homeopathyworks.com
www.homeopathyworks.com
This West Virginia division of Washington Homeopathic Products features bulk manufacturing and private labeling in a working museum setting. Full-line manufacturer offering special orders, tinctures, high potencies, poison ivy pills, kits, combinations, books, ointments, nosodes and sarcodes and more; over 1,700 single remedies; Pflueger USA products.

Related Organizations

Note: An asterisk (*) indicates that completion of this program alone does not grant a license or certification to pract.ice homeopathy.

United States

National Integrative Medicine Council
5151 E. Broadway Suite 1095
Tucson, AZ 85711
(520) 571-1110 phone
(520) 571-1177 fax
www.nimc.org
Founded by Dr. Andrew Weil, this nonprofit membership-based education and advocacy organization promotes a healing-oriented approach to health care.

Canada

British Columbia

Whole Health Now
59 Caton Pl
Victoria, BC V9B 1L1, Canada
(888) 722-5423 toll free
(250) 881-1252 phone
(250) 881-1251 fax
kim@whnow.com
www.wholehealthnow.com

Products include Synthesis Repertory, RADAR Homeopathic software and Encyclopedia Homeopathica; customer training and support.

Educational Organizations and Programs

Luminos Homeopathic Courses Ltd
Director: Louis Klein RSHom
F-31
Bowen Island, BC V0N 1G0, Canada
(604) 947-0757 phone
(604) 947-0764 fax
info@homeopathycourses.com
www.homeopathycourses.com

Has offered homeopathic education for everybody since 1995, from beginners to experienced practitioners. Currently available are the online foundation course, the homeopathic master clinician course as well as various seminars.*

Vancouver Homeopathic Academy
Box 34095 Station D
Vancouver, BC V6J 4M1, Canada
(604) 708-9387 phone
(604) 708-1547 fax
info@homeopathyvancouver.com
www.homeopathyvancouver.com

Four-year practitioner course: extensive clinical training, human sciences and in-depth curriculum in homeopathic philosophy, principles, *materia medica* and case management. One-year foundation course provides a systematic understanding of homeopathic principles and philosophy and how to apply them in first aid and acute situations.*

Ontario

Hahnemann Center for Homeopathy and Heilkunst
1445 St Joseph Blvd.
Ottawa, ON K1C 7K9, Canada
(613) 830-2556 phone
(613) 830-2056 fax
info@homeopathy.com
www.homeopathy.com

Comprehensive general and veterinary practitioner diplomas awarding the diploma in homeopathy and Heilkunst of the Hahnemann Center for Homeopathy and Heilkunst (DHHP), diploma in veterinary homeopathy and Heilkunst (DVHH), FHCH (fellowship of the Hahnemann Center for Heilkunst (FHCH).*

The School of Homeopathy Devon
(Correspondence Course)
Director Misha Norland FSHom
10620 Yonge St.
Richmond Hill, ON L4C 3C8, Canada
christine@homeopathyschool.com
www.homeoapthyschool.com

Comprehensive training in homeopathic philosophy and practice through North American flexible learning program. Tutored correspondence study is supported by seminars, clinical workshops and in-practice supervision. Anatomy & physiology and pathology & disease courses are also offered and required for completion.*

The Toronto School of Homeopathic Medicine
1246 Yonge St. Ste. 301
Toronto, ON M4T 1W5, Canada
(800) 572-6001 toll free
(416) 966-2350 phone
(416) 966-1724 fax
info@homeopathycanada.com
www.homeopathycanada.com

Three-year professional training program in homeopathy and sciences in a creative and supportive environment, with the emphasis on clinical proficiency.*

Quebec

Homeolab USA, Inc.
3025 De L'Assomption
Montreal, PQ H1N 2H2, Canada
(800) 404-4666 toll free
(514) 252-8911 phone
(514) 252-8919 fax
homeocan@videotron.ca
www.homeolab.com

Full-service manufacturer of pharmaceutical-grade homeo-pathic products. Maintains an extensive inventory of single remedies in pellets and oral dilutions as well as mother tinctures, combination remedies, creams and Essencia brand organic aromatherapy oils. HomeoLab offers private label service. ASG discount program available.

Canadian Academy of Homeopathy
1173 Blvd. du Mont Royal
Montreal, PQ H2V 2H6, Canada
(514) 279-6629 phone
(514) 279-0111 fax
cah@videotron.ca
www.homeopathy.ca
Offers video courses in homeopathy for health care professionals.*

India

New Delhi

B. Jain Publishers Overseas
1920/10 Chuna Mandi
Paharganj New Delhi 110 055
+91-11 3683100-3300 phone
+91-11 3670572 phone
+91-11 3683400 or (91-11) 3610471 fax
bjain@vsnl.com
www.bjainbooks.com
Homeopathic publishers/exporters; magazines, leather medicine kits, sugar globules, software.

New Zealand

Bay of Plenty College of Homeopathy
PO Box 784
Tauranga, New Zealand
+64-7-578-1331
+64-7-578-1369
bopcoh@wave.co.nz
www.homeopathycollege.com
Diploma of homeopathy training available by extramural video in New Zealand and internationally; diploma of homeopathy; animal health also available. Accredited by New Zealand Ministry of Education.

Appendix C: Resources

Ordering Flower and Gem Essences

Ordering from the Internet

Go to http://www.medicinegarden.com. Flower essences are clearly marked on the front page, or you can use the Search function and type in the name of the flower you are looking for. Place your order on a secure server. Most orders are sent out within 48 hours of receipt of your order.

Ordering by Mail

Mail your order in a letter to us. Flower essences are $10.95 each, plus shipping and handling. Send us a list of the names of what you would like (brandy base only please for the flower essences) and include your address and phone number. We take Visa or Mastercard. Simply send us your credit card number along with the expiration date. If we have any questions, we will call you. Most orders are sent within 72 hours of receiving them. Please send your mail order to:

Blue Turtle Publishing
PO Box 2513
Cottonwood, AZ 86326, USA

Ordering by Telephone

Just call Blue Turtle Publishing at (928) 634-5211; hours are Monday through Friday, 9 AM to 5 PM mountain standard time. If we don't answer, leave your name and phone number and we will return your call.

Free Catalog!

To request one (or more!) of our free catalogs, just email us at stoneman2@sedona.net or write to us at the Blue Turtle Publishing address mentioned above.

Flower Reports

What is your most favorite flower in the world? Did you know that it can help bring you back into balance and harmony with yourself? Yes, it can! What you love can help support you toward a more positive, integrated you. This has to do with the homeopathic law of similars: Like cures like. What you love can help you. It is that simple—and that profound.

All you have to do is ask yourself this question: What is my favorite flower? Then go to http://www.medicinegarden.com, click Flower Report on the home page and you will be whisked off to choose your report! (Starting in October 2004, you can also go to our flower reports website at http://www.WhatFlowerAreYou.com.) Not only that, we show you (partial) sample reports of what you can expect to receive. After getting your report and reading it, you may be inspired to order the essence as well! Because it comes from the flower you love most in the world, taking the essence will help you.

If you don't have access to the Internet, all you have to do is call us at (928) 634-9298, Monday through Friday, 9 AM to 5 PM (mountain standard time), and we'll take your order.

Locating a Shamanic Facilitator to Request a Soul Recovery and Extraction Journey for Yourself

On the Internet, go to http://www.medicinegarden.com. Click the Shamanic Facilitators tab on the home page to get to facilitators in all parts of the world who were trained by Eileen Nauman over the years. If you are from Europe, we suggest you go to the European page; if you are from Down Under, go to the Australia/New Zealand page; if you are from North or South America, we suggest the U.S. page. Just follow the instructions once you get to the page and that will put you in contact with the shaman of your choice.

You can also choose one of the shamans from the directory in the back of the book *Soul Recovery and Extraction* by Ai Gvhdi Waya (Eileen Nauman). Everyone getting a journey *must* first read the book; no facilitator will do a journey for you until you have read the book and understand it clearly.

You can order the book from http://www.medicinegarden.com. Just go to our Metaphysical Department and you will see it listed there for viewing purposes and ordering. Cost is $9.95, plus $2.00 for shipping and handling. You can also contact a shaman first, and the shaman will sell you the book.

If you do not have access to the Internet, you can order *Soul Recovery and Extraction* by mail. Send a letter to Blue Turtle Publishing, PO Box 2513, Cottonwood, AZ 86326. With your order, include your name, address and phone number and a personal check or Visa/Mastercard number and expiration date. The cost for one book is $9.95, plus $2.00 shipping and handling within the U.S., for a total of $11.95. Most orders for the book are filled within 72 hours of receipt of the order.

You can also place your order for *Soul Recovery and Extraction* by calling us at (928) 634-5211 Monday through Friday, 9 AM to 5 PM mountain standard time. We accept Visa/Mastercard or personal check.

Homeopathic Kits by Eileen Nauman

Eileen Nauman kits as well as individual homeopathic remedies are available from:

Hahnemann Laboratories Inc.
1940 Fourth Street
San Rafael, CA 94901
Hours: Monday–Friday, 9AM–1PM and 2PM–6PM PST
Call toll free: 1 (888) 427-6422
Fax: (415) 451-6981

The Nauman Traveler's Kit for the Treatment of Emerging Diseases with 50 remedies (2-dram bottle size, 30C potency) costs $119.95 and includes:

ACON AGAR ALL-C ANDROC ANT-T
APIS ARN ARS BAPT BELL
BELL-P CACT CALC-P CANTH CARB-V
CARB-AC CAUST CHINA CROT-H DIG
ELAPS FORMICA GLON HAM HEPAR
HYOS HYP IGN KALI-BI LACH
LAT-M LAUR LED MOSCH NUX-M
NUX-V PETR-ETHPHOS PYROG RHUST
RUTA SAMB SPONG STANN STAPH
STRAM SYMPHYT TARENT URT-U VERAT

Appendix D: Other Books by Eileen Nauman

Now available from Blue Turtle Publishing
PO Box 2513, Cottonwood, AZ 86326:

Ai Gvhdi Waya [Eileen Nauman], *Soul Recovery and Extraction*, 1992.
　　Ancient Native American healing technique, shamanism and how it can be utilized today to help us heal not only wounds of the spirit, but also emotional, mental and physical wounds. Eileen's father was part Eastern Cherokee and a shaman; he trained both Eileen and her brother, Gary Gent, to carry on this family healing tradition. Case histories, explanation of the technique and a directory of shamanic facilitators. $9.95.

Nauman, Eileen, *Medical Astrology*, 1982.
　　One of the world's best references on the topic; Part 1 discusses the astrology of medicine, and Part 2 offers a wealth of information for your health, including vitamins, minerals, Bach flower remedies, homeopathic remedies and much more. This book can be read and understood by both astrologer and non-astrologer. $29.95.

Nauman, Eileen, *Bach Flower Remedies and Astrology*, 1985.
　　A guide to using Dr. Bach's flower remedies, for the astrologer as well as the non-astrologer. Assignment of zodiac signs, planets and houses to the 38 remedies. An indispensable book that should be in everyone's medicine cabinet. Easy to understand and use. $6.95.

Nauman, Eileen, and Ruth Gent, *Colored Stones and Healing*, 1988.
　　The authors draw upon their Eastern Cherokee upbringing and experience and share Apache medicine woman Oh Shinnah

Fast Wolf's technique for healing with precious and semiprecious gemstones. Over 50 stones are given, with their healing properties, their symbols and which chakras they are to be used on. $9.95.

Nauman, Eileen, *Beauty in Bloom: Homeopathy to Support Menopause*, 2000.

You don't need to suffer from menopause symptoms! They can be cured naturally with homeopathy. The book explains how homeopathy works and that menopause is *not* a disease but a natural rhythm in women's lives. It discusses individual symptoms that may occur and what homeopathic remedies can help to make your transition comfortable. There is also information on vitamins and minerals as well as a *materia medica* of remedies so you know which one you need. $24.95.

Nauman, Eileen, *HELP! and Homeopathy: What to Do in an Emergency after You Have Called 911*, 1998.

This book will help you use homeopathy along with first-aid procedures. It will help you recognize signs, symptoms and indicators of an emergency injury or accident. It provides homeopathic information to utilize once the symptoms have been identified. Dosage and potency are specific for each emergency situation. Provides a *materia medica* of 50 remedies with specific symptoms to cross-reference with the injured person's symptoms in order to choose the correct homeopathic remedy. Provides useful information on conducting an examination of the injured person if 911 is slow in responding or not coming at all as well as basic first-aid information for the injured person. $16.95.

Nauman, Eileen, Crested Prickle Poppy Proving, 1997.

Eileen gave a flower essence from this powerful desert plant, *Argemone pleiacantha*, to 10 provers, to show homeopaths that a humble flower essence can evoke just as strong and clear symptoms as a homeopathically prepared, potentized proving remedy. This book covers the *materia medica*, botanical information, doctrine of signature as well as the history and repertory of that proving. $10.95.

Appendix E:
Homeopathic Software

I highly recommend what I feel is the best homeopathic software available for beginners as well as homeopathic professionals such as myself. This software will help you make informed decisions as to which remedy would be best for your symptoms. I own this program and love it because it is so easy to operate (I'm not a computer geek) and the visuals and photographs are stunningly beautiful. In case you have any questions, you will find that this company is Johnny-on-the-spot, there with swift help and support. It doesn't get any better than this.

In today's dangerous global environment, I feel that everyone needs to have homeopathic software on the computer at home. I have it both on my home computer and my laptop, which travels around the world with me. This is an insurance that will pay for itself time and time again. Think about it as a birthday gift, Christmas gift or a "just because" gift to yourself. Your health and the protection of your family in these times cannot be weighed in dollars and cents.

In North America, contact:

Chi Software
6061 E. Cave Creek Rd. Suite 2
Cave Creek, AZ 85331
(480) 488-2461 (phone)
(480) 488-1136 (fax)
www.chisoftware.com
support@chisoftware.com

Outside the U.S. contact:

Miccant Ltd.
14 Mulberry Close
West Bridgford

Nottingham
England NG2 7SS
+44 (0) 870 141 7053 (phone)
www.miccant.com

Homeopathic Software Offered by Miccant

ISIS

The latest offering from Miccant is a powerful, beautiful, easy-to-use and intuitive homeopathic software solution. ISIS is the only software that elegantly combines repertories, *materia medicas*, remedies and a homepathic dictionary in one fabulous interface. To take a tour of ISIS on the Internet, visit Miccant's or one of their distributors' sites.

Cara

This is the first homeopathic software program that was ever developed. It was originally designed for the London Homeopathic Hospital and continues to provide a comprehensive tool to both the student and the practicing homeopath.

Akiva

Akiva is the homeopathic advisor. It provides information on first aid and acute treatment using a question-and-answer format. Akiva offers advice on 64 common conditions and highlights 103 homeopathic remedies. It is perfect for home use.

Bibliography

Allen, H. H. *Allen's Keynotes to the Materia Medica.* 1898.

Allen, T. F., MD. *Pocket Characteristics Materia Medica.* 1894.

American Association of Blood Banks. Association Bulletin #03-08: "Recommended Guidance for Reporting West Nile Viremic Blood Donors to State and/or Local Public Health Departments and Reporting Donors Who Subsequently Develop West Nile Virus Illness to Blood Collection Facilities." American Association of Blood Banks, http://www.aabb.org/pressroom/in_the_news/ wnab03-8.htm.

American Psychiatric Assn. *Diagnostic and Statistical Manual of Mental Disorders.* Washington, DC, January 1995.

AP Wire Service. "West Nile Repertorized Symptoms." *The Alternative Newsletter* (July 2000).

Benveniste, J. "Human Basophil Degranulation Triggered by Very Dilute Antiserum against IgE." *Nature Magazine* 333 (1988): 816–18.

Benveniste, J., E. Davenas, and B. Poitevin. "Inserm U 200." *British Journal of Clinical Pharmacology* 25 (4) (April 1988): 439-44.

Berkow, R., MD. *The Merck Manual of Diagnosis and Therapy.* Rahway, NJ: Merc Research Labs, 1992.

Bernard, H., MD, *Bernard's Constipation.* Kent Homeopathic Associates. *Referenceworks Pro 3.0.* San Rafael, California, 2002.

"Biological Warfare Defense Information Sheet." *US Navy Manual on Operational Medicine and Fleet Support.*

Blackwood, A. L. *Diseases of the Kidney and Nervous System.* New Delhi, India: B. Jain Publishers, n.d.

Boericke, W. *Boericke's Materia Medica and Repertory.* Philadelphia: Boericke & Runyon, 1927.

Boger, C. M. *The Synoptic Key*, 1915.

Bowen, C., MD, BA. *Handbook of Materia Medica, Pharmacy and Therapeutics*. Philadelphia, PA: F. A. Davis, 1888.

Boenninghausen, C. von, MD. *The Lesser Writings of C.M.F.* New Delhi, India: B. Jain Publishers, 1991.

Brownlee, S. "The Disease Busters." *U.S. News & World Report* (March 27, 1995): 48-58.

Burnett, J. C., MD, FRGS. *Curability of Cataracts with Medicines*. London: The Homeopathic Publishing Company, 1880.

Butler, K., *The Biology of Fear*, July/August, 1996, The Family Therapy Neworker, Washington, D.C., 1996.

CARA homeopathic software, Miccant Ltd., England.

Cartier, François, MD. *Therapeutics of the Respiratory Organs*. New Delhi, India: B. Jain Publishers, 1991.

—. Transactions, Part "Essays and Communications." Paper presented at the International Homeopathic Congress, 1896.

CBS This Morning: "Ebola Virus." Interview with Alan Tomlinsin. July 18, 1995.

Centers for Disease Control and Prevention. "Bird Flu Fact Sheet." Centers for Disease Control and Prevention, http://www.cdc.gov/flu/avian/outbreak.htm.

—. *Detection of West Nile Virus in Blood Donations*. United States, 2003. MMWR 2003;52:769-72.

—. "West Nile Virus." Centers for Disease Control and Prevention, http://www.cdc.gov/ncidod/dvbid/westnile/.

Chappell, P., RSHom., BSc, FSHom. *Emotional Healing with Homeopathy: A Self-Help Manual*. Dorset, England: Element Books Ltd., 1994.

Clarke, J. H., MD, ME. *A Clinical Repertory to the Dictionary of Materia Medica*. N. Devon, England: Health Science Press, 1979.

—. *A Dictionary of Practical Materia Medica*. New Delhi, India: B. Jain Publishers, 1984.

Close, W. T., MD. *Ebola*. New York: Ivy Books, 1995.

Cooke, N. F., MD. *Instructions for the Use of N.F. Cooke's Family Medicines*, 1873.

Cournoyer, C. *What about Immunizations?* Santa Cruz, CA: Nelson's Books, 1991.

Department of Health and Senior Services. *West Nile Virus Encephalitis Fact Sheet*. Department of Health and Senior Services. http://www.state.nj.us/.

Derin-Kellogg, G., DOC. *Homeopathic Remedies for Ebola Virus*. May 1995.

—. "Remedies of War." Thesis, Hahnemann Homeopathic College, Albany, California, 1995.

Dixon, B. *Power Unseen: How Microbes Rule the World*. Oxford: Freeman, 1993.

—. "Return of the Killer Bugs." *New Statesman & Society* (March 17, 1995): 29-30.

Douglass, M. E. *Pearls of Homeopathy*. India, 1952.

Farrington, E. A., MD. *Therapeutic Pointers*. New Delhi, India: B. Jain Publishers, 2002.

Fields, B. N., and D. M. Knipe. *Virology*. New York: Raven Press, 1990.

Fisher, P., Dr., et al. "Fibrosistis." *British Medical Journal* 299 (1989): 365-366.

Garret, L. *The Coming Plagues*. New York: Farrar, Strauss & Giroux, 1994.

—. "The Plague Warriors." *Vanity Fair* (August 1995).

Geddes, N., and A. Lockie, MD. *The Complete Guide to Homeopathy: The Principles and Practice of Treatment*, Dorling Kindersley, New York, NY, 1995.

Gibson, D. *Studies of Homeopathic Remedies*. United Kingdom: 1987.

Guernsey, H. N. *Keynotes to the Materia Medica*. 1887.

—. Lectures.

Guess, G., MD. *Guess' Keynotes*. MacRepertory and ReferenceWorks software. San Rafael, CA: Kent Associates, 1999.

Gunavante, S. W. *Introduction to Homeopathic Prescribing*. New Delhi, India: B. Jain Publishers, 1982.

Healthtrak Infosource. "Colostrum: Nature's Infectious Disease Fighter." Healthtrak Infosource, http://www.colostruminfo .com/articles/disease_fighters.html.

Hering, C., MD. *The Guiding Symptoms Materia Medica*. 1879.

Hewitt, B., E. Stein, J. Wright, and M. Grant. "A Common Germ Turns Deadly." *People* (June 13, 1994): 103-104.

Hope-Simpson, R. E., FRCGP. *The Transmission of Epidemic Influenza*. New York: Plenum Press, 1992.

IBIS software. Portland, OR: Amar'ta, 1993.

Inglesby, T., D. Dennis, D. Henderson et al. 2000. "Plague as a Biological Weapon. Medical and Public Health Management." *The Journal of the American Medical Association*. 283(17):2281-2290.

Jouanny, J., MD. *The Essentials of Homeopathic Materia Medica,* Laboratoires Boiron. Boiron, France: 1984.

Julian, O. A. *Materia Medica of New Homeopathic Remedies.* United Kingdom: 1971.

Kane, J. *Famous First Facts.* New York: H.W. Wilson, 1981.

Karlen, A. *Man and Microbes; Disease and Plagues in History and Modern Times.* New York: Jeremy P. Tarcher/Putnam, 1995.

Kent Homeopathic Associates. *MacRepertory and Referencework software.* San Rafael, California, 2000.

Kent, J.T., MD. *Lectures on Homeopathic Materia Medica.* New Delhi, India: B. Jain Publishers, 1921.

Kiple, K. F., ed. *Cambridge World History of Human Disease.* New York: Cambridge University Press, 1993.

Farzad Mostashari et al. "Epidemic West Nile Encephalitis. Results of a Household-Based Serioepemiological Survey." *Lancet* (August 6, 2001) New York: 1999.

Lappe, M. *When Antibiotics Fail.* Berkely, CA: North Atlantic Books, 1986.

Laurie, J. *Elements of Homeopathic Practice of Physic.* 1865.

Leeser, O. *Textbook of Homeopathic Materia Medica.* United Kingdom: 1935.

Lemonick, MD. "The Invisible Invaders." *Readers Digest* (March 1995):79-82.

—. "Closing in on a Mysterious Killer." *Time* (December 6, 1993): 66.

—. "The Killers All Around." *Time* (September 12, 1994).

—. "Streptomania Hits Home." *Time* (June 20, 1994):54.

Leonardi, K., J. Matkovitch. *Research for Ebola Symptoms.* May 1995.

Lessell, C. B. *The World Travellers' Manual of Homeopathy.* Essex, England: C.W. Daniel Company, 1993.

LeRoux. *LeRoux's Acids.* Kent Homeopathic Associates. *Referenceworks Pro 3.0.* San Rafael, California, 2002.

Lilienthal, S. *Homeopathic Therapeutics.* 1878.

Lippe, A. von, MD. *Keynotes and Redline Symptoms of the Materia Medica.* Kent Homeopathic Associates. *Referenceworks Pro 3.0.* San Rafael, California, 2002.

Lockie, A., MD. *The Family Guide to Homeopathy.* New York: Simon & Schuster/Fireside, 1989.

Lovering, A. T., MD. *Hints in Domestic and Home Nursing.* Boston: Otis Clapp & Son Publishers, 1896.

Luckingham, B. *Epidemic in the Southwest 1918-1919.* El Paso, TX: Western Press, 1984.

MacFarlane, M. *Provings and Clinical Observations with High Potencies*, 1894.

Mathur, K. N., MD. *Principles of Prescribing—Collected from Clinical Experiences of Pioneers of Homeopathy.* New Delhi, India: B. Jain Publishers, 1981.

Medical and Surgical Reporter. March, 1873.

Medical News Today. "Whooping cough growing despite vaccinations in USA." *Medical News Today.* http://www.medicalnewstoday .com/index.php?newsid=6270.

Menear, V., MD. Telephone conversation. July 6, 1995.

Morrison, R., MD. *Desktop Guide to Keynotes and Confirmatory Symptoms.* Albany, CA: Hahnemann Clinic Publishing, 1993.

Morse, S. S., ed. *Emerging Viruses.* New York: Oxford University Press, 1993.

Murphy, R., ND. *Lotus Materia Medica.* Pagosa Springs, CO: Lotus Star Academy, 1995.

—. *Homeopathic Remedy Guide.* Colorado: The Hahneman Academy of North America, 2004.

Nash, E. B. *Leaders in Homeopathic Therapeutics.* 1899.

—. *Leaders in Respiratory Organs.* India: 1909.

Nauman, E., DHM. "The Coming Ebola Epidemic." *Sedona Journal of Emergence!* 5:9 (September 1995): 84-88.

New Jersey Health Department. *West Nile Virus Fact Sheet.* May 15, 2002.

Nichols, M. "Marauding Microbes." *Maclean's* 87 (June 17, 1994).

Nowak, R. "Flesh-Eating Bacteria: Not New, but Still Worrisome." *Science* 264 (June 17, 1994): 1665.

Pealer, L. N., A. A. Marfin, L. R. Petersen et al. "Transmission of West Nile virus through blood transfusion." United States, 2002. *New England Journal of Medicine* 2003;349:1236-1245.

Phatak, S. R. *A Concise Repertory of Homeopathic Medicines.* India: 1963.

Postgate, J. *The Outer Reaches of Life.* Cambridge, England: Cambridge University Press, 1993.

Preston, R. *Hot Zone.* New York: Doubleday, 1993.

—. "A Deadly Virus Escapes," *Time Magazine*, September 5, 1994: 66.

PROMED (Harvard Medical University). Promed@promed.isid. harved.edu, August 6, 2001, West Nile Virus update.

Pulte, J. H., MD. *Homeopathic Domestic Physician*. Cincinnati, OH: Moore, Wilstach, Keys & Co., 1856.

Raye, C. G., MD. *Special Pathology and Diagnostics with Therapeutic Hints*. Philadelphia, PA: F.E. Boericke, Hahnemann, 1885.

Ross, P. E. "A New Black Death?" *Forbes*, September 12, 1994: 240-250.

Royal, G., MD. *Textbook of Homeopathic Materia Medica*. Cooper Publishing, 1999.

Schmidt, M. A., L. H. Smith, and K. W. Schnert. *Beyond Antibiotics*. Berkely, CA: North Atlantic Books, 1993.

Schmookler, E., PhD. *Trauma Treatment Manual*. California, 1996.

Scott, P. T., J. B. Clark, and W. F. Miser. "Pertussis: An Update on Primary Prevention and Outbreak Control." *American Family Physician*. http://www.aafp.org/afp/970915ap/pertussis.html.

Simberkoff, M. S., MD. "Drug-Resistant Pneumococcal Infections in the United States." *JAMA (Journal of American Medical Association)* 271, no. 23 (June 15, 1994): 1875-1876.

Snelling, F. G., MD. *Snelling's Symptomology: Manual of the Homeopathic Materia Medica*.

Sterling Saunder, C., L.R. C. P., "Kali mur. with Special Reference to Its Antidotal Power Against Small Pox and Vaccine Poisoning, Etc." *Homeopathic World*, London, 1909.

Tarbell, J. A., MD, AM. *Homeopathy Simplified; Or, Domestic Practice Made Easy*. Boston: Otis Clapp & Son Publishers, 1890.

Taylor, M. A., and D. T. Reilly. "Is Homeopathy a Placebo Effect? Hay Fever Trial." *The Lancet* 2 (8512) (1986):8881-8886.

Thomas, C. L., MD, MPH. *Taber's Cyclopedic Medical Dictionary*. Philadelphia: F. A. Davis Co., 1997.

Tsai, T., MD. "West Nile Virus Infection." *Medscape* (October 9, 2000). http://www.medscape.com/.

Tyler, M., MD. *Pointers to Common Remedies*. India: 1939.

Underwood, B. F. *Underwood's Childhood Materia Medica*. Kent Homeopathic Associates. *Referenceworks Pro 3.0*. San Rafael, California, 2002.

Van Denberg, M. W. *Therapeutics of the Respiratory System*. 1916.

Vermeulen, F. *Synoptic Materia Medica*. Haarlem, Netherlands: Merlijn Publishers, 1996.

Vithoulkas, J. G. *Materia Medica Viva, Vol. 1*. Mill Valley, CA: Health and Habitat, 1992.

Voisin, H. *Concordant Materia Medica 2.* 1994.

Ward, J. F. *Ward's Repertory.* 1925.

Warkington, K.D., and M. Hourigan. *Referenceworks Pro 3.0.* San Rafael, CA: Kent Homeopathic Associates, 2002.

—. *ReferenceWorks software.* Farifax, CA: Kent Associates, 1992.

"West Nile Repertorized symptoms." *The Alternative Newsletter.* Phoenix, AZ. July, 2000.

Whitmont, E., MD. *The Alchemy of Healing.* 1993.

Wilson-Smith, A. "I'm Really Going to Make It." *Maclean's,* March 6, 1995: 14-15.

Index

O

P

PATH OF THE MYSTIC

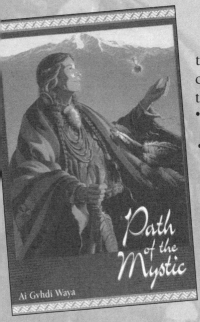

Ai Gvhdi Waya shares her own journey through Native American stories of her discovery—and how you can access the many teachers, too.

- Learn how to trust your own knowing and follow your heart.
- Walk the path of the mystic and understand how you can do that on a daily basis.
- Being a mystic gives us the opportunity to transform from chrysalis into butterfly. This gift is available to all of us.

11^{95} SOFTCOVER 114 P.
ISBN 0-929385-47-0

Chapter Titles:

- Our Own Best Teacher
- What Is Shamanism? Part 1
- What Is Shamanism? Part 2
- Sweat Lodge
- The Ant People
- Spirit Guides
- The Tree People

- Horse Medicine, Part 1
- Horse Medicine, Part 2
- Hummingbird Medicine
- Thunderbeings
- Vortexes of Mother Earth
- Temple Mounds

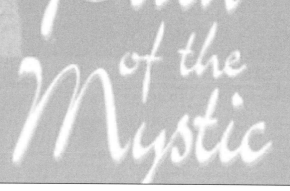

AI GVHDI WAYA

Eileen Nauman writing as Ai Gvhdi Waya. Born in an Eastern Cherokee household, member of the Wolf Clan, with a father who was one-quarter Cherokee. Ai Gvhdi Waya was trained, beginning at the age of nine, in the medicine path. She continues to work with native people of both North and South America.

SOUL RECOVERY AND EXTRACTION

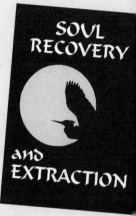

Putting Back the Pieces of Your Life
Soul Recovery is about regaining the fragments of one's soul energy that have been trapped, lost or stolen either by another person or through a traumatic incident that has occurred in one's life. Taking back control of your life is at the heart of this shamanic healing method.

- Depression • Obesity
- Memory loss, especially from your growing years
- Addictive behavior of any kind
- Codependence • Victim mentality
- Inability to release a person or situation
- Being controlled or manipulated by others

$9.95 **SOFTCOVER 85 P.**
ISBN 0-9634662-3-2

PUBLISHED BY
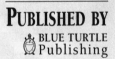
🐢 BLUE TURTLE
Publishing

Chapter Titles:

- **What Is Soul Loss and Recovery?**
- **Soul Recovery: The Beginning**
- **Case Histories of Soul Recovery and Extraction**
- **Integrating Your Returned Soul Pieces**
- **Spirit Guides:**
  Longterm
  Protection for a Client
- **Brief Biographies on Shamanic Facilitators**

Our best teachers

are inside

ourselves.

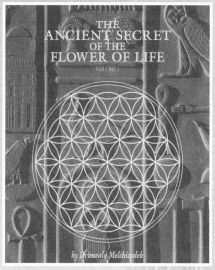
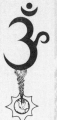
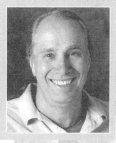

THE ANCIENT SECRET OF THE FLOWER OF LIFE
VOLUME 2

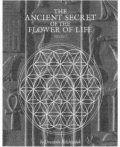

Softcover, 252 p.
ISBN 1-891824-21-X

$25⁰⁰

The sacred Flower of Life pattern, the primary geometric generator of all physical form, is explored in even more depth in this volume, the second half of the famed Flower of Life workshop. The proportions of the human body, the nuances of human consciousness, the sizes and distances of the stars, planets and moons, even the creations of humankind, are all shown to reflect their origins in this beautiful and divine image. Through an intricate and detailed geometrical mapping, Drunvalo Melchizedek shows how the seemingly simple design of the Flower of Life contains the genesis of our entire third-dimensional existence.

From the pyramids and mysteries of Egypt to the new race of Indigo children, Drunvalo presents the sacred geometries of the Reality and the subtle energies that shape our world. We are led through a divinely inspired labyrinth of science and stories, logic and coincidence, on a path of remembering where we come from and the wonder and magic of who we are.

Finally, for the first time in print, Drunvalo shares the instructions for the Mer-Ka-Ba meditation, step-by-step techniques for the re-creation of the energy field of the evolved human, which is the key to ascension and the next dimensional world. If done from love, this ancient process of breathing prana opens up for us a world of tantalizing possibility in this dimension, from protective powers to the healing of oneself, of others and even of the planet.

❂ **THE UNFOLDING OF THE THIRD INFORMATIONAL SYSTEM**
The Circles and Squares of Human Consciousness; Leonardo da Vinci's True Understanding of the Flower of Life; Exploring the Rooms of the Great Pyramid

❂ **WHISPERS FROM OUR ANCIENT HERITAGE**
The Initiations of Egypt; the Mysteries of Resurrection; Interdimensional Conception; Ancient Mystery Schools; Egyptian Tantra, Sexual Energy and the Orgasm

❂ **UNVEILING THE MER-KA-BA MEDITATION**
Chakras and the Human Energy System; Energy Fields around the Body; the Seventeen Breaths of the Mer-Ka-Ba Meditation; the Sacred Geometry of the Human Lightbody

❂ **USING YOUR MER-KA-BA**
The Siddhis or Psychic Powers; Programming Your Mer-Ka-Ba; Healing from the Prana Sphere; Coincidence, Thought and Manifestation; Creating a Surrogate Mer-Ka-Ba

❂ **CONNECTING TO THE LEVELS OF SELF**
Mother Earth and Your Inner Child; Life with Your Higher Self; How to Communicate with Everything; the Lessons of the Seven Angels

❂ **TWO COSMIC EXPERIMENTS**
The Lucifer Experiment and the Creation of Duality; the 1972 Sirian Experiment and the Rebuilding of the Christ Consciousness Grid

❂ **WHAT WE MAY EXPECT IN THE FORTHCOMING DIMENSIONAL SHIFT**
How to Prepare; Survival in the Fourth Dimension; the New Children

Available from your favorite bookstore or:
LIGHT TECHNOLOGY PUBLISHING
PO Box 3540
Flagstaff, AZ 86003
928-526-1345
800-450-0985
FAX 928-714-1132
Or use our online bookstore:
www.lighttechnology.com

3ᵒ LIGHT Technology
PUBLISHING

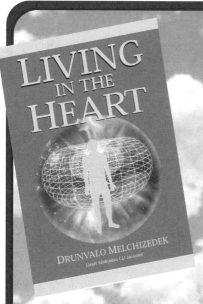

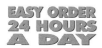

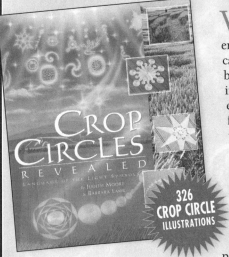

Book 1...
the EXPLORER RACE

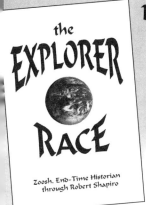

the EXPLORER RACE

Zoosh, End-Time Historian
through Robert Shapiro

You individuals reading this are truly a result of the genetic experiment on Earth. You are beings who uphold the principles of the Explorer Race. The information in this book is designed to show you who you are and give you an evolutionary understanding of your past that will help you now. The key to empowerment in these days is not to know everything about your past, but to know that which will help you now.

Your souls have been here on Earth for a while and have been trained in Earthlike conditions. This education has been designed so that you would have the ability to explore all levels of responsibility— results, effects and consequences—and take on more responsibilities.

Your number one function right now is your status of Creator apprentice, which you have achieved through years and lifetimes of sweat. You are constantly being given responsibilities by the Creator that would normally be things that Creator would do. The responsibility and the destiny of the Explorer Race is not only to explore, but to create.

$25.00 SOFTCOVER 574 P.
ISBN 0-929385-38-1

Chapter Titles:

THE HISTORY OF THE EXPLORER RACE
- The Genetic Experiment on Earth
- Influences of the Zodiac
- The Heritage from Early Civilizations
- Explorer Race Timeline, Part 1
- Explorer Race Timeline, Part 2
- The Experiment that Failed

GATHERING THE PARTS
- The ET in You: Physical Body
- The ET in You: Emotion and Thought
- The ET in You: Spirit

THE JOY, THE GLORY AND THE CHALLENGE OF SEX
- Emotion Lost: Sexual Addiction in Zeta History
- Sex, Love and Relationships
- Sexual Violence on Earth
- The Third Sex: The Neutral Binding Energy
- The Goddess Energy: The Soul of Creation

ET PERSPECTIVES
- Origin of the Species: A Sirian Perception
- An Andromedan Perspective on the Earth Experiment
- The Perspective of Orion Past on Their Role
- Conversation with a Zeta

BEHIND THE SCENES
- The Order: Its Origin and Resolution
- The White Brotherhood, the Illuminati, the New Dawn and the Shadow Government
- Fulfilling the Creator's Destiny
- The Sirian Inheritors of Third-Dimensional Earth

TODAY AND TOMORROW
- The Explorer Race Is Ready
- Coming of Age in the Fourth Dimension
- The True Purpose of Negative Energy
- The Challenge of Risking Intimacy
- Etheric Gene-Splicing and the Neutral Particle
- Material Mastery and the New Safety
- The Sterilization of Planet Earth

THE LOST PLANETS
- The Tenth Planet: The Gift of Temptation
- The Eleventh Planet: The Undoer, Key to Transformation
- The Twelfth Planet: Return of the Heart Energy

THE HEART OF HUMANKIND
- Moving Beyond the Mind
- Retrieving Heart Energy
- The Creator's Mission and the Function of the Human Race

THE EXPLORER RACE SERIES

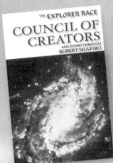

Book 7...

COUNCIL OF CREATORS

ROBERT SHAPIRO

The thirteen core members of the Council of Creators discuss their adventures in coming to awareness of themselves and their journeys on the way to the Council on this level. They discuss the advice and oversight they offer to all creators, including the Creator of this local universe. These beings are wise, witty and joyous, and their stories of Love's creation create an expansion of our concepts as we realize that we live in an expanded, multiple-level reality. SOFTCOVER 237 P. $14.95 ISBN 1-891824-13-9

Highlights Include:

- Specialist in Colors, Sounds and Consequences of Actions
- Specialist in Membranes that Separate and Auditory Mechanics
- Specialist in Sound Duration
- Explanation from Unknown Member of Council
- Specialist in Spatial Reference
- Specialist in Gaps and Spaces
- Specialist in Divine Intervention

- Specialist in Synchronicity and Timing
- Specialist in Hope
- Specialist in Honor
- Specialist in Variety
- Specialist in Mystical Connection between Animals and Humans
- Specialist in Change
- Specialist in the Present Moment
- Council Spokesperson and Specialist in Auxiliary Life Forms

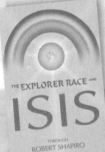

Book 8...

THE EXPLORER RACE AND ISIS

ROBERT SHAPIRO

This is an amazing book. It has priestess training, Shamanic training, Isis' adventures with Explorer Race beings—before Earth and on Earth—and an incredibly expanded explanation of the dynamics of the Explorer Race. Isis is the prototypical loving, nurturing, guiding feminine being, the focus of feminine energy. She has the ability to expand limited thinking without making people with limited beliefs feel uncomfortable. She is a fantastic storyteller, and all of her stories are teaching stories. If you care about who you are, why you are here, where you are going and what life is all about—pick up this book. You won't lay it down until you are through, and then you will want more. SOFTCOVER 317 P. $14.95 ISBN 1-891824-11-2

Highlights Include:

- The Biography of Isis
- The Adventurer
- Soul Colors and Shapes
- Creation Mechanics
- Creation Mechanics and Personal Anecdotes

- The Insects' Form and Fairies
- Orion and Application to Earth
- Goddess Section
- Who Is Isis?
- Priestess/Feminine Mysteries

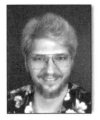

ROBERT SHAPIRO

SUPERCHANNEL ROBERT SHAPIRO can communicate with any personality anywhere and anywhen. He has been a professional channel for over twenty-five years and channels with an exceptionally clear and profound connection. Robert's great contribution to an understanding of the history, purpose and future of humanity is his epochal work, the Explorer Race series, *of which this book is number nine. The series includes Robert's channeling of beings from particles to creators to generators of pre-creation energy. He is also the channel of the six books in the* Shining the Light *series.*

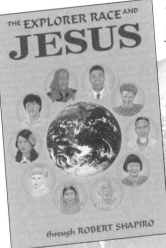

Book 9 of the EXPLORER RACE:

THE EXPLORER RACE AND JESUS
JESUS AND OTHES THROUGH ROBERT SHAPIRO

The core personality of that being known on the Earth as Jesus, along with his students and friends, describes with clarity and love his life and teaching 2000 years ago. He states that his teaching is for all people of all races in all countries. Jesus announces here for the first time that he and two others, Buddha and Mohammed, will return to Earth from their place of being in the near future, and a fourth being, a child already born now on Earth, will become a teacher and prepare humanity for their return. So heartwarming and interesting, you won't want to put it down.

16^{95} SOFTCOVER 354 P.
ISBN 1-891824-14-7

Each book weighs 1.07 lbs.
28 books per carton
30 lbs. per box

Chapter Titles:

- Jesus's Core Being, His People and the Interest in Earth of Four of Them
- Jesus's Life on Earth
- Jesus's Home World, Their Love Creations and the Four Who Visited Earth
- The "Facts" of Jesus's Life Here, His Future Return
- The Teachings and Travels
- A Student's Time with Jesus and His Tales of Jesus's Time Travels
- The Child Student Who Became a Traveling Singer-Healer

- The Shamanic Use of the Senses
- Other Journeys and the Many Disguises
- Jesus's Autonomous Parts, His Bloodline and His Plans
- Learning to Invite Matter to Transform Itself
- Inviting Water, Singing Colors
- Learning to Teach Usable Skills
- Learning about Different Cultures and People
- The Role of Mary Magdalene, a Romany
- Traveling and Teaching People How to Find Things

Light Technology Publishing • PO Box 3540 • Flagstaff, AZ 86003
Phone: 928-526-1345 or 800-450-0985 • Fax: 928-714-1132 or 800-393-7017

Visit our online bookstore: www.lighttechnology.com

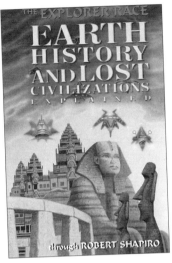

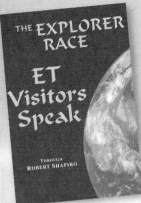

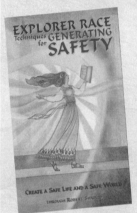

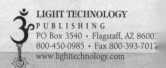

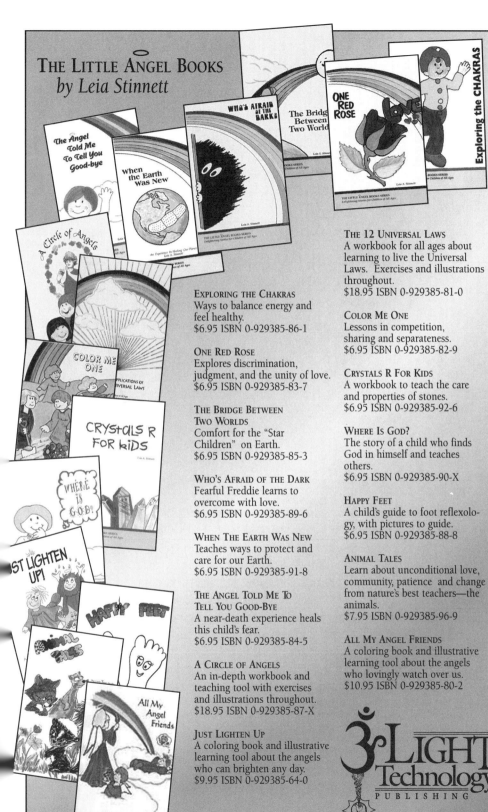

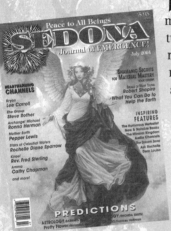
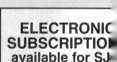